OXFORD MEDICAL PUBLICATIONS

Paediatric intensive care

Paediatric intensive care

Edited by

N.S. Morton

*Consultant in Paediatric Anaesthesia
and Intensive Care, Royal Hospital
for Sick Children, Glasgow, Scotland, UK*

OXFORD   NEW YORK   TOKYO
OXFORD UNIVERSITY PRESS
1997

This book has been printed digitally in order to ensure its continuing availability

OXFORD
UNIVERSITY PRESS

Great Clarendon Street, Oxford OX2 6DP

Oxford University Press is a department of the University of Oxford.
It furthers the University's objective of excellence in research, scholarship,
and education by publishing worldwide in

Oxford New York

Auckland Bangkok Buenos Aires Cape Town Chennai
Dar es Salaam Delhi Hong Kong Istanbul Karachi Kolkata
Kuala Lumpur Madrid Melbourne Mexico City Mumbai Nairobi
São Paulo Shanghai Singapore Taipei Tokyo Toronto
with an associated company in Berlin

Oxford is a registered trade mark of Oxford University Press
in the UK and in certain other countries

Published in the United States
by Oxford University Press Inc., New York

A catalogue record for this book is available from the British Library

Library of Congress Cataloging in Publication Data
(Data available)

ISBN 0-19-262511-X (Hbk)

Contents

List of contributors   vii

1   The spectrum of paediatric intensive care   1
J. Sinclair

2   Early recognition of the critically ill child   41
N.S. Morton

3   Resuscitation of infants and children   45
P.M. Cullen

4   Injuries to children   78
N.S. Morton

5   Airway management   81
D.N. Robinson

6   Paediatric ventilatory care   109
M. Kerr

7   Circulatory support   152
K.J. Millar

8   Fluid, nutritional, metabolic and haematological   184
support in critically ill children
N.S. Morton and F. Munro

9   Monitoring techniques in paediatric intensive care   212
M. Robson

10   Sedation and analgesia for critically ill children   241
T.G. Hansen and N.S. Morton

11   Stabilization and transport of the critically ill child   258
N.S. Morton

12   Nursing aspects of paediatric intensive care   267
     R. Macnab

13   Legal and ethical aspects of paediatric intensive care   288
     N.S. Morton

Index   293

List of contributors

P.M. Cullen, *Consultant in Paediatric Anaesthesia and Intensive Care, Royal Hospital for Sick Children, Glasgow, Scotland, UK*

T.G. Hansen, *Consultant in Paediatric Anaesthesia, Odense University Hospital, Odense, Denmark*

M. Kerr, *Research Fellow in Paediatric Respiratory Medicine, Department of Child Health, Royal Hospital for Sick Children, Glasgow, Scotland, UK*

R. Macnab, *Resuscitation Officer, Royal Hospital for Sick Children, Glasgow, Scotland, UK*

K.J. Millar, *Fellow in Paediatric Intensive Care, Royal Children's Hospital, Melbourne, Australia*

N.S. Morton, *Consultant in Paediatric Anaesthesia and Intensive Care, Royal Hospital for Sick Children, Glasgow, Scotland, UK*

F. Munro, *Senior Registrar in Paediatric Surgery, Edinburgh, Scotland, UK; formerly Fellow and Research Fellow, Paediatric Intensive Care Unit, Royal Hospital for Sick Children, Glasgow, Scotland, UK*

D.N. Robinson, *Specialist Senior Registrar in Paediatric Anaesthesia; formerly Fellow in Paediatric Intensive Care, Royal Hospital for Sick Children, Glasgow, Scotland, UK*

M. Robson, *Fellow in Paediatric Intensive Care, Royal Hospital for Sick Children, Glasgow, Scotland, UK*

J. Sinclair, *Consultant in Paediatric Anaesthesia and Intensive Care, Royal Hospital for Sick Children, Glasgow, Scotland, UK*

1

The spectrum of paediatric intensive care

J. Sinclair

A paediatric intensive care unit (PICU) is a facility specially designed, staffed and equipped for the treatment and management of critically ill children from early infancy to adolescence. Because PICUs are tertiary referral centres based at major paediatric teaching hospitals, large numbers of children are cared for, at least initially, outwith the tertiary centre in adult intensive care units (ICUs). The aims of this chapter are to introduce some of the wide spectrum of illnesses seen in the PICU, to highlight the differences between the management of patients in PICUs and adult ICUs, and to explain the reasons behind these differences. The spectrum of disease seen in any given PICU depends on the population from which it receives its patients. The presence of a cardiac surgery programme or organ transplant programme within the hospital will have major implications for the PICU.

For historical reasons the provision of intensive care for children has been fragmented. The neonatal special care baby unit overlaps with the surgical neonatal intensive care unit which in turn overlaps with the general PICU. A number of infants and children are cared for in specialist centres, such as neurosurgical and cardiac surgical centres, where the intensivists believe that there is more in common between adults and children with similar disease processes than between critically ill children with different illnesses.

To illustrate the range of workload, the diagnostic groups seen in the PICU at the Royal Hospital for Sick Children at Yorkhill in Glasgow, which has between 500 and 600 admissions per year, are shown in Fig. 1.1. Congenital heart disease accounts for 41% of admissions either in the immediate postoperative period or following an acute decompensation (usually related to respiratory tract infections). Children admitted with respiratory failure comprise 21% of admissions while postoperative elective ventilation following general or orthopaedic surgery is responsible for 9% of admissions. The majority of postoperative surgical neonates however are cared for in a separate surgical neonatal unit within the hospital. Trauma is responsible for only 7% of our admissions as many head-injured children are admitted to a regional neurosurgical adult ICU on a separate site. Seizures account for up to 5% of our admissions. These are usually children in status epilepticus or children with febrile convulsions who have received anticonvulsants and are failing adequately to protect their airway. We admit all children with suspected

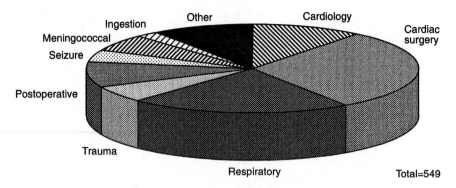

Fig. 1.1 Admissions to PICU, Royal Hospital for Sick Children, 1994

meningococcal disease to our unit for initial assessment and scoring. This accounts for nearly 5% of our admissions. The majority of children admitted to our PICU with accidental drug ingestions are admitted for cardiovascular monitoring following poisoning by tricyclic antidepressants.

The aim of paediatric intensive care is to monitor, support and eventually restore vital system function to critically ill or injured infants, children and adolescents. To attain this goal the paediatric intensivist must apply specialist knowledge and skills to ensure the optimal transfer of oxygen from the environment to the tissues. These principles of intensive care for infants and children are similar to those for adult intensive care. The difference is in the nature of the illnesses that cause children to become critically ill; the immaturity of the child's major organ systems, the presence of congenital abnormalities and the small physical size of neonates and infants. This requires special equipment, techniques and knowledge.

Studies are starting to show that the sickest children have an improved outcome if treated in tertiary paediatric intensive care facilities rather than in centres without a PICU.[1] If we compare the long-term outcome of children treated in PICUs with adults treated in adult ICUs we find that children admitted to PICUs are suffering from acute potentially reversible illness or injury which if treated appropriately can result in long productive lives. PICU patients have a low mortality and short stays. Adult ICU patients have a high mortality and reduced life-expectancy as the majority of patients are elderly. The cost of intensive care for each year of independent life saved in a child is about 1% of the cost of an adult.

To understand why infants, children, and adolescents are often treated in adult ICUs we need to look at the historical background of the development of PICUs. To understand why children fare better in dedicated PICUs we need to look at the special skills and knowledge that the PICU offers. It is the belief of paediatric intensivists, reinforced by recent reports on paediatric

intensive care, that the appropriate management of critically ill children cannot be extrapolated from knowledge of the care of acutely ill adults or of less acutely ill children.[2-5]

HISTORICAL PERSPECTIVE AND CURRENT STATUS

Paediatric intensive care is a young specialty less than 40 years old. Five fields were present at the birth of the subspecialty of paediatric intensive care in the 1950s and 1960s. These were the specialties of neonatal intensive care, paediatric general surgery, paediatric cardiac surgery, adult intensive care and paediatric anaesthesia. The first PICU was established by Goran Haglund, a paediatric anaesthetist, in Sweden in 1955. G. Jackson Rees, another paediatric anaesthetist, opened the first paediatric intensive care unit in the United Kingdom at Alder-Hey hospital in Liverpool in 1964. North America's first PICU was opened in the Children's Hospital Philadelphia in 1967 with J.J. Downes as director. The establishment of these PICUs and their training programmes led to a perceived improvement in the management of critically ill children and thus to the expansion of PICUs to most European and North American teaching centres during the 1970s and early 1980s.

In 1981 an important first step in the recognition of the developing specialty of paediatric intensive care was the creation of the Section on Paediatric Critical Care in the Society of Critical Care Medicine in the United States. In 1987 the American Board of Pediatrics created a board in critical care medicine and established a certifying exam. The same year in the United Kingdom the Paeditric Intensive Care Society was formed with the aim of promoting training and education in paediatric intensive care.

In 1983 in the United States the American Academy of Pediatrics and the Society of Critical Care Medicine provided guidelines on the organizing, staffing and equipping of PICUs which was subsequently updated in 1993. Similarly, in the United Kingdom the British Paediatric Association set up a working party to look at PICU facilities, organization, and staffing which reported in 1987 with updated recommendations from a multidisciplinary working party being published in 1993.

In the United Kingdom 12 822 children were identified as receiving intensive care in 1991. Of these children 51% received their care in a PICU, 28.6% were cared for in children's wards and 20.5% were cared for in adult ICUs. Thus 49% of the children in the United Kingdom requiring intensive care receive their care in units that are neither staffed nor equipped to provide this care.

A national survey of 235 PICUs in the United States in 1993 found that over 40% of PICUs had less than six beds, just over 25% had no paediatric intensivist and one-fifth had no medical school affiliation. These characteristics are believed to be associated with a poorer outcome although to date

studies of these characteristics are comparisons between single sites or extra-polations from adult ICU data.

Therefore at present and in the future large numbers of children will be cared for outwith teaching hospital affiliated PICUs.

CARDIOVASCULAR SYSTEM

The cardiovascular system exemplifies the differences between adult and paediatric intensive care medicine. An example of these differences can be seen by looking at the causes of cardiac arrests in children versus adults. In adults the commonest cause of cardiac arrest is secondary to ischaemic heart disease.[6] Rapid defibrillation of the patient in ventricular fibrillation (VF) is of paramount importance. Except in postoperative cardiac surgery patients, the incidence of VF in children is very low (children with the rare condition of long Q-T syndrome being one of the exceptions). A defibrillator plays little part in the resuscitation of the pulseless infant or child brought into the accident and emergency department. The thrust of paediatric resuscitation is to treat the antecedents of asystolic cardiac arrest.[7] The commonest under-lying cause of cardiac arrest in children is respiratory failure. Circulatory failure, caused by fluid loss, blood loss or septic shock, is the second most common reason for cardiac arrest in children.

Another example of the differences between adult and paediatric intensive care is the thermodilution catheter (used to measure cardiac output). The practicalities of inserting such a device in an infant in cardiac failure may make insertion impossible or alter the risk benefit ratio so far towards risk as to contraindicate its use. A more fundamental problem is that the majority of children with a primary cardiac problem suffer from congenital heart disease. In these children the underlying assumption, that the right-sided or pulmon-ary cardiac output is the same as the left-sided or systemic output, may be unfounded as intracardiac and extracardiac shunting may make the measured value of cardiac output meaningless.

The incidence of congenital heart disease is about 8:1000 livebirths. One-third of these children have mild anomalies that require no treatment and one-third present neonatally with cardiac failure, cyanosis or shock. In the general paediatric population 90% of children with primary cardiac failure will have initially presented before 1 year of age. Children presenting for the first time with cardiac failure, after this age, tend to have myocarditis or a cardiomyo-pathy. The transition from the intrauterine to extrauterine circulation, coupled with the rapid discharge of apparently healthy newborn babies from maternity units, can lead to the presentation of shocked infants to the accident and emergency department. These infants often have duct dependent congenital heart disease which has not been recognized and present as their duct closes.

Developmental cardiovascular physiology

To understand the pathophysiology of the cardiovascular system in infants and children we need to understand the normal transition that occurs in the cardiovascular system at the change from intrauterine to extrauterine life and the normal changes that occur in the heart as it matures. We also need a basic knowledge of some of the possible congenital defects that can occur as the heart develops *in utero* and their impact on the neonate, infant and child.[8]

The cardiovascular system changes dramatically at birth. It changes from a parallel circulation to a series circulation and from one with numerous central shunts to one with no central shunts. It also changes from a circulation with a low cardiac output, high pulmonary vascular resistance (PVR) and relatively low systemic vascular resistance (SVR) to one with relatively high cardiac output, low PVR and high SVR.

As the infant takes its first breaths, replacing the fluid in the alveoli with air, and establishes rhythmic ventilation, the PVR falls and pulmonary bloodflow increases. The increased pulmonary venous return to the left atrium increases left atrial pressure and functionally closes the foramen ovale (between the right and left atria).

Oxygenated blood in the ductus arteriosus (between the pulmonary artery and the aorta) leads to its functional closure in the first 24–96 h of life. With the removal of the placental circulation the systemic vascular resistance increases as does the cardiac output and the transition from the fetal parallel circulation to the adult series circulation is complete. The problem with this transitional period is that the changes are readily reversible. Hypoxia, hypercarbia, or acidaemia will increase PVR and reopen the ductus arteriosus. The rise in right-sided pressures caused by the increased PVR leads to right to left intra-atrial shunting and desaturation. If the pulmonary artery pressures are suprasystemic then right to left shunting will also occur at the ductus with systemic desaturation. An understanding of the transitional circulation is vital for the management of neonates in the PICU.

At birth the right ventricle is approximately the same size as the left ventricle. By early childhood the left ventricle is twice as heavy as the right in response to the increased volume and pressure load of the systemic circulation. The contractile mass of the neonatal heart is proportionally less than the adult and the neonatal heart is less compliant. It has difficulty increasing its stroke volume, as it sits high up on its Starling curve, with maximum contractility occurring at resting artrial pressures. The neonate is thus dependent on increases in heart rate to increase cardiac output. Bradycardia is therefore poorly tolerated and volume loading will not significantly alter cardiac output in the neonate.

The combination of a transitional circulation, immature cardiopulmonary physiology, and a bewildering variety of congenital cardiac defects makes the management of these children particularly challenging.

Congenital heart disease

Functionally the effects of congenital heart disease can either be to alter pulmonary bloodflow or to produce a volume or pressure load on the ventricles.

As the pulmonary vascular resistance falls after birth and right-sided pressures fall conditions such as a ventricular septal defect (VSD), an atrial septal defect (ASD), an atrioventricular (AV) canal defect, a patent ductus arteriosus (PDA) or a truncus arteriosus allow left to right shunting to occur and increase pulmonary blood flow. This increased flow leads to pulmonary artery hypertrophy and increased pulmonary vascular resistance. If this increased flow is prolonged, pulmonary vascular obstructive disease can develop.

Decreased pulmonary bloodflow occurs in conditions such as tetralogy of Fallot or pulmonary artery stenosis. Here some degree of cyanosis is present and the child adapts in severe cases by becoming polycythaemic.

Volume overload of the ventricles occurs when large shunts are present (VSDs, ASDs, AV canal defects, and PDAs) and inevitably leads to some ventricular dysfunction with dilation and hypertrophy. If these defects are repaired early in life residual dysfunction is less likely.

Pressure overload of the ventricles occurs when there is obstruction of the ventricular outflow tract. This leads to ventricular hypertrophy and failure. Examples include: coarctation of the aorta, aortic valve stenosis, pulmonary stenosis and following the Mustard repair of transposition of the great vessels—right ventricular (systemic) pressure overload. Unlike volume overload residual ventricular dysfunction seems to remain even when the pressure load is removed.

Infants in heart failure present with feeding difficulties, breathlessness and sweating. They may be peripherally shutdown, centrally cyanosed, be using accessory muscles of respiration, have hepatomegaly and tachycardia on examination and have cardiomegally on chest X-ray. In severe heart failure initial resuscitation includes airway control and oxygenation, assessment of adequacy of ventilation, assessment of adequacy of intravascular volume (remembering the commonest cause of acute circulatory failure in the infant and child is hypovolaemia) and correction of acid–base imbalances. Further treatment includes volume expansion if hypovolaemic, dopamine if normovolaemic or failing to respond to volume, and diuretics if the heart and liver are enlarged and a primary cardiac problem is suspected. Specific treatment depends on the underlying heart problem. Early consultation with a paediatric cardiologist and early echocardiography to establish the diagnosis are essential. Duct dependent lesions respond to prostaglandin E1 (PGE1 alprostadil), pulmonary hypertension responds to nitric oxide (NO) and balloon septostomies can be performed in the paediatric or neonatal ICU (NICU) to increase systemic and pulmonary atrial mixing.

RESPIRATORY SYSTEM

Again there are major differences in the diseases that are commonly treated in adult ICUs and those seen in the PICU. Chronic obstructive airway disease secondary to smoking is not a problem in the PICU. Infants however are vulnerable to infections, particularly viral infections, to which adults have an acquired immunity.

The anatomy of the infant's upper airway is also significantly different from that of the adult. The newborn larynx is designed to allow sucking of milk and breathing to go on virtually simultaneously. The infant larynx is more cephalad than the adults (opposite the 2nd and 3rd cervical vertebrae compared with the 4th cervical vertebra in adults) with a large epiglottis. The epiglottis with the vallecula rises during swallowing and seals off, at the soft palate, the mouth from the glottis. This allows air to pass from the nasopharynx to the trachea simultaneously to the swallowing of milk already lying in the lateral recess of the hypopharynx. Thus the infant can get on with the important business of feeding without interrupting breathing. This is particularly important as the infant's metabolic rate per kilogram is almost twice that of an adult and hence his caloric requirement and need to expire CO_2 is double the adult requirement. The infant larynx is funnel-shaped with the narrowest part at the cricoid ring. Unlike in an adult, it is possible to pass an endotracheal tube through the vocal cords that is too large to advance into the trachea. The ring-like cricoid cartilage means that cuffed endotracheal tubes are unnecessary in children until about 10 years of age. This allows a tube with a relatively larger internal diameter to be inserted. An air leak, at 30 cmH$_2$O positive pressure ventilation is essential to avoid subglottic oedema or loss of epithelium at the cricoid ring which may lead to stridor or obstruction on extubation.

Respiratory developmental physiology[9]

At birth the lungs are immature, although the bronchial tree is essentially complete by 16 weeks' gestation the number of alveoli continues to increase until about 8 years of age. The lung size increases 13-fold between birth and 6 years of age (mostly alveoli which increase from 24 million to 300 million) and a further threefold increase in size occurs between 6 years and adulthood (which is mainly an increase in alveolar size). Children under 5 years of age are more likely to develop respiratory failure in response to small airway disease. As the child has the same number of airway generations as the adult the physical size of these airways is much smaller than the adult. The airway resistance is thus higher in the child than the adult until about 5 years of age.

The child's lung is less compliant than the adult's due to the presence of immature alveolar buds and the lack of elastin. The child's cartilaginous thorax

is however more compliant. This combined with the decreased lung compliance would lead to atelectasis and decreased functional residual capacity if the child did not overcome this by tachypnoea and laryngeal braking. The infant's chest configuration with a more horizontal rib-cage is also mechanically less efficient than the adult's. The infant's intercostal and diaphragmatic muscles fatigue more easily than adult's as the child does not develop the adult number of type 1 low fatigue muscle fibres until approximately 2 years of age. Finally, as mentioned earlier, the basal oxygen consumption of 7–8 ml/kg/min in infants is twice the adult value and because of the limited ability to increase tidal volume respiratory rate is twice the adult value.

By birth the lungs are full of surfactant rich fluid. Surfactant consists of a mixture of phospholipids (85%), neutral lipids (5%) and protein (10%). The action of the phospholipid component of surfactant is to lower surface tension at the air–tissue interface stopping the collapse of small alveoli. It also increases the compliance of the lung reducing the work of breathing and prevents the transudation of fluid into the alveoli. The lack of surfactant in the preterm infant is the primary cause of respiratory distress syndrome of the newborn.

Bronchopulmonary dysplasia

The infant equivalent of the adult patient with chronic respiratory disease is the infant who has graduated from the neonatal intensive care unit (NICU) with bronchopulmonary dysplasia (BPD). This is a disease that was first described in 1967 and is associated with the ventilation of infants under 1500 g with respiratory distress syndrome. It is frequently seen in the NICU and is characterized by neonatal ventilation, oxygen dependence beyond the first 4 weeks of life and persistent respiratory symptoms. The typical radiological features are hyperinflation and diffuse areas of streaky opacification alternating with areas of increased lucency. It appears to be caused by the combination of preterm birth, oxygen toxicity and barotrauma. It is exacerbated by pneumonia (commonly *Ureaplasma urealyticum* or cytomegalovirus), a patent ductus arteriosus or meconium aspiration.

The severity of the BPD can range from minimal symptoms to a crippling disease that requires long-term ventilation and is complicated by recurrent episodes of pneumonia, sepsis and poor growth. When these infants are eventually extubated they may require long-term domiciliary oxygen. As the early months of life pass, the incidence of acute respiratory failure and infection decreases but the infant's lung function remains abnormal. They continue to complain of coughing, wheeze, and limited exercise tolerance. The commonest causes for admission of these children to a PICU are acute viral infections (particularly respiratory syncytial virus (RSV)), postoperatively, or for long-term ventilation.

The PICU management includes: oxygenation to avoid the development of pulmonary hypertension, the use of bronchodilators (as the peribronchial

smooth muscle is hypertrophied in BPD), and diuretics to decrease pulmonary interstitial fluid and oedema. General supportive measures include ensuring adequate nutrition and an adequate haemoglobin. Like the patient with congenital heart disease the early use of ribavarin in RSV infection may be indicated. The role of steroids, while well established in the initial NICU management of BPD (to try and stop respiratory distress syndrome developing into BPD), remains controversial in the treatment of the older infant with acute, often infective, exacerbations of BPD.

Laryngotracheobronchitis (croup)

Inspiratory stridor is the major feature of upper airway obstruction. The combination of preceding coryza, inspiratory stridor, hoarseness, barking cough, and respiratory distress typifies laryngotracheobronchitis (LTB) or croup. 95% of croup is viral with the parainfluenza virus being responsible for 75% of cases and RSV for 9%. The peak incidence is in children aged 6 months to 3 years. 5% of children with croup require intubation. *Staphylococcus aureus*, streptococci or *Haemophilus influenzae* type B (HIB) can be responsible for a bacterial tracheitis which is an uncommon but life threatening form of croup. With a bacterial tracheitis the child appears toxic, febrile and almost inevitably requires ventilation.

Treatment is supportive with humidified oxygen and good hydration to avoid drying of secretions. The use of nebulized adrenaline (1 in 1000 : 0.5 ml/kg to a max. of 5 ml) as a topical vasoconstrictor is used in the PICU, with electrocardiograph monitoring, to decrease stridor and can be repeated every 30 min. The benefit however tends to decrease with time and often heralds the need for intubation. Swelling of the tracheal mucosa may mean that a smaller than usual endotracheal tube is required. The largest uncuffed tube with a leak at 30 cmH$_2$O should be used. Steroids in non-intubated patients remain controversial. In intubated patients steroids reduce the duration of intubation and decrease the need for reintubation. Antibiotics have no role in the treatment of viral croup.

Acute supraglottitis (epiglottitis)

Epiglottitis typically presents as an acute infection over a number of hours in a child 2–6 years old who appears toxic, is sitting up, has increased work of breathing, is unable to swallow, is drooling saliva and is unable or reluctant to cough. HIB is the usual organism although with the introduction of the HIB vaccine epiglottitis may become rarer. Other organisms such as β haemolytic streptococcus, *Staphylococcus aureus*, pneumococcus and *Neisseria catarrhalis* may also cause epiglottitis.

The first priority is to secure the child's airway. The child is disturbed as little as possible while preparations are made either in theatre or the PICU for

gaseous induction of anaesthesia and intubation by an experienced paediatric anaesthetist. Intubation may be difficult because of the large cherry like swollen epiglottis. Some centres have an ear, nose and throat surgeon present at the induction to perform an emergency tracheostomy if intubation fails. Treatment with cefuroxime is commenced once IV access is gained and cultures have been taken. Typically the child is extubated within 24–48 h once a leak is detected around the endotracheal tube.

Pneumonia and bronchiolitis

Outwith the neonatal period bacteria cause less than 10% of all cases of lower respiratory tract infection. Different age groups have different susceptibilities (Table 1.1). In the school child the commonest non-viral pneumonia is mycoplasma pneumonia (the walking pneumonia) which typically is less severe than other bacterial pneumonias and rarely requires hospitalization.

The highly contagious respiratory syncytial virus is responsible for 75% of lower respiratory tract disease (bronchiolitis) in infants and young children. Bronchiolitis is the most common severe respiratory infection in childhood with 2–3% of all infants being admitted to hospital with this diagnosis. 1–2% of these children will require PICU admission. It is commonest in children under 2 years of age with virtually all children becoming infected with RSV by 3 years. The remaining 25% of bronchiolitis is caused by other respiratory viruses such as influenza, parainfluenza, adenoviruses, and occasionally mumps. The mortality rate in previously healthy children is low (less than 1%) but children who are immunosuppressed or suffer from conditions such as BPD, complicated congenital heart disease or cystic fibrosis have a higher mortality. The disease typically is self limiting resolving after 2–3 days, although respiratory function remains affected for several weeks.

The treatment is supportive with humidified oxygen and intravenous or nasogastric fluids. Ventilatory support is most commonly required for infants less than 3 months old who become fatigued due to the increased work of breathing. The role of bronchodilators is controversial. Bronchial smooth

Table 1.1 Community-acquired pneumonias

Age	Suspected bacterial agent	Antibiotics of choice
<3 months	*E. coli*, Streptococci, Staphylococci, *Chlamydia*, *Bordetella pertussis*	Ampicillin and gentamicin; add erythomycin if afebrile
3 months–5 years	Pneumococcus, *Haemophilus influenzae*, *Staphylococcus*	Cefuroxime
5–16 years	*Mycoplasma*, Pneumococcus, *Haemophilus influenzae*	Erythromycin and cefuroxime

muscle is poorly developed in these patients and the increased airway resistance is usually attributed to oedema. Antibiotics have no role in the treatment of a viral illness unless a superadded bacterial pneumonia is present. Ribavirin, a virustatic agent, is used in high-risk patients with proven RSV bronchiolitis but its role in ventilated patients remains controversial. Steroids are not indicated in the acute phase but may have a role when a severely affected child who has become RSV negative is failing to wean from ventilatory support.

Asthma

Acute exacerbations of asthma are one of the commonest causes of admission of children to hospital. Viral infections are responsible for up to 90% of the exacerbations in children. Only 1–2% will require PICU admission. In recent years the objectives of asthma management have changed. Previously the main aim was to prevent bronchospasm by treating acute exacerbations with broncholidators. Now the control of asthma with anti-inflammatory drug therapy, self evaluation and self management to prevent life-threatening deteriorations is the aim of therapy. Children with life-threatening asthma (Table 1.2) should be admitted to a PICU.

Oxygen, β agonists and steroids remain the cornerstones of the management of acute exacerbations. The first-line treatments are concurrent administrations of:

- oxygen by face mask, nasal cannulae or head box to achieve O_2 saturations greater than 95%

- nebulized salbutamol up to one dose (1 ml 0.5% solution diluted to 4 ml) every 20 min outside the PICU. Continuous nebulized (neat 0.5%) salbutamol is used in the PICU with ECG monitoring of heart rate (or a salbutamol intravenous infusion (1–5 micrograms/kg/min))

- corticosteroids (hydrocortisone 5 mg/kg IV 6 hourly).

Failure to respond to this therapy (a peak expiratory flow <30%, PCO_2 >45 mmHg (6.0 kPa), PO_2 <60 mmHg (8.0 kPa), evidence of confusion, exhaustion or other signs of impending respiratory arrest) is an indication for ventilation. Mechanical ventilation of the asthmatic patient is one of the most difficult ventilation problems in the PICU. The aim is to set realistic targets

Table 1.2 Features of life-threatening asthma

PEF <33% predicted or best
Cyanosis, a silent chest, poor respiratory effort
Fatigue or exhaustion
Agitation or reduced level of consciousness

for oxygenation and ventilation. The high airway pressures which may be needed to achieve adequate oxygenation may lead to a pneumothorax or pneumomediastinum. Muscle relaxants and sedation are used to minimize airway pressures. A high PCO_2 is well tolerated if acidosis (pH <7.20, H^+ >60 nmol/l) is avoided. Oxygen saturations of 85–95% are acceptable. Short inspiratory times and long expiratory times (I:E at least 1:2) allow time for expiration. Positive end expiratory pressure (PEEP) is usually avoided or is limited to 2–3 cmH_2O. Rarely, inhalational anaesthetic agents such as isoflurane may need to be used to manage severe refractory bronchospasm. Aminophylline seems to have nothing to add to β agonists and steroids. The reason for ventilation is usually exhaustion and respiratory muscle fatigue. Rapid weaning within 24 h is often possible once the bronchospasm has reduced.

Adult respiratory distress syndrome

Adult or acute respiratory distress syndrome (ARDS) is an acute lung injury that occurs in children as well as adults and carries the same mortality as in adults of about 60%.[10] The cause of the lung injury can be direct (such as pneumonia, aspiration, pulmonary contusion, near-drowning, or smoke inhalation) or indirect (such as sepsis, multiple trauma, drug overdose, post-cardiopulmonary bypass, or burns). The combination of diffuse fluffy infiltrates (without heart failure, fluid overload or chronic lung disease), one or more recognized risk factors for the development of ARDS and severe abnormalities in pulmonary gas exchange (PaO_2 (kPa): F_IO_2 of <20) defines ARDS.

The initial management is aimed at the underlying cause. Further management is supportive while the lung hopefully is recovering from the injury. It is important to aim for attainable goals. The lowest PEEP and F_IO_2 that give an arterial oxygen saturation of 85–90% are adequate when the haemoglobin is higher than 12 g/dl. Volume trauma to the small amount of relatively normal lung should be avoided by low peak inspiratory pressures, pressure controlled ventilation and PEEP (5–15 cmH_2O). Reverse ratio ventilation has been advocated by some workers. A CO_2 that gradually rises is well tolerated as long as severe respiratory acidosis (pH <7.20, H^+ >60 nmol/l) is avoided. The avoidance of overhydration is paramount as high lung water content is associated with poor outcome. It is better not to give the extra fluid than to give too much and then try to remove it with diuretics. Central venous pressure and in older children pulmonary capillary wedge pressure (PCWP) must be measured to determine the lowest cardiac filling pressures associated with an adequate cardiac output (i.e. one that avoids tissue hypoxia and acidosis).

CENTRAL NERVOUS SYSTEMS (CNS)

The comatose child is a medical emergency. Children commonly present in coma from head injuries or following diffuse metabolic insults. Hypoxia, seizures, central nervous system infections, sepsis, renal failure, hepatic failure, hypothermia and inborn errors of metabolism can all result in a child presenting to the PICU in coma.

Initial management is aimed at the basics of airway breathing and circulation. All comatose children should have a rapid bedside blood glucose determination and glucose should be given if the child is hypoglycaemic. In adult practice many experts recommend that thiamine and naloxone should be given to the comatose patient. Thiamine deficiency is not an issue in children and narcotic overdose is rare. While excluding hypoglycaemia the child's coma scale should be assessed and evidence of an intracranial mass or raised intracranial pressure (ICP) should be sought. Any focal abnormalities or brainstem reflex abnormalities are indications for consultation with a paediatric neurologist and for a rapid computed tomography (CT) scan. The commonest reason for admission of a comatose child to the PICU is following a convulsion. The CNS of the newborn infant and young child is immature and these children have a lower threshold for seizures.

Neurological development

At birth the neurological system is immature. In particular the immaturity of the cerebral vasculature of the periventricular capillary bed and immature autoregulation of cerebral bloodflow leads to a high risk of periventricular haemorrhage (PVH). It is the major cause of mortality and morbidity in the very low-birthweight infant and affects 20–30% of infants less than 1.5 kg. An increased risk of PVH is associated with hypoxaemia, hypercarbia, acidosis, high ventilatory pressure, pneumothoraces, respiratory distress syndrome, and hypertension.

In the child a knowledge of normal development is required to assess their neurological status. A 1-year-old with a best verbal response of unintelligible sounds is probably perfectly normal. The same finding in a 3-year-old is abnormal. The Glasgow Coma Scale has been modified for children (Table 1.3).

The debate over whether the infant can feel pain or not is now resolving with good evidence that infants respond to painful stimuli with neurohormonal, somatic, and autonomic changes.

Seizures

Status epilepticus is defined as either continuous seizure activity lasting for more than 30 min or two or more seizures occurring sequentially without full

Table 1.3 Glasgow Coma Scale

Sign	Evaluation: adult	Score	Evaluation: child	Score
Eye opening	Spontaneous	4	Spontaneous	4
	To speech	3	To speech	3
	To pain	2	To pain	2
	None	1	None	1
Best verbal response	Oriented	5	Oriented	5
	Confused	4	Words	4
	Inappropriate	3	Vocal sounds	3
	Incomprehensible	2	Cries	2
	None	1	None	1
Best motor response	Obeys commands	6	Obeys commands	6
	Localizes pain	5	Localizes pain	4
	Withdrawal to pain	4	Flexion to pain	3
	Flexion to pain	3	Extension to pain	2
	Extension to pain	2	None	1
	None	1		
	Maximum	15		14
	Severe injury requiring ventilation	≤8		
	Normal score for children			
	Birth–6 months	9		
	6 months–1 year	11		
	1–2 years	12		
	2–5 years	13		
	Older than 5 years	14		

recovery of consciousness between seizures. The first part of this definition is rather artificial as in practice antiepileptic drug administration is started on any patient seizing for more than 10 min. About 50% of cases of status epilepticus occur in young children with a significant morbidity and mortality. More than 60% of children with status epilepticus lasting more than 60 min will have irreversible brain damage. The mortality in adults is about 10% compared to 3% in children. The common causes in children are febrile convulsions (36%), missed or changed medication in a known epileptic (20%), metabolic (8%), congenital (7%), anoxia (5%), and trauma (3.5%).

Simple febrile convulsions occur typically in children aged between 6 months and 5 years who have no developmental or neurological abnormalities. They last for less than 20 min, have no focal features, are not repeated in the same episode and are associated with full recovery within 1 h. The prognosis for simple

febrile convulsions is excellent with less than 1% subsequently developing epilepsy. However up to a third of children will have further febrile convulsions. The initial management is as always in any unresponsive patient the support of airway, breathing and circulation. Oxygenation and intravenous (IV) access, to give diazepam, are priorities. Rectal diazepam may be given if IV access is not immediately available. Patients admitted to PICUs following a febrile convulsion tend to have had an atypical seizure which has failed to respond to this initial management.

In status epilepticus, severe hypoxaemia and cerebral hypoperfusion combine with an increased cerebral metabolic rate to accelerate the development of irreversible brain damage. Priorities in the management of status epilepticus are therefore airway, maintenance of ventilation, oxygenation and circulatory support. Stopping the seizure quickly and preventing further seizures should be addressed at the same time as the ABCs. Airway management and ventilation are easier once the seizure is controlled. The drug of choice in the initial management of the seizure is diazepam intravenously or rectally (0.25–0.4 mg/kg IV, 0.4 mg/kg PR) which can be repeated after 5 min. Rectal paraldehyde or intravenous phenytoin (18 mg/kg) at 1 mg/kg/min with ECG monitoring is the next line of management if diazepam fails to control the seizure. If the seizure is still not controlled phenobarbitone 20 mg/kg IV should be given and this can be repeated. Severe sedation and hypoventilation following any of the above drugs necessitate close monitoring of the child in a PICU. Seizures resistant to the above regimen may need to be controlled with a thiopentone infusion (muscle relaxation, ventilation and circulatory support will be required) with electroencephalography (EEG) monitoring to confirm burst suppression and seizure termination.

Investigations to identify the cause of the seizure include blood glucose, temperature, calcium, phosphate, magnesium, full blood count, urea, and electrolytes and gases. In young children with fever and status epilepticus CNS infection is a major concern. It has been suggested that a lumbar puncture (LP) should be carried out on all children less than 18 months old with febrile convulsions. Any child with atypical febrile convulsions or a febrile convulsion and signs of meningism, drowsiness, irritability, or systemic illness should also have an LP. Do *not* carry out an LP if you think the child has raised intracranial pressure.

Meningitis

Bacterial meningitis is an acute, life-threatening illness in children. In children outwith the neonatal period *Haemophilus influenzae*, *Streptococcus pneumoniae* and *Neisseria meningitidis* account for 95% of cases. With the introduction in 1992 in the United Kingdom of vaccination against the capsulated form of *Haemophilus influenzae* type b, which is responsible for most of the cases of *Haemophilus* meningitis, a marked decrease in *Haemophilus* meningitis can

Table 1.4 Bacterial meningitis

Age	Suspected bacterial agent	Antibiotic
Neonate	E. coli Group B *Streptococcus* Listeria Other streptococci	Ampicillin and cefotaxime, or ampicillin and aminoglycoside
1–3 months	Combination of neonates and older children	Ampicillin and cefotaxime
>3 months	Meningococcal Pneumococcal H. influenzae	Cefotaxime or ceftriaxone

be expected. In neonates the organisms most commonly associated with meningitis are group B streptococci and *Escherichia coli* (accounting for 80% of cases) with about 10% of cases being caused by listeria.

In the younger child the clinical picture is less specific. The classic signs in the neonate of fever, bulging fontanelle and head retraction are late signs of meningitis. A high index of suspicion is required with LP forming an essential part of any septic screen in the sick neonate. In older children the clinical features include fever, headache, vomiting, rash, neck stiffness and positive Kernig's sign. Initial management includes airway, breathing, circulation and antibiotics (Table 1.4). An LP should be performed unless there are signs of increased intracranial pressure, focal neurological signs, or if the patient is comatose. In these circumstances a CT scan should be performed prior to an LP. The question of whether steroids are indicated to decrease the incidence of deafness remains controversial.[11]

Meningococcal disease presents in two distinct forms: meningococcal meningitis and fulminant meningococcal septicaemia (see below). We initially admit all children with meningococcal disease to our PICU until the form of the disease is clear.

RENAL AND FLUID BALANCE

The number of children seen in a given PICU with renal failure depends to a large extent on the population that the unit serves. Those units with an active cardiac surgery programme tend to see larger numbers of children with acute renal failure. The commonest causes of acute renal failure seen in the PICU, except in the cardiac surgery patient, are septic shock and post cardiac arrest. If spontaneous recovery of renal function is going to occur it takes between

1 and 3 weeks (depending on the severity of the insult) during which time the child will need renal support. Healthy kidneys in children are just as capable as adult kidneys at maintaining fluid balance. The aim in the PICU is to give enough fluid to meet insensible and obligatory renal losses while in addition trying to ensure adequate nutrition without imposing an intolerable fluid load on the kidney.

Developmental physiology of the renal system (see Chapter 8)

Until birth the placenta acts as an efficient excretory organ for the infant. Even infants with bilateral renal ageneses (Potter syndrome) can survive to term. Normally however the kidneys actively excrete urine *in utero* adding to the amniotic fluid volume. Nephrogenesis starts in the first trimester and continues up to 36 weeks by which stage each kidney has approximately a million nephrons. At term, however, only the juxtamedullary nephrons extend deep into the medulla. Glomerular and tubular function rapidly mature over the first 5 months. Glomerular filtration rate (GFR) increases from approximately 20–30 ml/m^2/min at birth to 80 ml/m^2/min at 5–6 months and reaches adult levels of 120 ml/m^2/min by 2 years. The infant's low GFR means that he has difficulty coping with fluid loads and sodium loads. The infant is able to maintain a normal urea, despite the immaturity of the loops of Henle, as the action of the so-called 'third kidney' (the incorporation of up to 50% of dietary nitrogen into new tissue growth) means that the nitrogen load to the kidney is lower than expected. The concentrating ability of the kidney is limited, however. In summary then the neonate can regulate fluid and electrolyte balance within narrow limits but has little renal reserve to deal with stress.

Total body fluid can be divided into intracellular fluid and extracellular fluid. Extracellular fluid is further divided into interstitial fluid and intravascular fluid. As the child matures total body water as a percentage of body weight alters as do the relative volumes of the different spaces. At birth 70–80% of body weight is water. This drops to 65% by 1 year and to 55–60% in the adult. In the neonate the extracellular fluid is about 50% of total body fluid (40% body weight) compared to the adult in which it represents about one-third of total body fluid (20% body weight). Total circulating blood volume is 80–90 ml/kg in the neonate, dropping to 70–80 ml/kg by 3–6 months and 70 ml/kg in older children.

Paediatric fluid and electrolyte balance (see Chapter 8)

In 1957 Holliday and Segar[12] estimated children's daily fluid requirements based on their caloric requirement with the assumption that each kilocalorie requires 1 ml of fluid. This calculation has remained the standard in paediatric fluid balance. Pyrexia will increase fluid requirements by 10% per degree centigrade rise in temperature.

Fluid replacement for the first 10 kg of body weight is 4 ml per hour. The next 10 kg are replaced at half this value, 2 ml per hour, and the remainder is replaced at half this value again, 1 ml per hour. Thus, a 25 kg child receives 65 ml per hour of fluid: $(10 \times 4) + (10 \times 2) + (5 \times 1) = 65$. This calculated fluid requirement is adequate to replace insensible losses (about 20%), ensure adequate fluid for obligate urinary nitrogen losses (a further 20%) and is sufficient to allow a modest diuresis. In children with other ongoing fluid losses (e.g. from diarrhoea, vomiting or burns), additional fluid must be given.

Dehydration, usually following gastroenteritis, is commonly seen in paediatrics. Estimates of the extent of the dehydration can be made on clinical examination. Thirst, dry mouth, decreased urine output and loss of skin turgour occur at about 3–5% loss of body weight. By 10% loss of body weight, skin turgour is markedly depressed, eyes and fontanelle are sunken, the child is lethargic and heart rate and respiratory rate are increased. At 15% dehydration cardiovascular compensation has reached its limits and tachycardia, hypotension, peripheral vasoconstriction, oliguria, and CNS depression are present. In the 10 kg child with a 10% loss of body weight due to dehydration, a fluid deficit of 1000 ml (10 kg $\times$ 10/100 = 1.0 l) needs to be corrected. This can be corrected with initial boluses of 20 ml/kg of crystalloid (e.g. 0.9% saline) repeated until heart rate and blood pressure are normalized with a further slow correction of the remaining fluid deficit over 24 h to avoid rapid shifts in fluid. This is in addition to maintenance fluids as calculated above. This regime is tailored according to biochemistry results. The normal daily requirement for Na^+ is 2–6 mmol/kg/24 h and for K^+ 2–4 mmol/kg/24 h. For most children Na^+ and K^+ can be given at 2.5 mmol/100 ml of fluid.

If renal function is impaired or fluid restriction is indicated (cardiac failure, meningitis, cerebral oedema) a moderate fluid restriction of 60% of the calculated maintenance fluid will meet insensible losses and obligate urinary losses and allow some extra fluid for nutrition.

Acute renal failure (ARF)

Critically ill children commonly develop oliguria (<1 ml/kg/h). Oliguria can be secondary to obstruction or occlusion of the bladder, both ureters, both renal arteries or both renal veins. Ultrasound of the urinary tract will identify these structural causes of ARF. To differentiate between decreased renal perfusion, established post-insult ARF and increased antidiuretic hormone (ADH) secretion, urinary sodium, and osmolarity can be measured along with plasma osmolarity. The kidney responds to hypoperfusion by retaining sodium and fluid. A low urinary sodium (<10 mmol/l) and high urinary osmolarity (>500 mmol/l) therefore suggests decreased renal perfusion. In ARF following an acute renal insult both tubular function and glomerular filtration are lost. This leads to loss of renal concentrating ability (urinary osmolarity isotonic with plasma =300 mosm/l, urinary sodium >50 mmol/l)

and a rapid rise in urea and creatinine. In inappropriate ADH secretion a concentrated urine is produced (urinary osmolarity >500 mosm/l) despite a decreased plasma osmolarity and sodium is excreted by the kidney (urinary sodium >50 mmol/l) despite hyponatraemia.

In the child in ARF weighing is a sensitive measure of fluid balance. Replacing insensible losses, the previous hour's urine output and other losses (e.g. vomiting, diarrhoea) will prevent overhydration. Central venous pressure monitoring of children in ARF ensures that they do not become hypovolaemic with renal vasoconstriction exacerbating the ARF.

Hyponatraemia secondary to water retention and decreased renal sodium conservation is seen in post-hypoxaemic ARF. It is also seen in diabetic keto-acidosis and following inappropriate ADH secretion. Children and menstruant women are most likely to develop permanent brain injury with symptomatic hyponatraemia. Fluid restriction will allow Na^+ to slowly rise and is used in moderate hyponatraemia (Na^+ >120 mmol/l). If the sodium falls below 120 mmol/l convulsions may occur. Slow correction with 514 mmol/l sodium or dialysis is indicated. Rapid correction of the Na^+ deficit can lead to cerebral oedema (the aetiology of osmotic demyelinization syndrome or central pontine myelinoysis is controversial and may be related to hypoxaemia rather than rapid correction of hyponatraemia). A reasonable sodium to aim at is 130 mmol/l corrected to this level at no faster than 1 mmol/l/h with maximum correction of 25 mmol/48 h. Attempted diuresis with frusemide or dopamine may worsen the hyponatraemia by increasing urinary sodium losses.

Continuous arteriovenous haemofiltration (CAVH) has been used in paediatric patients in the management of ARF. In infants and young children vascular access is the limiting factor for CAVH. Complications include: vessel thrombosis, infection, and bleeding. CAVH also causes a significant arterio-venous shunt. The lower blood pressures in children and the smaller arteries may mean that the transmembrane pressures and the flow through the filter are inadequate. Increasingly continuous venovenous haemofiltration (CVVH) is being used. This requires the use of pumps and a bubble trap but has the advantage of predictably allowing fluid to be removed and thus allows adequate enteral or parenteral nutrition to be given.

Haemolytic uraemic syndrome

The commonest cause of acquired ARF in children is the haemolytic uraemic syndrome (HUS). In its milder forms it is managed outwith the PICU in renal wards. It is a multisystem disorder that occurs almost exclusively in children and presents with the three characteristic features of ARF, thrombocytopenia, and microangiopathic haemolytic uraemia. Endothelial injury and platelet aggregation with subsequent erythrocyte damage produces haemolysis and widespread occlusion of renal and other organ arterioles. CNS involve-ment, if present, typically presents with seizures. This may be secondary to

hyponatraemia or hypertension or directly caused by microthrombi leading to cerebral vasculitis and oedema. Gastrointestinal involvement with colonic gangrene, perforation and pseudomembranous colitis has been reported.

Typically HUS starts with a preceding gastrointestinal infection with a verotoxin producing *E. coli* 0157 or 0.26:H11 (other pathogens such as *Shigella* are also implicated in HUS). This produces a watery diarrhoea followed by a bloody diarrhoea. Management is supportive with careful fluid balance, early renal support, blood product administration (for coagulopathy and anaemia), and aggressive control of hypertension and seizures. Peritoneal dialysis or continuous arteriovenous haemofiltration is frequently needed in severe HUS with anuria.

HEPATIC AND GASTROINTESTINAL

Hepatic

Acute hepatic failure in children is uncommon with hepatitis B, non-A non-B hepatitis and drugs (e.g. paracetamol, phenytoin, methyldopa, halothane, isoniazid) accounting for over 90% of cases. The commonest cause of chronic hepatic failure in children is biliary atresia with a 3-year survival rate following portoenterostomy ranging between 35% and 65% and arguably early hepatic transplant being a reasonable alternative treatment. Other causes in childhood include neonatal hepatitis and α_1-antitrypsin deficiency.

Hepatic developmental physiology

Hepatic development begins as an outgrowth of the foregut at about 10 weeks gestation. At birth the functional development of the liver is immature, particularly in preterm and small for gestational age infants. The newborn infant rapidly uses up its hepatic glycogen stores after birth and remains vulnerable to hypoglycaemia if stressed for the first few weeks of life. The preterm liver is unable to handle protein loads. Protein synthesis at birth is variable. Albumin approaches adult values at birth but coagulation factors are depressed with synthesis of the vitamin K-dependent factors (II, VII, IX, and X) taking 2–3 months to mature fully. Protein catabolism is also immature at birth as is drug metabolism. Hyperbilirubinaemia (physiologic jaundice) occurs because among other reasons gluconyl transferase and a cytoplasmic protein called ligandin within the newborn liver are unable to conjugate fully the bilirubin load delivered to them. This jaundice peaks at about day 5 and then resolves by 1 week. The increased portal blood flow to the liver, as the ductus venosus closes and enteral nutrition is established, leads to rapid liver maturation with normal liver function occurring by 3 months.

Table 1.5 Grading of hepatic encephalopathy

Grade	Mental state
i	Mild confusion, slurred speech, altered sleep, euphoria or depression
ii	Drowsy but rousable, inappropriate behaviour
iii	Sleeps most of the time but rousable
iv	Unrousable, may not respond to painful stimuli

Fulminant hepatic failure

The combination of acute hepatic failure and encephalopathy is called fulminant hepatic failure. Hepatic encephalopathy is thought to be due to the impaired handling of ammonia, fatty acids, mercaptans, and phenols which damage the blood–brain barrier and reduce Na^+, K^+-ATPase activity. This leads to glial swelling and cerebral oedema. Table 1.5 shows a simple but useful clinical grading for hepatic encephalopathy. 80% of children with fulminant hepatic failure and grade iv encephalopathy die.

Therapy is mainly supportive: monitoring and treating abnormal oxygen saturations, blood glucoses, acid–base imbalances and electrolyte and coagulation defects. The coagulopathy is caused by a combination of decreased production of coagulation factors, vitamin K malabsorption, thrombocytopenia, and disseminated intravascular coagulation. Intravascular volume must be maintained to avoid renal impairment and impede the development of hepatorenal syndrome (as urea production is decreased creatinine is a better indicator of renal function than urea in hepatic failure). Treatment of encephalopathy and raised ICP is supportive. Sedation should be avoided. Toxin production can be decreased by restricting dietary proteins and giving lactulose. H_2 receptor antagonists are given prophylactically to decrease the incidence of gastrointestinal bleeding with its high (30%) mortality. ICP monitoring is usually instituted in children with stage iii encephalopathy. Mannitol, steroids, hyperventilation, haemodialysis and exchange transfusions have all been used with equivocal efficacy. These children are at high risk of infection because of neutrophil dysfunction and the seeding of blood by enteric organisms. Infection may present subtly with changes in conscious level. Broad-spectrum gram positive and negative cover is required.

Gastrointestinal system

Structural abnormalities during the development of the gastrointestinal system and the subsequent surgical correction or palliation result in infants and children being admitted to the PICU. Necrotizing enterocolitis (NEC) is a common problem affecting 1–5% of all neonates admitted to neonatal

intensive care units. Severe dehydration following diarrhoea is another common cause of PICU admission.

Development

The intestine begins as a hollow tube with the respiratory system appearing as an outgrowth from the foregut at about 3 weeks of age. By 4 weeks the septum transversum forms between the liver and the pericardium but leaves large openings on each side called the pericardioperitoneal canals. By about 5 weeks the pleuroperitoneal membrane closes over these canals thus forming the diaphragm. The midgut rapidly elongates producing a loop of bowel that temporarily outgrows the abdominal cavity by 6 weeks and herniates into the umbilical cord. During this period it rotates counterclockwise by 270° before returning to the abdominal cavity at the end of the third month. Failure of the midgut to return to the abdominal cavity is termed an omphalocele. Malrotation during its return to the abdominal cavity can lead to volvulus, obstruction or infarction. At about 7–10 weeks parts of the lumen of the gastrointestinal tract are temporarily obliterated but recanalize by means of vacuolization shortly thereafter. Failure of this recanalization leads to duodenal atresia.

Tracheoesophageal fistula

Tracheoesophageal fistulae (TOF) represent a failure of the respiratory tract to completely separate from the gastrointestinal tract and usually present in infancy as feeding difficulties with coughing and cyanosis. The commonest type (85%) has a blind upper oesophageal pouch with a distal tracheoesophageal fistula. 5% of tracheoesophageal fistulae are the so called 'H' type with a patent trachea and oesophagus and a fistula between them at the thoracic inlet. Aspiration, from fluid in the pharnyx which cannot be swallowed or continued soiling of the trachea in the 'H' type, leads to an aspiration pneumonitis. Diagnosis is made by failure of passage of a nasogastric tube with chest X-ray showing the tube lying in the oesophageal pouch. It is confirmed by barium and endoscopy. The 'H' type is more difficult to diagnose and may present in an older infant with feeding difficulties, coughing, choking, and recurrent episodes of pneumonitis. Ventilatory support of infants with tracheoesophageal fistulae can lead to rapid gastric dilatation with splinting of the diaphragm, making ventilation difficult. The position of the endotracheal tube may be critical. Intubation of a blind pouch within the trachea may lead to obstruction of ventilation. Conversely, advancing the tube beyond the TOF may be essential to allow ventilation without excessive gastric distension.

Diaphragmatic hernia

Failure of the pleuroperitoneal membrane to close the pericardioperitoneal canals leads to formation of a congenital diaphragmatic hernia with loops of bowel lying usually in the left hemithorax. The lung is hypoplastic, with a wide spectrum of severity depending on the size of the lung. Symptoms range from minimal to severe hypoxia, hypercarbia, and acidosis at birth. Both lungs tend to be affected. Controversy exists as to whether the underlying pathology is failure of normal lung maturation stopping the closure of the diaphragm or whether bowel within the hemithorax is responsible for the hypoplastic lung.

Stabilization of the infant in the intensive care unit rather than emergency closure of the diaphragm is the first priority.[13] Congenital diaphragmatic hernia presenting within the first 12 h of life has a 50% mortality. These children appear to fall into two groups. (1) A *low* mortality group in whom normal or low $PaCO_2$ can be achieved without high inflation pressures and rates. The preductal right arm O_2 saturation is higher than the post-ductal saturation suggesting adequate oxygenation with a high pulmonary artery pressure producing shunting at a ductal level. (2) The *high* mortality group remain hypercapnic despite high inflation pressures and respiratory rates and have severe pre and postductal hypoxaemia. The shunting here is occurring pre-ductally in the hypoplastic lungs or through a patent foramen ovale in the heart secondary to high right artrial pressures. At post-mortem examination this group has severely hypoplastic lungs. The patients in group one once stabilized can have early closure of their diaphragmatic hernia and with careful management can be weaned from ventilation in 48–72 h. The patients in group 2 will become increasingly acidotic on conventional ventilation. High-frequency oscillation (HFO) and extracorporeal membrane oxygenation (ECMO), with correction of the defect on ECMO, are currently under investigation for patients in this high-mortality group.

Necrotizing enterocolitis (NEC)

This is a common problem, affecting 1–5% of neonates in intensive care units and carries a 10% mortality (20% in infants who perforate). It is associated with preterm birth, hypoxaemia and stress. It is characterized by ulceration of the small bowel and colon and is assumed to be caused by bowel hypo-perfusion which decreases mucosal integrity and allows infection with gas-forming organisms to occur.

The untreated disease typically starts with abdominal distension, feeding intolerance, and bloody stools progressing to abdominal obstruction and per-foration over a period of days (hours in the fulminant form). The abdominal X-ray is normal in mild cases but progresses to thickening of the bowel wall with dilated bowel loops and eventually pneumatosis intestinalis (gas bubbles in the bowel wall) and perforation with free gas in the abdomen in severe NEC.

Management is aimed at treating the underlying cause of the hypoperfusion (and if possible preventing the disease in the first place), 'resting the gut' by giving parenteral nutrition and nasogastric suctioning (for at least 7–10 days) and treating the mucosal infection with antibiotics (e.g. ampicillin, gentamicin, and metronidazole). Late intestinal obstruction is seen at 2–6 weeks in 5–10% of cases.

Diarrhoea

Children may present with severe dehydration following gastrointestinal tract infections. Viral diarrhoea is responsible for an estimated 5 million preschool deaths worldwide.

Group A rotaviruses produce a watery diarrhoea and are the major cause of dehydration with a viral diarrhoea in children aged between 6 months and 2 years. Treatment is supportive with oral rehydration solutions (typically containing 60 mmol Na^+ and 100 mmol glucose per litre) or breast milk for infants and children with mild to moderate dehydration. Severely dehydrated children should be given IV fluids along with oral fluids. In bacterial diarrhoeas (commonly *E. coli, Salmonella, Shigella, Campylobacter*), the management is again mainly supportive with antibiotics rarely indicated unless stool samples are positive for *Clostridium difficile* or *Giardia* or the child is severely ill with *Campylobacter* or *Shigella* infections.

Nutrition

Nutrition in the critically ill child has undergone a profound rethink in the last 5 years. The hazards of total parenteral nutrition (TPN) combined with the realization that the gastrointestinal tract requires a luminal source of nutrition to maintain its integrity has led to the enteral feeding of the majority of patients in the PICU despite critical illness, muscle relaxants and morphine. The importance of enteral nutrition compared to parenteral nutrition is that it preferentially maintains the integrity of the gut mucosa, stopping the translocation of bacteria through the gut wall. Even if the enteral nutrition is inadequate for total body caloric requirements it is started to ensure substrate is available for the gastrointestinal mucosa.[14]

Infants and children have decreased fat and protein stores compared to adults and tolerate stressed starvation poorly. Enteral feeding should be started as soon as possible and can be introduced as quarter-strength or half-strength feeds. Basal calorific requirements are calculated as per Holliday and Segar.[1] To these requirements a stress factor is added ranging from 10% for surgery to 100% for large burns. Expressed breast milk has about 0.7 kcal/ml, as do most standard infant milk formulas. Pediasure which is used from about 1–5 years of age has 1.0 kcal/ml. After this age adult isotonic formula can be used with typical caloric values of 1.0 kcal/ml.

Current TPN solutions are low in glutamine and arginine. Glutamine is used by replicating cells and is the preferred energy source for enterocytes helping to maintain gastrointestinal integrity. Arginine is used to increase NO production, an important cellular messenger, and is a semiessential amino acid (being required for growth). In the future the new concept of nutritional therapy rather than nutritional support may be increasingly important. Nutritional therapy is giving nutritional supplements such as glutamine, arginine, omega 3 fatty acids (to enhance prostaglandin synthesis) or uracil (to improve cellular immunity) to decrease the incidence of nosocomial infections.

INBORN ERRORS OF METABOLISM, REYE'S SYNDROME AND SUDDEN INFANT DEATH SYNDROME[15]

Inborn errors of metabolism are being increasingly recognized as more centres can perform diagnostic tests and paediatricians are increasingly aware of the presenting symptoms. Many cases of Reye's syndrome and sudden infant death syndrome (SIDS) are now recognized as inborn errors of organic acid, urea cycle, or amino-acid metabolism. Although each different type of inborn error of metabolism is rare the large number of different types (at least 58 presenting in the newborn period) means that PICUs in major teaching centres see two or three cases per year. The definitive diagnosis is difficult for the non-specialist. The initial management and resuscitation of these children, however, follows basic principles until the definitive diagnosis is reached.

Those inborn errors presenting with acute life-threatening illness tend to present in the neonate or young infant as protein is introduced into the diet. Initially vomiting is characteristic with the later development of seizures, coma, apnoea, respiratory distress, cardiovascular collapse, or sepsis. The presence of hypoglycaemia and severe metabolic acidosis should warn of the possibility of an inborn error of metabolism and trigger checking of the child's ammonia and lactate levels.

Hyperammonaemia (more than three times normal) suggests a urea cycle defect. Hyperammonaemia in combination with severe acidosis suggests an organic acid metabolism defect. Lactic acidosis and hypoglycaemia suggest a problem in carbohydrate metabolism. Blood for amino-acid screening and carnitine levels and urine for ketones and organic acid analysis should be taken at the initial presentation. The more usual bloods for gases, electrolytes, glucose, ammonia, lactate, liver function tests and a coagulation screen are also needed.

Intravenous glucose must be given to correct the hypoglycaemia and a continuous glucose infusion will be required. Peritoneal dialysis or haemofiltration is an effective therapy for hyperammonaemia until appropriate specific therapy can be started (e.g. protein restriction, arginine supplementation, and

the use of alternative pathways for nitrogen excretion in the urea cycle defects or the use of carnitine in medium chain acyl-coA dehydrogenase (MCAD) deficiency to enhance acetyl-coA metabolite excretion). Early discussion of the child with a paediatrician who has an interest in inborn errors of metabolism is essential.

The incidence of Reye's syndrome is one to six cases per million in children. It is usually preceded by an acute viral illness such as influenza or chickenpox. Reye's syndrome is an unexplained, non-inflammatory encephalopathy in a child under 16 years of age with serum hepatic transaminases or blood ammonia concentrations greater than three times the upper normal limit. Hepatic histopathology shows swollen and pleomorphic mitochondria. The incidence in the United Kingdom has fallen recently for two reasons. First, warnings issued in 1986 abut the association between Reye's syndrome and aspirin ingestion in children has led to the withdrawal of paediatric formulations of aspirin. Second, up to a quarter of children initially diagnosed as suffering from Reye's syndrome are subsequently recognized as having an inborn error of metabolism.

The management of Reye's syndrome is aimed initially at correcting the hypoglycaemia, correcting the acidosis, rehydrating the child and treating the raised ICP with a thiopentone infusion to maintain a cerebral perfusion pressure >40 mmHg.[16]

Up to 5% of children dying from SIDS may have an MCAD deficiency. These children, however, tend to be unwell for 24–48 h prior to presentation. Again, as in Reye syndrome, a public health campaign ('back to sleep') has resulted in a marked fall in the incidence of SIDS. In 1989 there were 1337 cot deaths in England and Wales compared with 442 in 1993. Deaths are most common (60%) in the first 3 months of life, are more common in winter than summer and are strongly associated with parental smoking.

DIABETIC KETOACIDOSIS

Most children with diabetic ketoacidosis (DKA) are satisfactorily treated outwith the PICU. It is, however, a life-threatening condition with a 15% mortality and a number of children need PICU monitoring (Table 1.6). The combination of polyuria, polydipsia, dehydration and Kussmaul respiration with laboratory confirmation of hyperglycaemia, ketosis and acidosis should lead to the rapid treatment of the diabetic ketoacidosis. Initial therapy, as always, is management of the Airway, Breathing and Circulation. Airway and ventilation problems are usually associated with depressed conscious level. All children with a Glasgow Coma Score less than 8 should have their airway secured. All children with DKA are dehydrated. Treatment of the dehydration with isotonic saline or Ringer's lactate with repeated boluses of 10–20 ml/kg is required until the patient is cardiovascularly stable. An insulin infusion is

Table 1.6 Reasons for admitting child to PICU or tertiary-care centre

Circulatory shock	Cerebral oedema
Severe acidosis (pH <7.1, H⁺>80 nmol/l)	Young age (<2 years)
Cardiac dysrhythmias	Hospital unfamiliar with management
Coma	of child with diabetic ketoacidosis
Respiratory failure	

started at 0.1 units/kg/h until the blood glucose falls below 15 mmol/l. At this point 5 or 10% glucose can be started to maintain the blood glucose in this range while the ketosis is resolving.

Electrolyte imbalances include hyperkalaemia, hypokalaemia and hypophosphataemia. Severe acidosis is a combination of lactic acidosis and ketoacidosis. Treatment with bicarbonate is usually withheld unless the pH is less than 7.1 (H^+ >80 nmol/l) or the patient is hyperkalaemic. Cerebral oedema may be a potentially fatal complication of therapy. Subclinical brain-swelling has been identified in children treated for diabetic ketoacidosis and may be an unavoidable result of treatment. In the hyperosmolar state the brain protects itself from dehydration by producing osmoprotective molecules. If the serum osmolarity is subsequently rapidly decreased, by giving the patient relatively hypotonic solutions or by rapidly dropping the serum glucose or sodium, the brain swells and brain herniation and death may occur. Fluid should be limited to 4 l/m²/24 h and serum sodium, which should rise as the serum glucose falls, should be closely monitored.[17]

SEPSIS SYNDROME AND SEPTIC SHOCK[18]

Septic shock is an exaggerated host response to bacteria and their cell wall components rather than a direct action of the bacteria itself on the host. The host response to bacterial invasion of tissues is to activate a complex combination of humoral and cellular defences to destroy the bacteria. Some local tissue damage is the acceptable cost to the host of the eradication of the infection. In systemic infections these same mechanisms, globally activated, are responsible for the widespread pathophysiologic changes seen in sepsis syndrome and septic shock.

The terminology for different stages of shock has until recently been confused. Consensus statements for definitions of severity of septic shock in adults and children have recently been published. The systemic inflammatory response syndrome (SIRS) describes the spectrum of disease caused by a variety of immunological, traumatic, surgical or septic insults which may lead to multiple organ dysfunction syndrome (MODS) and death. In SIRS, caused

by infections, the progression is from sepsis to sepsis syndrome to early septic shock to refractory septic shock to MODS and death (Table 1.7). This progression can be extremely rapid, over no more than a few hours, as occurs in fulminant meningococcal septicaemia.

Tumour necrosis factor (TNF) and interleukin-1 (IL-1) are cytokines released by macrophages and endothelial cells in response to exposure to bacteria and their breakdown products. These cytokines with numerous other mediators (e.g. arachidonic acid metabolites, platelet activating factor, interferons, and interleukins) lead to a cellular and a humoral response. The activation of polymorphonuclear leukocytes is thought to be responsible for the vascular injury in septic shock. Complement further activates polymorphs and causes histamine release from mast cells. A direct interaction between endotoxin and factor XII (Hageman factor which also takes part in bradykinin production) activates the intrinsic pathway while cytokines interact with factor vii to activate the extrinsic pathway. Together this leads to the development of disseminated intravascular coagulation. Endogenous opiates are thought to regulate peripheral responses by acting as neurotransmitters in sepsis and septic shock but their exact role is unknown.

The aim of intensive care management of sepsis is to ensure the optimal transport of oxygen from the environment to the tissues by ensuring adequate ventilation and oxygenation and by supporting the circulation with fluids and vasoactive inotropes. Treating the underlying cause with appropriate antibiotics and drainage of known purulent foci is essential if MODS is to be avoided. Early volume resuscitation is essential as restoring the circulating volume early in sepsis maintains cardiac output and hence oxygen delivery to the tissues. A large volume of fluid, at least 100 ml/kg of crystalloid in fulminant meningococcal septicaemia, is required in early septic shock to try and prevent the development of refractory septic shock. Central venous monitoring is essential. Volume resuscitation should be started before inotropes or vasoconstrictors as 'flogging an empty heart' is pointless. Dopamine is often the inotrope/vasoconstrictor of first choice as arguably it combines α and β adrenergic actions in a dose-dependent fashion. As the early septic shock progresses to refractory septic shock adrenaline or noradrenaline may need to be added to maintain adequate renal and cerebral perfusion pressures. As MODS develops venovenous haemofiltration may be required.

In paediatric practice the age of the child, the origin of the bacteria (community versus hospital acquired) and the immunological status of the patient are important factors in the correct choice of empiric antibiotic (Table 1.8).

Meningococcal septicaemia[19]

The overall case fatality rate for meningococcal disease is 5–10%. No vaccine is available for the commonest organism in the United Kingdom, the group B meningococcus. Fulminant meningococcal septicaemia presents classically

Table 1.7[18] Definitions of the stages of the systemic inflammatory response syndrome (SIRS)

Sepsis ⟶ Sepsis syndrome ⟶ Early septic shock ⟶ Refractory septic shock ⟶ Multiple organ dysfunction syndrome (MODS)

Sepsis	Sepsis syndrome	Early septic shock	Refractory septic shock	Multiple organ dysfunction syndrome (MODS)
Infection with: hyperthermia/ hypothermia tachycardia tachypnoea abnormal WBC	Sepsis with at least one of: acute mental changes hypoxia lactate raised oliguria	Sepsis syndrome with: hypotension or poor capillary refill responding to fluids or drugs	Sepsis syndrome with: hypotension or poor capillary refill lasting for more than 1 hour despite fluids, drugs, and inotropic support	Any combination of: DIC ARDS Acute renal failure Acute hepatic failure Acute CNS dysfunction

WBC = white blood cell count; DIC = disseminated intravascular coagulation; ARDS = adult respiratory distress syndrome; CNS = central nervous system.

Table 1.8 Choice of antibiotic for community acquired and nosocomial infections by age groups

Age	Suspected bacterial agent	Antibiotics
Neonate Community acquired	Group B streptococci Enterococci *Listeria pseudomonas* E. coli	Ampicillin + gentamicin
Nosocomial	Staphylococci	add flucloxacillin (vancomycin if known to be resistant)
1–3 months	Above + below	Ampicillin + cefotaxime
>3 months Community acquired	*Haemophilis influenzae* Pneumococcus Meningococcus	Cefotaxime or ceftriaxone
Nosocomial	Staphylococci	Add flucloxacillin (vancomycin if known to be resistant)

with purpura, shock, and coma in previously well children, under 5 years of age. Rapid deterioration to MODS and death is common. Fulminant meningococcal septicaemia represents one end of a spectrum of disease with a benign self-limiting infection at the other extreme. Septicaemia with meningitis seems to be a good prognostic factor while meningococcal meningitis on its own has the best prognosis.

Meningococcal septicaemia is one of the most challenging disease processes to treat in the PICU but can also be one of the most rewarding as full recovery is common in survivors. The early treatment with antibiotics preferably before admission to hospital and the use of scoring systems, such as the Glasgow meningococcal septicaemia prognostic score (GMSPS), to identify rapidly the children with meningococcal infection who will need aggressive intensive care support are associated with improved outcome.

Antibiotics (ceftriaxone or cefotaxime) and early fluid loading (up to 100 ml/kg of crystalloid in 10–20 ml/kg aliquots) with CVP monitoring is required initially to try and prevent the development of refractory septic shock. Children failing to respond to these measures with high scores on the GMSPS should be intubated and ventilated. Inotropes such as dopamine, dobutamine, enoximone, noradrenaline, or adrenaline may be required to maintain adequate tissue perfusion. The insertion of a pulmonary artery flotation catheter, although difficult in small children, allows the measurement of

pulmonary artery occlusion pressures and cardiac outputs. This allows fluid loading and inotropic support to be modified so as to optimize tissue perfusion. The early initiation of haemofiltration allows fresh frozen plasma and platelet replacement therapy to be given if required for disseminated intravascular coagulation without volume overloading the child.

Raised ICP combined with poor cerebral perfusion can lead to severe brain damage in an otherwise intact child. Keeping the head in a neutral position with a slight head up tilt with hourly neurological observations to detect changes in pupillary reactions is essential. Mannitol and hyperventilation may temporarily decrease cerebral swelling and allow the underlying hypoperfusion problem to be addressed. The role of ICP monitoring in the management of the most severely ill children is controversial.

The acute course of fulminant meningococcal septicaemia is usually quite short with improvement or demise within the first 48 h.

Toxic shock syndrome

The combination of high fever (>38.9 °C), hypotension, diffuse macular erythroderma with secondary desquamation and MODS is typical of toxic shock syndrome. This is caused by a toxin-producing strain of *Staphylococcus aureus* or occasionally a group A *Streptococcus*. Antibiotic cover with flucloxacillin and a third generation cephalosoporin combined with a determined effort to identify a source of infection is required in addition to the normal supportive measures in the septicaemic patient.

Haemorrhagic shock encephalopathy

This syndrome presents in a previously healthy child usually aged between 2 and 10 months with the rapid onset of shock, fever, seizures, coma, hepatorenal dysfunction, and disseminated intravascular coagulation (DIC). The aetiology is unknown but appears to be non infectious and may be related to hyperpyrexia. It is associated with a 50% mortality and severe neurological deficits in the survivors despite aggressive ICU management.[20]

TRAUMA

Trauma is the major cause of death in children older than 1 year of age in the United Kingdom. It is responsible for 22% of deaths in the 1- to 4-year-olds and 34% of all deaths in the 5- to 14-year age group. Paediatric trauma differs from adult trauma in a number of ways. A far higher proportion of children are pedestrians or cyclists. Falls and road traffic accidents account for almost 80% of all paediatric trauma. Trauma in the paediatric patient tends to be blunt with multisystem injury the rule rather than the exception. About 50%

of deaths could be avoided by simple preventative measures with optimal post-injury management saving an additional 5% of children. Non accidental injury is a feature of paediatric trauma which requires a high index of suspicion by the clinician and must be constantly examined for. The injured child has a significant chance of full recovery even following devastating injuries to solid viscera and extremities as long as he has not received a significant head injury.

Head injury in the child is responsible for 25% of all deaths in children aged 5–15 years. Head injuries, if associated with severe CNS injury, never fully recover and can condemn the child to severe long-term disability. The concept of the 'golden hour' established by adult trauma surgeons is compressed to a few 'golden moments' in the head-injured child. Little can be done about the primary effects of the head injury which occur at the moment of the trauma and consist of contusion, intracranial bleeding and neuronal shearing. As extracranial causes of secondary injury are more common than intracranial the secondary brain injury can be minimized by ensuring adequate cerebral tissue perfusion and oxygenation. The rapid application of the ABCs at the site of the accident by advanced trauma life support (ATLS), paediatric advanced life support (PALS) or advanced paediatric life support (APLS) trained personnel offers the best hope of decreasing the secondary injury. The intracranial causes of secondary injuries are cerebral oedema, neuronal swelling, cerebral hyperaemia and haematomas which lead to raised ICP and decreased cerebral perfusion. Prompt evacuation of haematomas is associated with decreased mortality and morbidity. Indications for a neurosurgical opinion and for CT scan have been published (Table 1.9). Head injuries continue to kill and cripple children.

Early traumatic epilepsy is common in children, especially in infants and only rarely signifies an intracranial haematoma. Seizures are usually self-limiting with phenobarbitone or phenytoin being given to control the frequency and duration of subsequent seizures. The management of generalized brain swelling is controversial but in patients with a Glasgow Coma Scale <8, moderate hyperventilation to a $PaCO_2$ of 25 mmHg (3.2 kPa), a CT scan to exclude focal lesions and intracranial pressure monitoring is common practice. Control of low cerebral perfusion pressure by hypothermia, barbiturate

Table 1.9 Criteria for CT scan and referral to neurosurgical unit

Acute	Urgent
Skull fracture + any neurological sign	Confusion persisting for >6 hours
Coma persisting after resuscitation	Compound depressed skull fracture
Deterioration in conscious level	Suspected cerebrospinal fluid leak (nose or ear)
Focal pupillary or limb signs	Persisting or worsening headache or vomiting

coma, mannitol, inotropes, fluid restriction, and the use of specific neurotoxic mediator antagonists remain to be fully evaluated.[21,22]

Blunt thoracic trauma is common in children usually associated with multi-system injury. The most common injuries are pulmonary contusion, haemo or pneumothoraces, and rib fractures. Major thoracic vascular injuries following trauma are relatively rare but are associated with a high mortality, occurring in about 8% of fatalities.

The vast majority of abdominal injuries in the paediatric patient are caused by blunt trauma. The success of conservative management of hepatic and splenic disruption is now well established in paediatric practice. The indication in paediatric patients for peritoneal lavage is thus diminished as a positive lavage does not necessarily result in operative exploration of the abdomen. The early involvement of the paediatric surgeon who will eventually be looking after the child, combined with frequent monitoring and observation of the child's haemodynamics and fluid balance is essential.

Near-miss drowning

Drowning is the third most common cause of death in children in the United Kingdom. About one-third of children admitted unconscious to hospital will die or be severely neurologically disabled. Prompt retrieval from the water and on-site resuscitation is associated with a good outcome. On admission to hospital the best sign of a good outcome is established spontaneous respiration. By 6 h post-immersion all children who fully recover have normal sustained pupillary responses.

In the United Kingdom most outdoor drownings are associated with water temperatures of less than 20 °C. The protective effect of hypothermia (<32 °C) is more pronounced in children as their large surface area in relation to body weight leads to rapid even cooling. The aphorism that 'you are not dead until you are warm and dead' is particularly apt in the near-drowned child as up to one-third of hypothermic children with fixed dilated pupils will make a full recovery. Aggressive resuscitation of the hypothermic child is thus warranted. Active warming with warm fluids, warmed and humidified gases, peritoneal lavage, and cardiopulmonary bypass if available is advocated. The further PICU management includes ventilation, correction of fluid and electrolyte imbalances and ICP monitoring. Raised ICP is associated with a poor outcome. Aggressive resuscitation of the child who is normothermic, and has suffered a cardiac arrest or has fixed dilated pupils, is associated with severely neurologically disabled survivors.

Child abuse (non-accidental injury)

Again the difference between adult ICU practice and PICU practice can be seen in this uniquely paediatric syndrome. A child is considered to be abused

Table 1.10 Child abuse

Features of non-accidental injury
Delay in seeking medical help
Details of accident vague or alter with each telling
Accident incompatible with injury
Parental affect abnormal
Parents may be hostile, rebut imagined accusations or leave before being seen by a consultant
Abnormal interactions between child and parents
Child may reveal abuse

if he or she is treated by an adult in a way that is unacceptable in a given culture at a given time. Non accidental injury or physical abuse is only one type of abuse. Neglect, sexual abuse and emotional abuse also occur. About 4% of children under the age of 12 years are notified to the authorities in the United Kingdom because of suspected child abuse. Commonly the abuser is a parent or cohabitant who is not related to the child. Often the abuser was abused as a child.

As in most diagnosis the history is often the most important part of the examination (Table 1.10). Some injuries such as cigarette burns, fingertip bruising, and frenulum tears are virtually diagnostic of child abuse. It is the commonest cause of severe head injury in the first year of life. In the infant the combination of coma and retinal haemorrhages should be assumed to have been caused by shaking. The history from the carers as to the cause of the injury will usually be misleading and will often understate the severity of the insult. The presence of subdural haemorrhages in an infant or toddler strongly suggests physical abuse. A simple fall or normal playful activity is not compatible with this finding.

The role of the intensivist is not to make a definitive diagnosis of child abuse. The intensivist, by having a high index of suspicion and a low threshold for referral, should ensure that all children who may have suffered from child abuse are referred to a consultant paediatrician or in tertiary paediatric referral centres are notified to the appropriate multidisciplinary team. The diagnosis of child abuse will never be made if it is never considered. Failure to consider the diagnosis may have major implications for the future welfare of the child and may be a matter of life or death for the infant.[23]

PHARMACOKINETICS AND PHARMACODYNAMICS

In 1992 the unexpected deaths of five children, aged between 4 weeks and 6 years, following propofol infusions highlighted again the difference in drug handling which occurs in paediatric patients. A large number of drugs used in the PICU are not licensed for use in paediatrics. Simple extrapolation from the adult data to the critically ill child without consideration of the differing physiology of the child is hazardous. The basic concepts of pharmacokinetics and pharmacodynamics are helpful in allowing the rational use of drugs in the PICU.

The pharmacokinetics of a drug is a description of the relationship between the drug dosage and the resulting concentration of the drug at the site of measurement (what the body does to the drug). It is usual to consider the absorption, distribution, metabolism, and excretion of the drug. In the PICU most drugs are given intravenously and absorption is essentially complete.

Distribution of water-soluble drugs, such as muscle relaxants, will vary markedly with the age of the child. In the preterm child total body water represents 85% of its weight but drops to 65% by 1 year and to 55% by adolescence. To achieve a given plasma concentration of a water-soluble drug a higher initial dose per kilogram must be given to the infant than to an adult. Reciprocal changes are occurring in fat, muscle and organ weight during maturation. Body fat content rises from 12% at birth to 30% at 1 year and settles at 10–15% in adolescent males and between 20 and 30% in females.

Drug metabolism is also age-dependent. Lipid-soluble drugs must first be metabolized to more water-soluble compounds before excretion in the bile or urine. Drugs are metabolized by phase 1 reactions, phase 2 reactions or both. Phase 1 reactions occur in the microsomal enzyme systems in the liver and are responsible for oxidation, reduction, and hydrolysis of drugs. These systems although present in neonates have reduced activity. During infancy and childhood these enzyme systems seem to be induced, when compared to the adult, leading to an increased capacity for clearance of drugs by children. The consequence of the changes in this enzyme system can be seen with phenobarbitone. The normal adult dose of phenobarbitone given on a weight basis to a neonate will lead to toxic blood levels. A similar dose calculated on a weight basis in a 2-year-old results in subtherapeutic levels. Conjugation or phase 2 reactions are markedly depressed in the neonate. Paracetamol and chloramphenicol both undergo hepatic conjugation which is deficient in the neonate and reduced doses should be used in the infant. Glucoronidization reaches adult values by 3 months.

Most drugs are excreted by the kidneys which are functionally and structurally immature at birth (see above). Thus most drugs have a decreased clearance and an increased half-life in infancy. Antibiotics and digoxin, for example, will need higher loading doses in the infant (because of the increased body water content) but lower subsequent doses or longer dosing intervals.

Renal function peaks at about 3 years of age and then steadily declines. In the critically ill child renal function may be impaired or non existent with marked cumulation of drugs occurring.

The pharmacodynamics of a drug is a description of the pharmacological response a given concentration of the drug produces (what the drug does to the body). The concentration of free drug at its site of action is dependent on the pharmacokinetics of the drug and amount of drug binding to albumin, α_1-acid protein (AAG) and other proteins. Not only are these proteins lower in infants than in children and adults but they also appear to have diminished binding capacity. The amount of free drug at a given total drug plasma concentration is thus higher in the neonate and infant.

The interaction between pharmacodynamics and pharmacokinetics is seen in the use of muscle relaxants. The infant seems to be more sensitive to the action of vecuronium in that the plasma concentration of vecuronium required to produce muscle relaxation is lower than in the child or adult. However, because of the increased volume of distribution of vecuronium in the infant the initial dose of vecuronium is similar to the adult dose. The increased volume of distribution combined with increased efficacy of the drug at lower plasma concentrations leads also to prolongation of its action.

Close monitoring of plasma levels of drugs (e.g. antibiotics, anticonvulsants and digoxin) combined with daily biochemistry to monitor renal and hepatic function allows rational prescribing in critically ill children.

Poisoning

Since the introduction in 1976 of child-resistant containers there has been a steady fall in the incidence of accidental poisoning (16 deaths in 1989) despite the fact that 20% of children under the age of 5 years can open these containers. Poisoning represents less than 3% of the admissions to the PICU at the Royal Hospital for Sick Children in Glasgow, with most being admitted for observation following the ingestion of tricyclic antidepressants. The treatment of accidental ingestion of drugs or other poisonous substances is based on the ABCs of resuscitation combined with general supportive measures, attempts to decrease further absorption, attempts to enhance elimination and specific therapy when appropriate. The local poisons information service should be contacted for advice on specific management of the particular agent ingested and to ascertain the toxic dose in children. The role of ipecac and gastric lavage is controversial. In particular, ipecacuanha should not be given to children who are not fully alert or if corrosives have been ingested. If more than 4 h have elapsed since ingestion then its value is limited unless the drug is known to decrease gastric emptying. Its use can also make subsequent treatment with activated charcoal or polyethylene glycol ineffectual. Activated charcoal acts by binding the drug to the charcoal and decreasing its absorption. The use of a combination of activated charcoal and a

cathartic such as sorbitol should be limited to a single dose. The role of whole gut lavage with isotonic preparations such as polyethylene glycol to flush out the bowel remains controversial. Specific therapies include the use of digoxin specific antibodies, desferrioxamine in iron poisoning and acetylcysteine in paracetamol poisoning. General supportive measures nowadays also extend to the use of ECMO following tricyclic ingestion or lignocaine overdosage.[24–27]

NOSOCOMIAL INFECTIONS

A nosocomial infection is an infection that was acquired in hospital and was not present or incubating upon admission. The overall mortality attributed to nosocomial infections is approximately 11% in NICUs and PICUs. The reported incidence of nosocomial infections varies widely (3–24%) depending on the type of PICU (neonatal, cardiac or general) and definitions of infection. An infection implies the multiplication of the organism within the host compared to colonization which suggests that the organism is multiplying on a body surface without evidence of an immune response.[28,29]

In general the incidence of nosocomial infection increases with:

- the length of patient stay (<1% at 72 h but >50% by 35 d)

- the severity of illness (3.4% if Paediatric Risk of Mortality Score (PRISM) <10 but 10.8% if PRISM >10)

- the age of the child (13.4% in neonates compared to 3.8% in children >10 years, and up to 25% in children under 2 years)

- invasiveness and duration of procedures (2.7% of arterial lines infected at 6 d but 100% infected by 34 d).

Bacteraemias and pneumonias are the commonest types of nosocomial infection encountered in the PICU. The most common nosocomial organisms in bacteraemias are coagulase-negative staphylococci and *Staphylococcus aureus*. They are almost invariably intravascular cannulation related. Ensuring sterility at the time of insertion and minimizing the number of 'break-ins' may decrease the incidence of infections. The type of fluid being infused, the presence of a surgical wound or the presence of infection elsewhere in the patient are also important determinants of catheter-related infections. The use of antibiotics with activity against normal upper-respiratory flora, H_2 blockers which allow colonization of the stomach with gram-negative bacilli, nasogastric tubes which allow organisms to reflux to the oropharynx, and endotracheal intubation which bypasses the normal barriers against respiratory tract infection, all combine to increase the likelihood of developing nosocomial pneumonias. Nosocomial pneumonias with gram-negative organisms are the commonest fatal noscomial infections with a mortality ranging from 20 to

70% depending on the organism. The use of sucralfate instead of H_2 blockers and minimizing the duration and indiscriminate use of broad-spectrum antibiotics may help to minimize the incidence of nosocomial pneumonias. Close consultation with a bacteriologist to target antibiotic therapy will decrease the indiscriminate use of, and frequent changes between different, broad-spectrum antibiotics which leads to the selection of resistant noso-comial bacteria and fungi. Other important causes of nosocomial infections are urinary catheters which should be removed as soon as possible, naso-tracheal intubation which is associated with sinusitis and otitis media (pre-sumably by direct obstruction of drainage from the sinuses and by causing dysfunction of the Eustachian tube). Hand-washing is the most important means of decreasing the transmission of organisms between patients and must be strictly enforced. RSV and *Clostridium difficile* will however defeat simple hand-washing and need barrier nursing as both are transmittable from en-vironmental surfaces surrounding the patient.

PSYCHOLOGICAL ASPECTS

The parents, child, extended family and staff of the PICU experience psy-chological stress when a child is critically ill or dying. In Western countries in the late twentieth century children are not expected to die. The death of a child produces the most intense grief reaction in parents. The five stages of grief—denial, anger, bargaining, depression, and acceptance—also apply to anticipatory grief. Recognizing these stages allows staff to support the parents through the early stages of their grief. Parents find particularly stressful periods when their child cannot communicate with them or when they see their child in pain or frightened. Parents need to receive accurate information which is frequently updated. They also need to be with their child so that they can continue their parenting role. Parents should be allowed liberal access to their child and should be afforded the opportunity to be with their child after his or her death.

Support for the parents may be available from extended family members, religious organizations, community mental health services or social services. An opportunity should also be given to the parents to talk to the PICU consultant some 6–8 weeks later to allow the parents a chance to ask questions and clear up concerns or feelings of guilt. The results of a post-mortem exam-ination can also be communicated to the parents at this time. Parents often feel they have failed their child even when the illness is outwith their control. Follow-up questions should be asked at this time to help screen for depression in the family.

The nursing and junior medical staff must make prompt and appropriate decisions in an extraordinarily stressful environment. Emotional detachment from the child can be perceived as cold and uncaring, while over-involvement

is emotionally draining, may impair the staff's judgment and may be detrimental to the care of other patients in the unit. Regular team meetings to ensuring appropriate positive feedback, ongoing education and to vent anxiety and offer support are important to decrease job-related stress. Unfortunately it is these areas which are often the first to be sacrificed when the unit is at its busiest and most stressful.[30]

LEARNING POINTS

1. The spectrum of diseases is different in paediatric intensive care compared with adult intensive care but the basic principles of management are the same.

2. The initial management of the child will continue to be outwith paediatric tertiary referral centres and so resuscitation skills must be taught and maintained.

3. The early transport of children following resuscitation and stabilization to a PICU will ensure optimal management of the critically ill child.

REFERENCES

1   Pollack MM, Alexander SR, Clark N *et al.* Improved outcomes from tertiary centre pediatric intensive care; a statewide comparison of tertiary and non tertiary care facilities. *Critical Care Medicine* 1991; **19**: 150–159.
2   Crone RK. Pediatric and neonatal intensive care. *Canadian Journal of Anaesthesia* 1988; **35**: S30–S33.
3   Shann F. Pediatric intensive care around the world: Australia. *Critical Care Medicine* 1993; **21**: S405–S406.
4   Downes JJ. The future of pediatric critical care medicine. *Critical Care Medicine* 1993; **21**: S307–S310.
5   Downes JJ. The historical evolution, current status and prospective development of pediatric critical care. *Critical Care Clinics of North America* 1992; **8**: 1–22.
6   European Resuscitation Council. Guidelines for advanced life support. *Resuscitation* 1992; **24**: 111–121.
7   European Resuscitation Council. Guidelines for paediatric life support. *Resuscitation* 1994; **27**: 91–105.
8   Soifer SJ. *Developmental cardiovascular physiology.* Pediatric Critical Care Clinical Review Series, The Society of Critical Care Medicine, Baltimore, 1990.
9   O'Rourke PP. *Developmental pulmonary physiology.* Pediatric Critical Care Clinical Review Series, The Society of Critical Care Medicine, Baltimore, 1989.
10 Beale R, Grover ER, Smithies M *et al.* Acute Respiratory Distress Syndrome (ARDS): no more than a severe acute lung injury. *British Medical Journal* 1993; **307**: 1335–1339.
11 Wald ER. Dexamethasone therapy for children with bacterial meningitis. *Pediatrics* 1995; **95**: 21–28.

12   Holliday MA, Segar WE. The maintenance need for water in parenteral fluid therapy. *Pediatrics* 1957; **19**: 823–832.

13   Bohn D, Tamura M, Perrin D *et al*. Ventilatory predictors of pulmonary hypoplasia in congenital diaphragmatic hernia, confirmed by morphologic assessment. *Journal of Pediatrics* 1987; **111**: 423–431.

14   Aitkinson S, Bihari D. The benefits of enteral nutrition in the critically ill patient. *Current Opinion in Anaesthesiology* 1994; **7**: 131–135.

15   Burton BK. Inborn errors of metabolism: the clinical diagnosis in early infancy. *Pediatrics* 1987; **79**: 359–369.

16   Glasgow JFT, Moore R. Reye's syndrome 30 years on: possible marker of inherited metabolic disorders. *British Medical Journal* 1993; **307**: 950–951.

17   Kecskes SA. Diabetic ketoacidosis. *Pediatric Clinics of North America* 1993; **40**: 355–363.

18   Saez-Llorens X, McCracken GH. Sepsis syndrome and septic shock in pediatrics: Current concepts of terminology, pathophysiology and management. *Journal of Pediatrics* 1993; **123**: 497–508.

19   Nadel S, Habibi P, Levin M. Management of meningococcal septicaemia. *Care of the Critically Ill* 1995; **11**: 33–38.

20   Editorial. Haemorrhagic shock and encephalopathy. *Lancet* 1985; **2**: 535–536.

21   Gentleman D, Dearden M, Midgley S *et al*. Guidelines for resuscitation and transfer of patients with serious head injury. *British Medical Journal* 1993; **307**: 547–552.

22   Arnaik AP, Lieh-Lai MW. Transporting the neurologically comprised child. *Pediatric Clinics of North America* 1993; **40**: 337–343.

23   Carty H, Ratcliffe J. The shaken infant syndrome. *British Medical Journal* 1995; **310**: 344–345.

24   Koren G. Medications which can kill a toddler with one tablet or teaspoonful. *Clinical Toxicology* 1993; **31**: 407–413.

25   Fine JS, Goldfrank LR. Update in medical toxicology. *Pediatric Clinics of North America* 1992; **39**: 1031–1053.

26   Phillips S, Gomez H, Brent J. Pediatric gastrointestinal decontamination in acute toxin ingestion. *Journal of Clinical Pharmacology* 1993; **33**: 497–507.

27   Vale JA, Proudfoot AT. How useful is activated charcoal?: Studies have left many unanswered questions. *British Medical Journal* 1993; **306**: 78–79.

28   Stein F, Trevino R. Noscomial infections in the pediatric intensive care unit. *Pediatric Clinics of North America* 1994; **41**: 1245–1257.

29   Goldmann DA. Infection control in pediatric intensive care. *Current Opinion in Pediatrics* 1992; **3**: 444–454.

30   Todres DI, Earle M, Jellinek MS. Enhancing communication. *Pediatric Clinics of North America* 1994; **41**: 1395–1403.

2

Early recognition of the critically ill child

N.S. Morton

It is as important that people working with children are able to recognize the *early* signs of failure of the respiratory, circulatory and central nervous systems as it is for them to be able to treat cardiac arrest in children (see Chapter 3). This is because the outcome from established paediatric cardiorespiratory arrest is so poor. It is particularly important to prevent progression to cardio-respiratory arrest whenever possible and, unfortunately, the compressed time-scale of deterioration in children is often not appreciated. Decompensation can occur in *seconds* in the seriously ill child.

So a scheme for assessing children must be equally quick and capable of being carried out simultaneously with basic life support manoeuvres. The aim is to sort out children in less than 30 s into (1) those who are stable, (2) those who have early signs of potential respiratory, circulatory or neurological failure, (3) those who have clear evidence of respiratory, circulatory or neurological failure, and (4) those who have arrested. In all but the first group, treatment should be started at once to prevent further deterioration.

RAPID ASSESSMENT OF CHILDREN

To decide whether vital systems are working properly should take less than 60 s and relies very much upon clinical observation. As in resuscitation, the priorities are to assess the airway, breathing and circulation with a rapid neurological assessment.

Simultaneously look to see if the child is making breathing movements, listen and feel for air movement and feel for a pulse. Is the child awake, only responding to sound or pain, or is he/she unresponsive?

If the child is making breathing movements, are these of a normal rate, pattern, and excursion with air moving in and out without extra work or added noises? If so, then the child's respiration is likely to be adequate provided the airway is open and the circulation and neurological status are normal. If not, then the child has the potential for respiratory, circulatory or neurological failure.

Rapid respiratory rate is a sign of airway or lung disease or is a response to a metabolic acid load. Slow respiratory rate is a sign of exhaustion, central nervous system depression, poisoning or raised intracranial pressure.

Is the child working hard to breathe? If so, then he/she is at risk of respiratory, circulatory or neurological failure. The pattern of breathing is a useful sign: a see-sawing of chest and abdominal breathing movements indicates increased work of breathing due to airway obstruction or decreased lung compliance. It is especially noticeable in young children in whom the rib-cage is very soft and compliant and breathing is mainly diaphragmatic. The attachments of the diaphragm pull inwards causing intercostal, subcostal and sternal recessions. In addition the child may use the accessory neck strap muscles to try to increase the rib excursion and may want to sit up and forward in a tripod position to use these muscles to greater advantage. This extra tug results in suprasternal and supraclavicular recessions.

Added noises such as stridor, wheezing, or grunting are important warning signs. Inspiratory stridor usually indicates upper airway obstruction, while expiratory stridor usually indicates intrathoracic airway obstruction. Expiratory wheeze indicates lower airway obstruction or narrowing and often results in a long expiratory time. If stridor or wheeze disappears, this may be very bad. It suggests that no air is moving in or out because airway obstruction is now complete or the child has become exhausted and is unable to maintain ventilation or has become apnoeic. *The silent chest is always a cause for alarm.*

Grunting may be heard in small infants with stiff lungs as they try to maintain their small airways and alveoli open during expiration. They breathe out against partially closed vocal cords to generate end expiratory positive pressure and this expiratory braking effect helps to prevent distal lung collapse.

In small infants who are obligate nasal breathers, flaring of the nostrils is a sign of increased work of breathing.

Periodic breathing is usually a sign of brain dysfunction, raised intracranial pressure or can occur in preterm or ex-preterm infants.

Cyanosis of the lips, tongue and skin can give warning of respiratory or circulatory failure but can be misleading and is often a late sign. For example, anaemia may prevent clinical cyanosis becoming evident despite profound hypoxaemia as the concentration of deoxygenated haemoglobin must be at least 5 g/dl.

Peripheral perfusion can be judged to be poor from the presence of cool, pale or mottled peripheries. Trends can be followed clinically by reassessing whether the line of demarcation moves centrally over time (indicating deterioration in perfusion) or peripherally (indicating improving perfusion). The capillary refill time in the periphery gives similar information with delayed refill in poorly perfused children.

Some skin rashes may give a 'spot diagnosis', for example the petechial rash of meningococcal disease is characteristic but confirmation by Gram staining

of scrapings from the lesions will assist differentiation from, for example pneumococcal septicaemia.

If a pulse is felt at the initial assessment, the rate is a helpful sign with very fast rates indicating high circulating catecholamines as may occur in shock or hypoxaemia, or due to increased metabolism as in pyrexia. Slow heart rate is nearly always secondary to hypoxaemia but can also occur in children with raised intracranial pressure. The presence of good volume central pulses in the absence of peripheral pulses indicates a circulation compensating for relative hypovolaemia by vasoconstriction. Weak central pulses indicate very poor cardiac output and profound hypotension. Absent femoral pulses may indicate aortic coarctation. A murmur, triple cardiac rhythm, irregular pulse or enlarged liver may suggest primary cardiac disease.

Depression of conscious level, pupillary dilatation or inequality, decorticate or decerebrate posturing or seizures are all important signs of primary or secondary neurological failure. Irritability or agitation are often associated with hypoxaemia.

AUGMENTED RAPID ASSESSMENT OF CHILDREN

To gain additional information quickly it is helpful to assess the arterial oxygen saturation by pulse oximetry (SpO_2), the arterial blood pressure using an automated non-invasive machine, the electrocardiograph, the core and peripheral temperatures and the estimated hourly urine output. Capillary or arterial blood samples can help in assessing the adequacy of ventilation, acidosis, serum electrolyte and blood sugar values. Repeated samples guide treatment. In most hospital situations results are available very quickly. A chest X-ray can be helpful in diagnosing gross lung pathologies. Children with airway obstruction should not be sent to the X-ray department for soft-tissue X-rays of the neck. If these are deemed necessary, they should be done in the paediatric intensive care unit.

All these techniques have problems in interpretation and should not be used in isolation or instead of the clinical assessments. Children have a tremendous capacity to compensate their physiological values until they suddenly decompensate. Examples are maintenance of blood pressure in shock, or maintenance of oxygenation and CO_2 elimination in airway obstruction.

REASSESSMENT AND TRENDS

A cycle of regular reassessment to follow the trends towards improvement or deterioration is essential and must be frequent in children and sometimes continuous.

LEARNING POINTS

1. Rapid deterioration can occur in children and assessment must be quick, thorough and concurrent with treatment.

2. Clinical signs should allow triage of children within 30 s.

3. Electronic monitoring, blood samples and imaging can all assist the recognition of critical illness but must not be used in isolation from the clinical findings.

FURTHER READING

Advanced Paediatric Life Support Group. *Advanced paediatric life support.* BMJ Publishing Group, London, 1993.

3

Resuscitation of infants and children

P.M. Cullen

Each year in the United Kingdom, approximately 7500 children die. About 50% will die in the first month of life, and a further 20% by the age of 1 year (Table 3.1). The causes of death vary with age.[1] In the neonatal period, birth asphyxia, congenital abnormalities, and factors associated with preterm birth such as respiratory distress syndrome, periventricular haemorrhage, and sepsis are the main killers. In infants less than 1 year, sudden infant death syndrome (SIDS) is the most common cause of death, followed by congenital abnormalities and infections. After 1 year trauma is the most frequent cause of death, and remains so well into adult life. Neoplasms are also an important cause of death in older children (Table 3.2).

The aetiology of cardiac arrest in children differs from that in adults. The commonest underlying cause in children is respiratory failure. This may result from upper or lower airway disease such as croup, bronchiolitis, pneumonia, asthma, and foreign body aspiration. Respiratory depression caused by prolonged convulsions, raised intracranial pressure, neuromuscular disease, or drug overdose may also lead eventually to cardiac arrest. The second commonest pathway to cardiac arrest is through circulatory failure due to fluid loss or fluid maldistribution. Cardiac arrest of primary cardiac origin, e.g. arrhythmias and pump failure are uncommon in childhood and are most frequently seen in the paediatric intensive care unit. The pathways leading to cardiac arrest in children are summarized in Fig. 3.1.

Asystole is the commonest recorded rhythm (77%), with ventricular fibrillation being relatively rare (9%).[1] This would help explain the poor prognosis compared with adults. In adults, most arrests are caused by a primary cardiac event, e.g. ventricular fibrillation.

The poor long-term outcome from cardiac arrests in childhood is easily understood if consideration is given to the aetiology. In the majority of children, the previously healthy heart continues to function until increasing hypoxia and acidosis produce progressive bradycardia and ultimately asystole. Anoxia sensitive organs such as brain and kidney may suffer massive insult before the heart finally stops. Often the child will be resuscitated, only to die of multi-organ failure in the intensive care unit. The worst possible outcome is to survive with severe neurologic deficit. Efforts to improve outcome are best directed to the early recognition and prevention of cardiac arrests.

Table 3.1 Number of deaths by age group (England and Wales, 1992. From the Office of Population Census and Surveys)

Age group	Number of deaths
0–28 days	2955
4–52 weeks	1584
1–4 years	874
5–14 years	1167

Table 3.2 Common causes of death in childhood (England and Wales, 1991)

	4–52 weeks	1–4 years	5–14 years
Cot death	42%	0%	0%
Trauma	4%	22%	34%
Infections	14%	15%	5%
Neoplasms	1%	12%	21%
Congenital abnormalities	18%	20%	10%

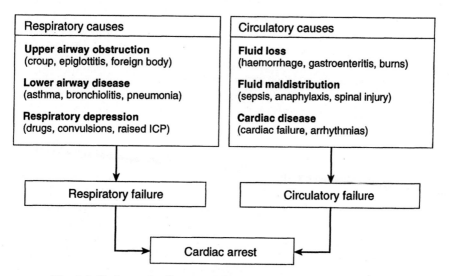

Fig. 3.1 Pathways leading to cardiac arrest in infants and children.

RECOGNITION OF THE SERIOUSLY ILL CHILD (SEE CHAPTER 2)

Cardiac arrest in infants and children is rarely a sudden event. It is more often preceded by progressive deterioration in respiratory and circulatory function. In many situations potential asystolic cardiac arrests may be averted by early recognition of the child in distress and prompt intervention. It is as important to recognize the signs of impending cardiopulmonary arrest, as it is to treat the arrest once it happens. In order to detect abnormalities, it is essential to be familiar with the normal physiological variables for that age (Table 3.3).

Respiratory failure is clinically characterized by inadequate ventilation or oxygenation. This can be assessed by looking at the work of breathing. Increased work of breathing will show as tachypnoea, recession, use of accessory muscles, grunting, and tachycardia. An inspiratory noise when breathing (stridor) is a sign of upper airway obstruction whilst wheezing denotes lower airway disease. Decreased effectiveness of breathing shows as a reduction in air movement on chest auscultation despite good effort.

Pulse oximetry is useful to measure oxygen saturation. The hypoxic and/ or hypercapnic child will be agitated and/or drowsy. As respiratory failure progresses the child becomes exhausted, respiratory effort decreases leading to acidosis, hypoxia and cardiac arrest.

Circulatory failure (shock) is characterized by inadequate perfusion of organs and tissues. Clinical signs may vary depending on the underlying cause (sepsis, hypovolaemia, cardiac failure). Tachycardia, decreased pulse volume, and poor peripheral perfusion (cool periphery, absent peripheral pulses, reduced capillary refill) are all important signs. Hypotension is a late and pre-terminal sign. Early agitation and then drowsiness leading to unconsciousness are characteristic. Oliguria and anuria may also be present.

Potential cardiopulmonary failure is present in any child with progressive respiratory failure, a reduced level of consciousness and/or evidence of shock. Bradycardia, hypotension, and irregular respirations are late, ominous signs. Every doctor who works with sick children should be able to recognize potential cardiopulmonary failure based on a rapid assessment (Table 3.4). The assessment should take less than 30 s to complete and allows the child to be

Table 3.3 Physiological variables by age group

Age (years)	Respiratory rate (breaths per min)	Heart rate (beats per min)	Systolic blood pressure (mmHg)
<1	30–40	110–160	70–90
2–5	20–30	95–140	80–100
5–15	15–20	80–120	90–110
>12	12–16	60–100	100–120

Table 3.4 Rapid cardiopulmonary assessment

A:	Airway	Patency
B:	Breathing	Respiratory rate
		Work of breathing
		Stridor/wheeze
		Air entry
		Skin colour
C:	Circulation	Heart rate
		Pulse volume
		Capillary refill
		Skin temperature
		Mental status

categorized as (1) stable, (2) potential respiratory or circulatory failure, (3) established respiratory or circulatory failure or (4) cardiopulmonary failure. This initial assessment should allow a systematic approach to treatment based on clinical findings.

RESUSCITATION TECHNIQUES

The cardiopulmonary resuscitation (CPR) sequence and general resuscitative principles are similar for infants, children and adults. However, priorities and techniques differ somewhat for different age groups.

A somewhat artificial line is generally drawn between infants (<1 year) and small children less than 8 years. Resuscitation of the critically ill child requires a rapid and systematic response that is well rehearsed. The team approach works best, with each member taking responsibility for different tasks. The team leader should be identified and take responsibility for directing the resuscitation. Ideally a minimum of four people should attend each arrest. Resuscitation must begin immediately and must not await the arrival of equipment. A single operator can support the vital respiratory and circulatory functions of a collapsed child without equipment.

Resuscitation is divided into two stages. Basic life support is defined as resuscitation without equipment while advanced life support is resuscitation using equipment and drugs. Both are required for optimum resuscitation. In the hospital setting basic life support may be required if drugs and equipment are not immediately available.

BASIC LIFE SUPPORT

On arrival at the arrest a rapid cardiopulmonary assessment should be performed to identify immediate life-threatening problems (Table 3.4). It includes evaluation of the airway, breathing and circulation (ABC). As in any resuscitation the ABC sequence should be adhered to. If trauma is suspected, the cervical spine must be completely immobilized, and neck extension, flexion, and rotation prevented. When the child is moved, the head and body must be held and turned as a unit.

AIRWAY

An obstruction airway may be the primary problem and correction of the obstruction can result in recovery without further intervention.

Relaxation of the muscles and passive posterior displacement of the tongue may lead to airway obstruction in the unconscious victim. This is relieved by the head tilt–chin lift manoeuvre. One hand is placed on the child's forehead and the head tilted back gently into a neutral or slightly extended position. The fingers of the other hand are placed along the bony margins of the chin lifting the mandible upwards and outwards (Fig. 3.2). Care must be taken to avoid closing the mouth or pushing on the soft tissues in the floor of the mouth as these will further obstruct the airway. In infants, an optimal airway is maintained with the head lying in the neutral position. In older children the neck should be slightly extended.

It should be remembered that infants are primarily nose-breathers and this is the child's built-in mechanism for overcoming obstruction caused by a relatively large tongue. If a neck injury is suspected, head tilt should be avoided, and the airway opened by jaw thrust. In this manoeuvre, two or three fingers are placed under each side of the lower jaw at its angle and the jaw lifted forward (Fig. 3.3).

Having opened the airway, we need to check that it is not obstructed by an obvious cause, e.g. vomit or a foreign body. Blood, mucus, and vomit should be removed by gentle suction. If a foreign body is present it should be removed carefully with a pair of forceps. The finger sweep technique used in adults should not be used in children as it may cause trauma and bleeding which will worsen the situation. Furthermore, foreign bodies may be forced further down the airway and become lodged below the vocal cords. Not all upper-airway obstructions are due to foreign bodies; infections of the upper airway such as epiglottis may rapidly produce total obstruction.

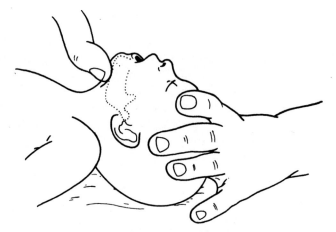

Fig. 3.2 Head tilt chin lift.

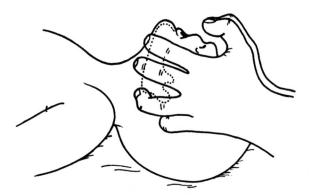

Fig. 3.3 Jaw thrust.

BREATHING

After the airway is opened, we next must determine if the child is breathing. This is done by looking for chest movement, listening for breath sounds and feeling for exhaled air over the mouth and nose. If the child is not breathing despite an adequate airway then ventilation should be started. If equipment is not immediately available, mouth-to-mouth ventilation will be required. Holding the airway open, the rescuer covers the mouth and nose of the infant or the mouth only of the older child with his or her mouth. Slow breaths are

given, pausing after each breath to take a breath, whilst watching for chest movement. By giving the breaths slowly, an adequate volume will be delivered at the lowest possible pressure thereby avoiding gastric distension. The correct volume for each breath is the volume that causes the chest to rise. Initially five breaths should be given before checking the pulse.

CIRCULATION

In infants, the brachial or femoral pulses are most easily felt,[2] whereas in the older child the carotids should be palpated. If the pulse is absent or slow or extremely weak, chest compressions should be started. For effective cardiac massage the child must be placed lying flat on a firm surface. In infants compression should be applied one finger's breadth below an imaginary line between the nipples at a rate of 100 beats/min and a depth of 2 cm.[3,4] Cardiac massage can be performed with the hands compressing the sternum with the thumbs (the encircling method) (Fig. 3.4). Alternatively, the sternum is compressed using two fingers (traditionally the ring and middle fingers are used). The former method is associated with a better cardiac output and blood pressure and is therefore the preferred technique.[5-7]

In older children compression is applied one or two finger-breadths above the xiphoid process, using the heel of the hand to a depth of 3 cm and a rate of 100 beats/min. For infants and small children, it is recommended that one ventilation is given for every five compressions. The combination of external chest compression and expired air ventilation is known as basic life support. The basic life-support sequence for the infant and older child is summarized in Fig. 3.5.

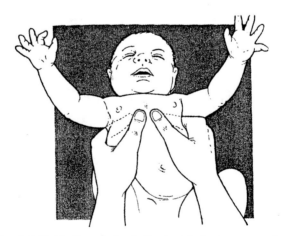

Fig. 3.4 Encircling method of external chest compression.

Paediatric Basic Life Support

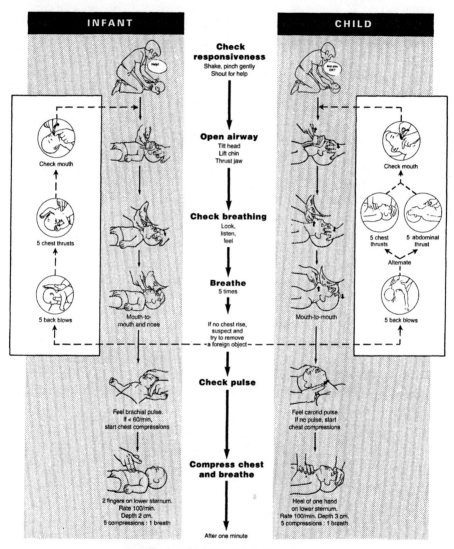

Fig. 3.5 Basic life support sequence.

THE CHOKING CHILD

The vast majority of deaths from foreign body aspiration occur in preschool children; 65% of these are infants. In the infant the larynx is conical, the narrowest part is at the level of the cricoid cartilage, hence foreign bodies tend to impact at this level. In older children and adults the larynx is cylindrical; the narrowest part is the laryngeal inlet above the vocal cords, hence foreign bodies tend to lodge at the inlet or pass into the lower airways. Virtually anything can be inhaled. The diagnosis should be suspected in infants and children experiencing acute respiratory[8] distress associated with coughing, gagging or stridor. If foreign body aspiration is witnessed, the child should be encouraged to cough as long as the cough remains forceful. Relief of obstruction should only be attempted when there are signs of complete upper-airway obstruction. Blind finger sweeps are not recommended as they simply impact the foreign body deeper in the airway.

In infants there are two techniques recommended for dislodging foreign bodies. The infant is supported in the prone position straddling the rescuer's forearm, with the head lower than the trunk. Five sharp blows can then be administered between the shoulder blades. Alternatively, with the infant lying supine along the forearm, five chest thrusts are given, using the same landmarks as for cardiac compression.

In children the Heimlich manoeuvre can also be used. Here the rescuer stands behind the victim and passes his or her arms around the victim's body. One hand is formed into a fist, covered by the other hand, and placed against the child's abdomen above the umbilicus and below the xiphisternum. A series of sharp inward tugs is then applied. In this age group, back blows can be applied with the child lying prone across the rescuer's lap or abdominal thrusts with the victim lying supine. After five back blows and five chest thrusts, the mouth should be checked and any visible foreign body removed. Ventilation should be attempted. If the obstruction remains we can repeat the sequence until the airway is cleared (Fig. 3.6). If all efforts fail then an artificial airway will be required (Table 3.5).

ADVANCED LIFE SUPPORT

Airway

As soon as skilled help and equipment arrives advanced life support should be started. Bag-valve-mask ventilation should replace expired air ventilation and the highest possible oxygen concentration should be administered. A soft closely fitting mask that is large enough to enclose the nose and mouth should be used. It should be applied firmly to the child's face whilst maintaining

Paediatric Advanced Life Support

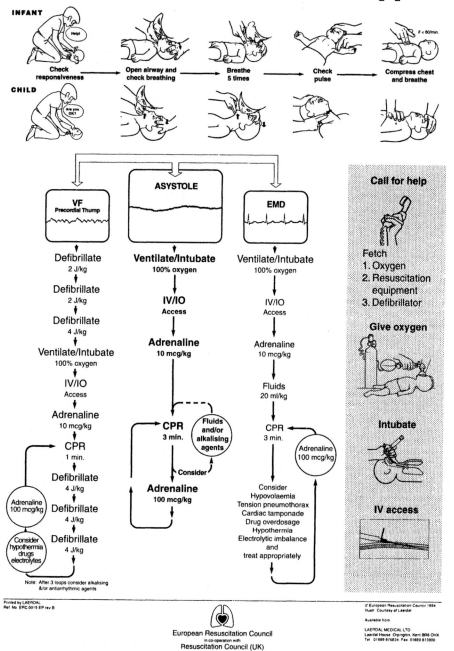

Fig. 3.6 Advanced life support sequence.

Table 3.5 The choking infant or child

CHOKING	
Infant	Child
Blind finger sweep is contraindicated	5 back blows
↓	↓
5 back bows	5 chest thrusts
↓	↓
5 chest thrusts	Check airway
↓	↓
Check airway	5 back blows
↓	↓
Repeat	5 abdominal thrusts
	↓
	Check airway
	↓
	Repeat

correct airway position. Semi-transparent face masks with cushioned rims provide the best seal.[9] The round masks (e.g. Laerdal) are particularly useful as they fit a range of ages (Fig. 3.7). During mask ventilation it may be necessary to gently move the head and neck through a range of positions to achieve optimum ventilation. If effective ventilation is not achieved, reposition the head, ensure the mask is fitted snugly against the face, lift the jaw, and consider suctioning the airway. Inflation of the stomach frequently occurs during

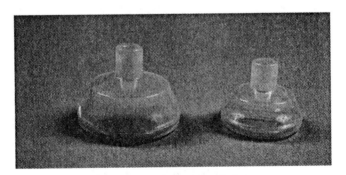

Fig. 3.7 Laerdal face masks.

mask ventilation especially when the airway is partially obstructed. Gastric distension should be avoided or promptly treated since it predisposes to regurgitation and aspiration of stomach contents.

The simplest airway adjunct is the Guedel oropharyngeal airway. Sizes vary from 000 to 4, and the correct size must be selected to be effective. The selection of too small a size will force the tongue backwards into the pharynx, causing airway obstruction. Too large a size may cause trauma, bleeding, or laryngospasm. The correct size is that which extends from the centre of the mouth to the angle of the jaw when laid on the child's face. They should not be used in the awake or semi-conscious child as they may provoke vomiting or laryngospasm.

Endotracheal intubation is the most effective method of securing the airway during CPR. It allows optimum ventilation, protects the airways from aspiration of gastric contents, and provides an optional route for drug administration. Intubation should only be attempted when the correct equipment is at hand, and should include a full range of tracheal tube sizes, suction catheters, laryngoscopes, stylets, and Magill forceps. Prior to intubation the child should be ventilated with 100% oxygen. The oxygen saturation and heart rate should be monitored. Intubation attempts should not last longer than 30 s. If unsuccessful, revert to bag and mask ventilation. A straight laryngoscope blade is recommended in infants and young children as this will allow elevation of the epiglottis with the tip of the blade (Fig. 3.8). In the emergency situation, intubation can be achieved in any age group by the skilled operator using an adult blade. Visualization of the cords may be difficult in the infant because of the relatively large tongue, more cephalad position of the larynx, and the large floppy epiglottis.[10] Having successfully intubated the child, correct positioning of the endotracheal tube should be checked by auscultation for equal breath sounds on both sides of the chest. Estimating endotracheal size and

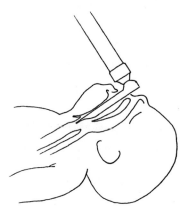

Fig. 3.8 Intubation with straight bladed laryngoscope.

length in an emergency is aided by a number of rules of thumb. Perhaps the simplest is the internal diameter of the tube which corresponds to the width of the child's little finger. Age-related formula are:

- internal diameter (mm) = 4 + age (years)/4
- length (oral)   = 12 cm + age (years)/2
- length (nasal)   = 15 cm + age (years)/2.

Another useful tip for correct tube length is to ensure that the length mark in centimetres placed at the level of the vocal cords corresponds with the internal diameter in millimetres. The tip of the tube is then invariably at mid-tracheal level. Uncuffed tracheal tubes are used in children up to 8 years of age. During resuscitation the oral route is preferred as it allows more rapid intubation. Once the child is stable the position of the tube should be confirmed by chest X-ray.

Breathing

If the child is not breathing adequately then ventilation should be assisted with a resuscitation bag attached to a face mask or endotracheal tube. Resuscitation bags are of two types: (1) self-inflating, and (2) gas-filled-anaesthetic T-piece. The self-inflating bag is manufactured in three sizes: infant, child and adult (Fig. 3.9). Most are supplied with a pressure-release valve, thus preventing enthusiastic overinflation of the lungs. The self-inflating bag delivers room air unless an oxygen source is attached. At an oxygen flow of 10 l/m, paediatric self-inflating bags deliver 30–80% oxygen without an oxygen reservoir. To deliver consistently high oxygen concentrations, a reservoir bag should be attached. Self-inflating bags are not ideal for the spontaneously

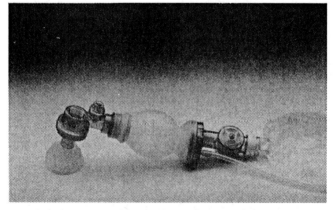

Fig. 3.9 Laerdal self-inflating resuscitator with reservoir.

breathing infant, because many small children cannot generate the increased inspiratory effort required to open the outlet valve.

The anaesthetic T-piece is preferred by skilled personnel as it allows 100% oxygen to be delivered (Fig. 3.10). Experience is necessary to use this system as it requires the operator to partially occlude the open tail of the reservoir bag whilst squeezing the bag. Similarly, it must be released during expiration. It has the advantage of giving the operator more control over peak inspiratory pressure, end tidal pressure (PEEP), and the duration of inspiration and expiration. Overventilation and overinflation can be achieved very easily. Also, the anaesthetic T-piece needs to be connected to a gas supply which, if it fails, will render the circuit useless.

Circulation

The circulation has been solely supported by external cardiac massage and monitoring of circulation has been by finger palpation of the major artery during basic life support. Monitoring equipment should now be available, electrocardiograph (ECG) leads, a non-invasive blood pressure cuff, and an oxygen saturation probe should be attached. If ventricular fibrillation is present, immediate defibrillation should be attempted. Further support of the circulation is dependent on gaining vascular access.

Rapid vascular access is critical in paediatric resuscitation for drug and fluid administration. In small children this may be extremely difficult because of the intense peripheral vasocontriction.[11] There are several options. Central venous drug administration is preferred since higher peak levels of drug are delivered more rapidly to the central circulation.[12,13] In practice, the largest

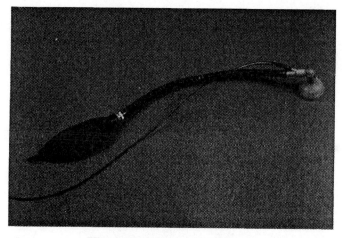

Fig. 3.10 Anaesthetic T piece.

visible vein is used and the biggest cannula possible inserted. Attempts at peripheral venous access should be limited to 90 s.[14] Useful central venous routes during resuscitation include the femoral vein, and the external jugular vein, which is often distended during a cardiac arrest. The internal jugular, subclavian and intracardiac routes mean interruption of external cardiac massage for significant periods and are prone to serious complications in young children.

When venous access is not possible, the intraosseous route is safe, rapid, and effective.[15-18] Drugs and fluids can be administered by this route and gain rapid access to the central circulation. The intraosseous route uses the rich vascular network of the long bones to transport drugs and fluids from the medullary cavity to the central circulation.

The most popular site for intraosseous needle insertion is the proximal tibia; other possible sites include the distal tibia and distal femur. The needle is inserted using a screwing action at right angles to the bone surface (Fig. 3.11). When the marrow cavity is entered a loss of resistance is felt and in some cases marrow can be aspirated. Correct positioning can be confirmed by lack of resistance to a bolus and absence of local swelling. Complications have been reported in less than 1% of cases, most of these can be avoided by careful insertion techniques.[19,20] Drugs given by this route should be followed by a bolus of fluid to facilitate rapid delivery to the central circulation. Fluid resuscitation by this route is most successful when given as repeated boluses using a syringe attached to a length of extension tubing.

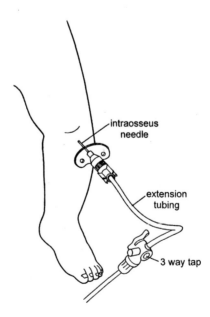

Fig. 3.11 Correct placement of an intraosseous needle.

Endotracheal intubation is often achieved early in the resuscitation and is therefore a useful route for drug administration. Lipid-soluble drugs, adrenaline, lignocaine, naloxone, and diazepam are suitable for use by this route.[21] However, animal studies suggest that peak blood levels are only about one-tenth of those achieved by the intravenous route, hence a ten fold increase in adrenaline dosage is recommended.[21-24] The dosage of other drugs given by this route will also need to be increased. The drug should be diluted in 2 ml of saline, using a fine-bore suction catheter, it should be instilled as distal as possible into the lungs, followed by a period of hyperventilation. The presence of intracardiac shunting and increased lung water may further affect pulmonary drug absorption in the newborn period. We should therefore not rely solely on this route but continue to seek more reliable access during resuscitation.

Drug usage during CPR (Table 3.6)

The majority of cardiac arrests in children are primarily respiratory in origin, therefore, ventilation with 100% oxygen is the first priority.

Adrenaline

Adrenaline is the most useful drug during resuscitation. It is a directly acting sympathomimetic agent with both alpha and beta adrenergic effects. During resuscitation, it is the alpha effects that are of primary importance. An increase in systemic vascular resistance elevates aortic diastolic pressure thus increasing coronary perfusion pressure which facilitates the return of spontaneous cardiac contractions.[25, 26] In the animal model of cardiac arrest, adrenaline increases the blood supply to the heart and brain. As the action of adrenaline is short lived, it should be repeated every 3 min of the arrest until the return of spontaneous cardiac activity. The currently recommended dose is 10 micrograms/kg for the first dose and 100 micrograms/kg for all subsequent doses. Recent evidence suggests that high doses (200 micrograms/kg) may be beneficial during asystolic cardiac arrest.[27,28]

Sodium bicarbonate (1 ml/kg 8.4% solution)

The use of sodium bicarbonate is recommended only during prolonged resuscitation and to treat documented metabolic acidosis. Bicarbonate administration in the absence of adequate oxygenation and perfusion will worsen intracellular acidosis by the production of carbon dioxide:

$$HCO_3^- + H^+ - H_2CO_2 - CO_2 + H_2O$$

The carbon dioxide diffuses readily across cell membranes and the blood–brain barrier causing an intracellular and cerebrospinal fluid (CSF) acidosis. The evidence for beneficial effects of bicarbonate during cardiac arrest is inconclusive at best.[29, 30]

Table 3.6 Paediatric resuscitation chart (from the Royal Hospital for Sick Children, Yorkhill, Glasgow)

	Neonatal/ 3.5 kg	3 months/ 5 kg	1 year/ 10 kg	3 years/ 15 kg	6 years/ 20 kg	8 years/ 25 kg	12 years/ 40 kg
Endotracheal tube							
Size (mm) Internal diameter	3.0	3.5	4.0	5.0	5.5	6.0	7.0
Length, oral (cm)	9	10	11	13	14	15	17
Length, nasal (cm)	11	13	14	16	19	20	22
Adrenaline 1:10 000 (IV, ET★, IO)							
1st dose 10 µg/kg (0.1 ml/kg)	0.3 ml	0.5 ml	1 ml	1.5 ml	2 ml	2.5 ml	3 ml
Repeat dose 100 µg/kg (1 ml/kg)	3 ml	5 ml	10 ml	15 ml	20 ml	25 ml	30 ml
Sodium bicarbonate 8.4%							
1 ml/kg (IV, IO)	3 ml	5 ml	10 ml	15 ml	20 ml	25 ml	40 ml
Atropine 100 µg/ml (IV, ET★, IO)							
20 µg/kg (0.2 ml/kg)	0.6 ml	1 ml	2 ml	3 ml	4 ml	5 ml	6 ml
Calcium chloride 10% (IV, IO)							
10 mg/kg (0.1 ml/kg)	0.2 ml	0.5 ml	1 ml	1.5 ml	2 ml	2.5 ml	3 ml
Defibrillation (J/KG)							
VF 2–4 J/kg	6–12	10–20	20–40	30–60	40–80	50–100	60–120
SVT 0.5 J/kg	2	3	5	7	10	12	15
Volume of fluid (colloid/crystalloid)							
20 ml/kg, repeat × 2–3 PRN	60	100	200	300	400	500	600

Drug infusion: Adrenaline / Isoprenaline / Noradrenaline — 0.3 mg/kg in 50 ml (1 ml/h = 0.1 microgram/kg/min)

Dopamine / Dobutamine — 3 mg/kg in 50 ml (1 ml/h = 1.0 microgram/kg/min)

*For endotracheal administration give ×10 intravenous dose. N.B. All drugs and fluids may be administered via the intraosseus route.

The mixed metabolic and respiratory acidosis during cardiac arrest is best treated by hyperventilation with 100% oxygen, and treatment of shock to increase tissue perfusion.

Calcium (0.1 mg/kg of 10% solution)

Calcium is essential for excitation-contraction coupling. In the normal heart calcium increases myocardial contractile function. In the ischaemic heart energy sources are depleted and calcium accumulates in the cytoplasm causing toxic effects. Studies have shown that calcium entry into the cell cytoplasm is the final common pathway in cell death, and calcium administration during cardiac arrest may actually cause injury.[31,32] Calcium administration causes coronary spasm and may produce cardiac arrest in systole unresponsive to further drug therapy. Calcium may also cause spasm of the cerebral vessels and so increase post-arrest neurological deficit. Calcium may be of use in specific situations, cardiac arrest related to hyperkalaemia, suspected hypocalcaemia, or overdosage with calcium channel blocking drugs.

Other drugs

Atropine is a parasympatholytic drug used to treat bradycardia caused by vagal stimulation. It has been shown to be ineffective during the acute phase of resuscitation. There is a scarcity of information about the use of anti-arrhythmic drugs during paediatric resuscitation. Ventricular arrhythmias are infrequent in children and are best treated by treating the underlying cause. Anti-arrhythmic drugs tend to be negatively inotropic and to increase the fibrillation threshold. The dose of lignocaine is 1 mg/kg followed by an infusion of 0.1 mg/kg/min iterated as required.

Glucose (2 ml/kg of 25% glucose)

Small infants and chronically ill children have limited glycogen stores that may be rapidly depleted during stressful situations. Since the clinical signs of hypoglycaemia mimic those of hypoxia, the blood sugar of all children should be checked frequently during resuscitation.

Fluid resuscitation

Expansion of the circulating blood volume is a critical component of paediatric advanced life support in children who have sustained trauma and acute blood loss.[33] It may also be life-saving in shock due to sepsis or other conditions causing fluid depletion (diabetic ketoacidosis, gastroenteritis). Early restitution of circulating blood volume in the child with circulatory shock is important to prevent progression of shock to overt circulatory failure and

cardiac arrest. Volume expansion is usually achieved with colloid initially, e.g. 5% albumin solution, haemacel, or gelofusine. An initial bolus of 20 ml/kg is given, the circulatory status is then reassessed, repeat boluses are given until improvement is seen. Further fluid resuscitation may be given as crystalloid or blood, whichever is the more appropriate.

Treatment algorithms

Asystole (Fig. 3.12)

This is the commonest cardiac arrest rhythm in children and is usually preceded by a long period of hypoxia and acidosis. The initial treatment as with any cardiac arrest is to start basic life support: airway, breathing, and circulation. Effective ventilation with 100% oxygen and chest compressions are the first priority. Drugs are given as per protocol in Fig. 3.12. Adrenaline is the most important drug after oxygen in asystole. The initial dose is 10 micrograms/kg (0.1 ml of 1:10 000) by the intravenous or the intraosseous route or 100 micrograms/kg (0.1 ml of 1:1000) down the endotracheal tube. The second dose of adrenaline and all subsequent doses should be 100 micrograms/kg (0.1 ml of 1:1000). Adrenaline is repeated every 3 min until the return of spontaneous cardiac activity. Sodium bicarbonate is no

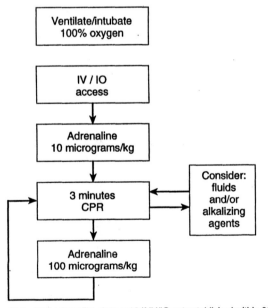

Note: ETT adrenaline dose × 10 if IV/IO not established within 90 s.

Fig. 3.12 Treatment protocol, asystole. (From *Guidelines for Paediatric Life Support Resuscitation* 1994; 27: 91–105.)

longer recommended during short cardiac arrests. It should only be considered for the treatment of severe metabolic acidosis associated with prolonged cardiac arrest. In the non-witnessed cardiac arrest it may be considered when there is no response to adrenaline. CPR is continued at compressions to ventilation of 5:1. If cardiac arrest is secondary to circulatory failure fluid therapy is indicated. A standard bolus of 20 ml/kg should be given if there is no response to the first dose of adrenaline. Either normal saline or 5% albumin can be used. The prognosis is very poor if more than two doses of adrenaline are required.

Ventricular fibrillation (VF) (Fig. 3.13)

This rhythm is uncommon in the paediatric age group and is documented in about 10% of children where terminal rhythm is recorded. Small infants lack the critical mass of ventricular muscle to sustain fibrillation potentials. The treatment is similar to that for adults. If the VF arrest is witnessed, a precordial thump is indicated, on the basis that it is quick to perform, it is unlikely to do any harm and may terminate the arrhythmia. The definitive treatment for VF is prompt defibrillation.

The first three shocks are given in rapid succession, two at 2 J/kg and the third at 4 J/kg. If the initial three shocks fail to produce defibrillation, cardiac compression should be commenced, and the child intubated and hyperventilated with 100% oxygen. An intravenous cannula should be sited and adrenaline given, followed by three further DC shocks at 4 J/kg. This sequence of adrenaline followed by three DC shocks at 4 J/kg and 1 min of CPR is continued until either VF stops or resuscitation is abandoned. If after 12 DC shocks, spontaneous rhythm has not returned, the prognosis is very poor.

The underlying cause of the arrhythmia should be considered, hypothermia or drug overdose will require specific therapy and continued aggressive resuscitation. The use of bicarbonate (1 mmol/kg) or an anti-arrhythmic agent (lignocaine 1 mg/kg: bretylium 5 mg/kg if >12 years) should also be tried. If there is still no response, different paddle positions or another defibrillator may be successful.

The paddle selected should be the largest size that allows good chest contact over the entire paddle surface and separation between the two paddles.

Infant paddles (4.5 cm) are recommended for infants up to a year of age (10 kg) and adult paddles for the rest. The larger the paddle size the lower the transthoracic impedance.[34] The anterior-posterior paddle position is theoretically superior but impractical during CPR. In the standard electrode position, one paddle is placed on the upper right chest below the clavicle and the other to the left of the nipple in the left anterior axillary line. If infant paddles are not available, adult paddles may be used by placing one on the infant chest and the other on the back.[35]

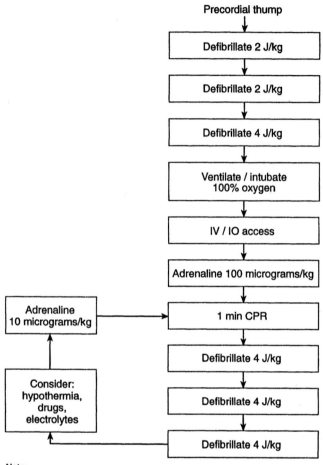

Precordial thump

Defibrillate 2 J/kg

Defibrillate 2 J/kg

Defibrillate 4 J/kg

Ventilate / intubate
100% oxygen

IV / IO access

Adrenaline 100 micrograms/kg

Adrenaline
10 micrograms/kg

1 min CPR

Defibrillate 4 J/kg

Consider:
hypothermia,
drugs,
electrolytes

Defibrillate 4 J/kg

Defibrillate 4 J/kg

Note:
1. ETT adrenaline dose × 10 if IV/IO not established within 90 s.
2. After 3 loops consider alkalizing and/or antiarrhythmic agents.

Fig. 3.13 Treatment protocol, ventricular fibrillation. (From *Guidelines for Paediatric Life Support Resuscitation* 1994; 27: 91–105.)

Electromechanical dissociation (Fig. 3.14)

This is the absence of a palpable pulse despite the presence of recognizable complexes on the ECG monitor, otherwise known as pulseless electrical activity (PEA). Causes include hypoxia, severe acidosis, hypovolaemia, tension pneumothorax, and pericardial tamponade. Other potential causes are hyperkalaemia, profound hypothermia, and drug overdose (tricylic anti-depressants, β blockers, and calcium antagonists).

The treatment is similar to that for asystole: establish basic life support, give 100% oxygen and administer adrenaline. A thorough search is made for

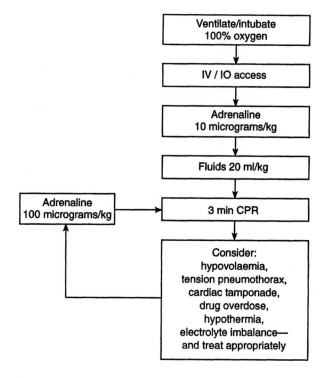

Note:
ETT adrenaline dose ×10 if IV/IO not established within 90 s.

Fig. 3.14 Treatment protocol, electromechanical dissociation. (From *Guidelines for Paediatric Life Support Resuscitation* 1994; 27: 91–105.)

the underlying cause, for example, a tension pneumothorax in a trauma victim. Hypovolaemia is the most common cause in children, therefore, following the first dose of adrenaline, a fluid bolus (20 ml/kg) should be given. Calcium is reserved for suspected hypocalcaemia, hyperkalaemia or poisoning with calcium channel blockers. While treatable causes are being excluded, treatment should continue as for asystole.

Arrhythmia management
Supraventricular tachycardia is the most common arrhythmia seen in children.

Synchronized cardioversion 0.5–2 J/kg is the treatment of choice if the child is in shock. Intravenous adenosine is rather like giving a 'medical shock' and is used in preference to DC shock as the first-line treatment.[36–38] The dose is 50 micrograms/kg, increasing over three doses to 500 micrograms/kg. The half-life of the drug is about 6 s, so it should be given as close to the heart as possible. Brief asystole is often seen, but sinus rhythm usually follows.

Discontinuing resuscitation

Currently there are no guidelines for discontinuing resuscitation. The prognosis for the child who has suffered a cardiac arrest is poor, especially if the arrest occurs outwith the hospital. In successful resuscitations there is usually a return of spontaneous circulations within a few minutes. If there is no cardiac output after 30 min of cardiopulmonary resuscitation the likelihood of a successful outcome approaches zero. It is therefore reasonable to stop resuscitation after 30 min if there is no evidence of cardiac activity. Exceptions to this rule include hypothermia, in which resuscitation should continue until the core temperature is 32 °C, and drug overdose with cerebral depressant drugs.

Neonatal resuscitation (Fig 3.15)

Approximately 6% of newborn infants require some form of assistance immediately after birth, and in those whose birthweight is less than 1500 g, this figure rises to 80%.[39] It is estimated that 70% of infants requiring resuscitation come from predictably high-risk situations. The most common predisposing factors are antepartum or intrapartum asphyxia. Other causes include maternal drug administration, sepsis and trauma. Virtually all drugs used as analgesics, sedatives, or general anaesthetics during labour can cross the placenta and in theory depress the newborn infant's respiratory centre.[40] It is important to anticipate these problems as it allows time to summon appropriately skilled staff and check resuscitation equipment. An organized and physiologically appropriate approach to resuscitation of the asphyxiated newborn is essential for a successful outcome.

Assessment

The Apgar scoring system (Table 3.7) has been widely used as a method of assessing the condition of the newborn infant. Five physical signs are examined and the score computed at 1 and 5 min after birth. It is a poor indicator of the degree of fetal acidosis, especially in the premature infant, and does not intuitively suggest a sequential, physiological approach to resuscitation.[41-43] For these reasons, assessment and intervention should be based on the ABCs of resuscitation and should never be delayed while awaiting the 1-min Apgar score.

The infant will generally fall into one of the following categories:

- vigorous crying infant (90–95%)

- gasping with a heart rate >80 beats/min (5–6%)

- pale, apnoeic and bradycardic (0.5%)

- stillborn.

Initial assessment

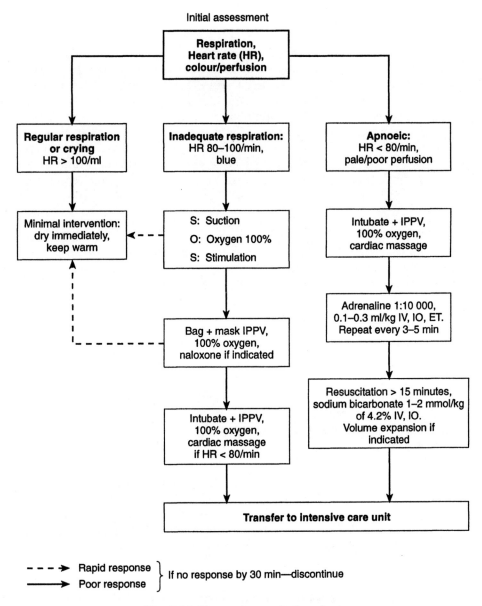

Fig. 3.15 Neonatal resuscitation chart.

Table 3.7 APGAR score

Clinical features	Score		
	0	1	2
Heart rate	0	<100	>100
Respiration	Absent	Gasping or irregular	Regular or crying
Colour	White	Blue	Pink
Response to pharyngeal suction	Nil	Grimace	Cough
Muscle tone	Limp	Diminished	Active

The initial assessment must also include an estimation of gestational age. Premature infants have a higher incidence of birth asphyxia and there is evidence that elective intubation and ventilation improves survival.[44] A decision not to resuscitate may be made in cases of extreme immaturity or gross congenital abnormality incompatible with life.

A suggested protocol for resuscitation of the newborn infant is shown in Fig. 3.15. The principles of resuscitation of the newborn infant are similar to those for adults, namely airway management, the provision of effective ventilation and circulatory support. The correct sequence may be remembered by the mnemonic ABC.

Equipment for resuscitation should be readily available and should be checked regularly to ensure that it is in good working order when required. Equipment used during resuscitation should always be replaced.

Resuscitation technique

Immediately after delivery of the head but prior to the first breath, the infant's mouth and nose should be gently aspirated. The infant is then delivered, the umbilical cord clamped and cut and the baby transferred to a pre-warmed resuscitaire. It is very important to keep the baby warm. Hypothermia increases metabolic rate and oxygen consumption, causing acidosis and hypoglycaemia and predisposes to coagulation abnormalities. The baby should be quickly dried and wrapped in a warm blanket to prevent heat loss during assessment.[45] The temperature of the delivery room should be as high as staff can tolerate and an overhead radiant heater should always be used during resuscitation.

A pink crying baby requires no further help. In the remainder, respiratory effort, heart rate, and colour should be assessed. Oxygen should be administered while the neonate is being assessed for need of additional resuscitative measures. Initially oxygen can be delivered by free-flow through a face mask attached to an anaesthetic breathing system or through a mask or funnel attached to an oxygen source set to deliver 5 l/min. Self-inflating bags should not be used as they will not deliver sufficient flow passively.

For the same reason they are unsuitable for oxygen delivery in the spontaneously breathing neonate. It is quite safe to administer 100% oxygen even to tiny premature infants for short periods during resuscitation.

If on initial assessment the newborn infant's heart rate is greater than 80/min, gentle suction and stimulation should be tried to induce respiration. The nose and buccal cavity should be gently suctioned with a soft 8F or 10F catheter and a maximum pressure of 100 mmHg. Suctioning should continue for no more than 5 s at a time whilst monitoring the heart rate. Deep suctioning of the oropharynx may result in bradycardia and apnoea.[46] If there is evidence of meconium staining, thorough suctioning of the mouth, nose, and posterior pharynx should be performed as soon as the head is delivered. Immediately after delivery, further suctioning under direct vision will be required. If the meconium is thick or the infant depressed, direct endotracheal suctioning, using the endotracheal tube as a suction catheter, should be performed. Tracheal suctioning should be repeated until no further meconium can be aspirated.

Drying and suctioning cause enough stimulation to induce spontaneous respiratory activity in most newborn infants. Gentle slapping of the feet or rubbing the back are also permissible. If by the age of 1 min such manoeuvres have not led to the baby breathing spontaneously, bag and mask ventilation should be commenced.

The recognized way of inflating the newborn lung has been to use an inflation pressure of 30 cmH$_2$O maintained for 1 s, and an I:E ratio of approximately 1:1. This currently recommended inflation pressure of 30 cmH$_2$O may be inadequate to expand the lungs artificially in the apnoeic infant and pressures of 40 or even 50 may be required in the initial stages. It has also been shown that it may be necessary to hold the lungs inflated for more than 3 s to obtain an adequate functional residual capacity.[47-49] In the apnoeic newborn infant, gradual inflation of the lungs to a peak pressure of 20–40 cmH$_2$O over 3–5 s once or twice is best. Once the lungs have expanded lower pressures will be required for effective ventilation. The recommended respiratory rate is 30–40 breaths per min (bpm). Fast rates in excess of 60 bpm do not allow an adequate inspiratory time for expansion of the poorly compliant newborn lungs.

Bag and mask ventilation is often a futile endeavour in the baby who has never drawn breath. Tidal volumes of only one-third the value seen after intubation were obtained for the same inflation pressure using bag-mask ventilation. If this form of resuscitation fails to achieve adequate air entry or

if the heart rate falls to less than 80 bpm, intubation will be required. Early intubation is recommended in the severely asphyxiated newborn infant. Ventilation is of primary importance in neonatal resuscitation and most bradycardias will respond to ventilation alone. If bradycardia continues for more than 30 s after intubation, cardiac massage should be started. The recommended rate of cardiac compressions combined with ventilation is 120/min and a ratio of three compressions to each ventilation.[50] The methods of chest compression have been described earlier in this chapter.

Drugs in neonatal resuscitation

With the exception of naloxone, drug therapy is rarely required during newborn resuscitation. Naloxone (0.1 mg/kg) is used to reverse narcotic-related depression only. The drug is short acting and may need to be repeated, thus continued monitoring is necessary after administration. By antagonizing endogenous opiods, naloxone may increase the severity of the neonatal asphyxial insult, perhaps by increasing catecholamines.[51] Care should be taken when administering naloxone to the newborn infants of narcotic addicts, since this may precipitate an acute withdrawal episode.

The indications for the use of adrenaline and sodium bicarbonate are similar to those for older children. The recommended dose of adrenaline in this age group is 10–30 micrograms/kg. The efficacy and safety of higher doses have not been evaluated in the newborn infant. A major concern, especially in the preterm infant, is the high risk of periventricular haemorrhage following systemic hypertension.[52]

Sodium bicarbonate is considered much less important than in the past.[53,54] It should only be given when there is documented severe metabolic acidosis. The dose is 1–2 mmol/kg of 4.2% given slowly. Excessive sodium bicarbonate have been implicated in the aetiology of periventricular haemorrhage in the sick neonate.[55,56] Volume expansion is recommended when there is a strong suspicion of hypovolaemia in a neonate unresponsive to other resuscitative efforts. Colloid, crystalloid, or blood may be used, and should be given in 10 mg/kg increments over 5–10 min as required. The umbilical vein is the preferred route for vascular access in the immediate newborn period. A 3.5 or 5 FG catheter should be inserted until there is free flow of blood. This prevents inadvertent infusion of hypertonic solutions into the liver. Other useful routes include peripheral vein, umbilical artery, femoral vein, and intraosseous. The endotracheal route is useful for the administration of adrenaline and naloxone.

There are a number of studies which show that babies who take up to 20 min to respond, even after the most intensive resuscitation, can subsequently develop entirely normally.[57–59] Such an outcome is rarely seen in babies who fail to make any respiratory efforts after 30 min. Certainly, if an infant with poor circulatory function has no spontaneous respiratory activity after 30 min despite adequate resuscitation, then resuscitation should be stopped.[60,61]

Before discontinuation of resuscitation one must be absolutely certain that respiratory depression is not due to sedation from maternal narcotics, over-ventilation or inherited neurological disorder. The more difficult problem is the infant whose circulation picks up but fails to breathe. These babies may be ventilated for 24–48 h and many will die from severe asphyxial encephalopathy or multi-organ failure. There is currently some dispute about the number of these babies who will be normal, and estimates range from 30% to 85%.[62]

POST-RESUSCITATION CARE

Following a successful resuscitation, a clear history of the arrest and preceding events should be obtained. This may provide useful information about the possible aetiology of the arrest, and aid definitive treatment. Post-resuscitation care consists of frequent assessments of cardiopulmonary function to detect improvement or deterioration with treatment, even if the child's condition initially appears stable. Appropriate investigations should be sent including arterial blood gases, electrolytes, blood glucose, full blood count, blood cultures, and a coagulation screen. A chest X-ray should be performed to check the position of the endotracheal tube and exclude complications. Treatment should continue to correct residual hypovolaemia, ongoing metabolic acidosis and seizure activity.

In the post-arrest period, it is common to have poor cardiac function, and inotropic support is often required. The choice of inotropic drugs will be determined by the underlying cause of the cardiac arrest. In septic or ana-phylactic shock, drugs which increase systemic vascular resistance (adren-aline, noradrenaline) will prove most useful. Whilst in cardiogenic shock, drugs which induce vasodilation and decrease myocardial oxygen requirements (dobutamine, enoximone) may be preferred. Most children will benefit from a period of controlled hyperventilation in the immediate post-arrest situation. Controlled ventilation will help ameliorate cerebral oedema and correct the mixed respiratory and metabolic acidosis resulting from the arrest.

Once the child has been stabilized, a thorough secondary survey should be performed in a systematic manner to assess other potential problems. This should consist of a complete head to toe examination, looking for bruising, lacerations, swelling, or deformity.

In trauma victims, care should be taken not to move the cervical spine during the assessment, and X-rays of skull, cervical spine, and pelvis should be requested. Continued monitoring of pulse, blood pressure, oxygen saturation, pupil size and reactivity, and Glasgow Coma Score are mandatory.

With the exception of a brief respiratory arrest following over-enthusiastic analgesia, all children who have suffered a cardiorespiratory arrest should be

transferred to an intensive care unit. For some children this will mean transfer to a tertiary referral centre. Ideally all such hospitals should have an organized paediatric support service. Transport of the critically ill or injured child is best performed by an experienced team, even if this results in some delay.

OUTCOME

The initial survival rate from true cardiac arrests is about 33% of all attempts, but when long-term survival is considered this falls to 15%.[63-65] Outcome from pure respiratory arrests is much better, with long-term survival rates in excess of 75%.[66] Survivors have a significantly shorter interval to commencement of resuscitation. If the cardiac arrest occurs outside the hospital, the chances of successful outcome are remote and many of the survivors will be neurologically damaged. Children who respond in the first few minutes of resuscitation have a much better outcome than those requiring prolonged efforts. The chances of successful outcome are negligible if there is no response after 30 min of resuscitation.

Survival rate for neonates are even lower than those for older children, with an initial survival rate of 14% and only 7% after 1 year. Factors associated with poor outcome include preterm birth, sepsis and intraventricular haemorrhage.

LEARNING POINTS

1. The aetiology of cardiac arrest in infants and children differs from that in adults. In children, the arrest usually follows a long period of profound hypoxaemia and acidosis, whilst, in adults, it is most often a sudden cardiac event.

2. The vast majority of arrests in children are preventable, therefore, awareness of precipitating factors, early recognition of the child in distress and rapid intervention are essential.

3. The general resuscitative principles are similar for infants, children and adults, and follow the ABC sequence.

4. The outcome from asystolic cardiac arrest is very poor, whilst the outcome from the more frequently occurring respiratory arrests is much better.

5. The real benefit of paediatric resuscitation training is the early treatment of potential respiratory or circulatory failure, thus preventing true cardiac arrests.

REFERENCES

1   Eisenberg M, Bergner L, Hallstrom A. Epidemiology of cardiac arrest and resuscitation in children. *Annals of Emergency Medicine* 1983; **12**: 672–674.
2   Cavallaro DL, Melker RJ. Comparison of two techniques for detecting cardiac activity in infants. *Critical Care Medicine* 1983; **11**: 188–190.
3   Philips GW, Ziderman DA. Relation of the infant heart to the sternum; its significance in cardiopulmonary resuscitation. *Lancet* 1986; **i**: 1204–1025.
4   Orlowski JP. Optimum position for external cardiac massage in infants and children. *Critical Care Medicine* 1984; **12**: 224.
5   Thaler MM, Stobie GH. An improved technique of external cardiac compressions in infants and young children. *New England Journal of Medicine* 1963; **269**: 606–610.
6   Todres ID, Rogers MC. Methods of external cardiac massage in the newborn infant. *Journal of Pediatrics* 1975; **86**: 781–782.
7   David R. Closed chest cardiac massage in the newborn infant. *Pediatrics* 1988; **81**: 552–554.
8   Committee on Pediatric Emergency Medicine. First Aid for the choking child. *Pediatrics* 1993; **92**: 477–479.
9   Palme C, Nystron B, Tunell R. An evaluation of the efficiency of face masks in the resuscitation of newborn infants. *Lancet* 1985; **ii**: 207–210.
10 Westhorpe RN. The position of the larynx in children and its relationship to the ease of intubation. *Anaesthesia and Intensive Care* 1987; **15**: 384–388.
11 Rossetti VA, Thompson BM, Aprahamian C *et al*. Difficulty and delay in intravascular access in pediatric arrests. *Annals of Emergency Medicine* 1984; **13**: 406.
12 Hedges JR, Barsan WB, Doal LA *et al*. Central versus peripheral intravenous routes in cardiopulmonary resuscitation. *American Journal of Emergency Medicine* 1984; **2**: 385–390.
13 Emerman CL, Pinchak AC, Hancock D *et al*. Effect of injection site on circulation times during cardiac arrest. *Critical Care Medicine* 1988; **16**: 1138–1141.
14 Kanter RK, Zimmerman JJ, Strauss RH *et al*. Pediatric emergency intravenous access: evaluation of a protocol. *American Journal of Diseases of Children* 1986; **140**: 132–134.
15 Rosetti VA, Thompson BM, Miller J *et al*. Intraosseous infusion: an alternative route of pediatric intravascular access. *Annals of Emergency Medicine* 1985; **14**: 885–888.
16 Valdes MM. Intraosseous fluid administration in emergencies. *Lancet* 1977; **i**: 1235–1236.
17 Orlowski JP, Porembka DT, Gallagher JM *et al*. Comparison study of intraosseous, central intravenous and peripheral intravenous infusions of emergency drugs. *American Journal of Diseases of Children* 1990; **144**: 112–117.
18 Kersall AWR. Resuscitation with intraosseous lines in neonatal units. *Archives of Disease in Childhood* 1993; **68**: 324–325.
19 Orlowski JP, Julius CJ, Petras RE *et al*. The safety of intraosseous infusions: risks of fat and bone marrow emboli to the lungs. *Annals of Emergency Medicine* 1989; **18**: 1062–1067.
20 Heinild S, Soderguard T, Tudvad F. Bone marrow infusions in childhood: experience from a thousand infusions. *Journal of Pediatrics* 1947; **30**: 400–411.

21 Johnston C. Endotracheal drug delivery. *Pediatric Emergency Care* 1992; **8**: 94–97.

22 Quinton DN, O'Bynne G, Aitkenhead AR. Comparison of endotracheal and peripheral intravenous adrenaline in cardiac arrest: is the endotracheal route reliable? *Lancet* 1987; **i**: 828–829.

23 Mullett CJ, Kong JQ, Romano JT *et al.* Age-related changes in pulmonary venous epinephrine concentration, and pulmonary vascular response after intratrachael epinephrine. *Pediatric Research* 1992; **31**: 458–461.

24 Orlowski PJ, Gallagher JM, Porembka DT. Endotrachael epinephrine is unreliable. *Resuscitation* 1990; **19**: 103–113.

25 Kosnik JWè, Jackson RE, Keats S *et al.* Dose related response of centrally administered epinephrine on the change in aortic diastolic pressure during closed-chest massage in dogs. *Annals of Emergency Medicine* 1985; **14**: 204–208.

26 Otto CW, Takaitis RW, Blitt CD. Mechanism of action of epinephrine in resuscitation from cardiac arrest. *Critical Care Medicine* 1981; **9**: 321–324.

27 Mark G, Goetting MD, Norman A *et al.* High dose epinephrine in refractory pediatric cardiac arrest. *Critical Care Medicine* 1989; **17**: 1258–1262.

28 Barton C, Callaham M. High-dose epinephrine improves the return of spontaneous circulation rates in human victims of cardiac arrest. *Annals of Emergency Medicine* 1991; **20**: 722–725.

29 Graf H, Leach W, Arieff AI. Evidence for a detrimental effect of bicarbonate therapy in hypoxic lactic acidosis. *Science* 1985; **227**: 754–756.

30 Ritter JM, Doktor HS, Benjamin N. Paradoxical effect of bicarbonate on cytoplasmic pH. *Lancet* 1990; **335**: 1243–1246.

31 Katz AM, Reuter H. Cellular calcium and cardiac cell death. *American Journal of Cardiology* 1979; **44**: 188–190.

32 Strueven HA, Thompson B, Aprahamian C *et al.* Lack of effectiveness of calcium chloride in refractory asystole. *Annals of Emergency Medicine* 1985; **14**: 626–629.

33 Carillo JA, Davis AL, Zaritsky A. Role of early fluid resuscitation in pediatric septic shock. *Journal of the American Medical Association* 1991; **9**: 1242–1245.

34 Atkins DL, Sirna S, Kieso R *et al.* Pediatric defibrillation; importance of paddle size in determining transthoracic impedance. *Pediatrics* 1988; **82**: 914–918.

35 Atkins DL, Kerber RE. Pediatric defibrillation; current flow is improved by using adult paddle electrodes. *Circulation* 1992; **86**(Supp.): 1235.

36 Overholt ED, Rheuban KS, Gutgusell HP *et al.* Usefulness of adenosine for arrhythmias in infants and children. *American Journal of Cardiology* 1988; **61**: 336–340.

37 Rossi AF, Burton DA. Adenosine in altering short-and-long-term treatment of supraventricular tachycardia in infants. *American Journal of Cardiology* 1989; **64**: 685–686.

38 Till J, Shinebourne EA, Rigby ML *et al.* Efficacy and safety of adenosine in the treatment of supraventricular tachycardia in infants and children. *British Heart Journal* 1989; **62**: 204–211.

39 Roberton NRC, ed. *Textbook of neonatology*, 2nd edn, pp. 173–195. Churchill Livingstone: Edinburgh, 1992.

40 Barrier G, Sureau C. Effects of drugs on labour, fetus and neonate. *Clinics in Obstetrics and Gynaecology* 1982; **9**: 351–367.

41 Editorial. Is the APGAR score outmoded? *Lancet* 1989; **i**: 591–592.

42 Silverman F, Suidan J, Wasserman J *et al.* The APGAR score: is it enough? *Obstetrics and Gynaecology* 1985; **66**: 331–336.

43 Sykes GS, Molloy PM, Johnson P *et al.* Do APGAR scores indicate asphyxia? *Lancet* 1982; **ii**: 494–496.

44 Drew JH. Immediate intubation at birth of the very low birth weight infant. *American Journal of Diseases of Children* 1982; **136**: 207–210.

45 Dahm LS, James LS. Newborn temperature and calculated heat loss in the delivery room. *Pediatrics* 1972; **49**: 504–513.

46 Cordero L, Hon EH. Neonatal bradycardia following nasopharyngeal stimulation. *Journal of Pediatrics* 1971; **78**: 441–447.

47 Vyas H, Field D, Milner AD *et al.* Determinants of the first inspiratory volume and functional residual capacity at birth. *Pediatric Pulmonology* 1986; **2**: 189–193.

48 Boon AW, Milner AD, Hopkin IE. Lung expansion, tidal volume and formation of functional residual capacity during resuscitation of asphyxiated neonates. *Journal of Pediatrics* 1979; **95**: 1031–1036.

49 Vyas H, Milner AD, Hopkin IE *et al.* Physiological response to prolonged and slow rise inflation. *Journal of Pediatrics* 1981; **99**: 635–639.

50 Guidelines for cardiopulmonary resuscitation and emergency cardiac care. Neonatal resuscitation. *Journal of the American Medical Association* 1992; **268**: 2276–2281.

51 Young RSK, Hessert TR, Pritchard GA *et al.* Naloxone exerbrates hypoxic-ischaemic brain injury in the neonatal rat. *American Journal of Obstetrics and Gynecology* 1984; **150**: 52–56.

52 Burchfield DJ, Berkowitz ID, Berg RA *et al.* Medications in neonatal resuscitation. *Annals of Emergency Medicine* 1993; **22**: 435–439.

53 Hein HA. The use of sodium bicarbonate in neonatal resuscitation: help or harm? *Pediatrics* 1993; **91**: 496–497.

54 Howell JH. Sodium bicarbonate in the perinatal setting revisited. *Clinics in Perinatology* 1987; **14**: 807–816.

55 Wheeler AS, Sadri S, Gutsche BB *et al.* Intracranial hemorrhage following intravenous administration of sodium bicarbonate or saline solution in the newborn lamb asphyxiated in utero. *Anaesthesiology* 1979; **51**: 517–521.

56 Simmons MA, Adcock, EW, Bard H *et al.* Hypernatremia and intracranial hemorrhage in neonates. *New England Journal of Medicine* 1974; **291**: 6–10.

57 Scott H. Outcome of very severe birth asphyxia. *Archives of Disease in Childhood* 1976; **51**: 712–716.

58 Erglander U, Eriksson M, Setterstrom R. Severe birth asphyxia: incidence and prediction in Stockholm area. *Acta Paediatrica Scandinavica* 1983; **72**: 321–325.

59 Koppe JG, Kleinerd AG. Severe asphyxia and outcome of survivors. *Resuscitation* 1984; **12**: 193–206.

60 Milner AD. Resuscitation of the newborn. *Archives of Disease in Childhood* 1991; **66**: 66–69.

61 Roy RN, Betheras FR. The Melbourne Chart—A logical guide to neonatal resuscitation. *Anaesthesia and Intensive Care* 1990; **18**: 348–357.

62 Levine MI, Sands C, Grindulis H *et al.* Comparison of two methods of predicting outcome in perinatal asphyxia. *Lancet* 1986; **i**: 67–71.

63 Eisenberg M, Bergner L, Hallstrom A. Epidemiology of cardiac arrests and resuscitation in children. *Annals of Emergency Medicine* 1983; **12**: 672–674.

64 Freinen RM, Duncan P, Tweed WA *et al.* Appraisal of pediatric cardiopulmonary resuscitation. *Canadian Medical Association Journal* 1982; **126**: 1055–1058.

65 Barzily Z, Somakh E, Sagy M *et al.* Pediatric cardiopulmonary resuscitation outcome. *Journal of Medicine* 1988; **19**: 229–241.

66 Thompson JE, Bonner B, Lower GM Jr. Pediatric cardiopulmonary arrest in rural populations. *Pediatrics* 1990; **86**: 302–306.

FURTHER READING

European Resuscitation Council. Guidelines for Paediatric Life Support. *Resuscitation* 1994; **27**: 91–105.

4

Injuries to children

N.S. Morton

ASSESSMENT AND RESUSCITATION

The priorities are assessment of the airway while neck control is carried out, assessment of breathing and the circulation while controlling bleeding, assessment of the level of consciousness and an overall assessment for other injuries. This scheme can be carried out very quickly and is easily remembered as an alphabetical list:

- airway and neck control

- breathing

- circulation and bleeding control

- disability

- exposure

The details of this scheme are similar to the rapid assessment of any critically ill child but you must assume the cervical spine is injured until proven otherwise and you must actively look for injuries other than the most obvious. Treatment should start during the initial rapid assessment if this is appropriate. So control of the neck with a hard collar in the conscious or uncooperative child or with in-line manual stabilization, a semi-rigid collar, sandbags, and tape in the unconscious child. Particular care of the neck needs to be taken during intubation, when turning or on moving the child. Immediate intubation and ventilation may be needed in severe head, face, chest or abdominal injuries, in smoke inhalation or burns or if the child is shocked.

Circulatory access with intraosseous needles, large bore peripheral venous cannulae, or central venous lines should be performed as required and surgical cut downs may be needed. Upper limb access is preferable in trauma. It is safe to give a traumatized child 20 ml/kg of colloid or 0.9% saline as a bolus. If there is no improvement, this volume can be repeated. If further fluid is needed, blood should be used and surgical help sought urgently.

Blood samples for cross-matching, haematology and biochemistry should be taken early and X-rays or scans organized. A gastric tube and urinary catheter should be passed, with care being exercised in children with suspected

basal skull fracture (use an orogastric tube not a nasogastric one) and pelvic fractures (remember urethral or bladder damage). Pain relief should be titrated intravenously and appropriate local anaesthetic blocks can quickly be performed (e.g. femoral nerve block in the child with a fractured shaft of femur, intercostal nerve blocks in the child with fractured ribs).

It is also very important to get an accurate and detailed history of the injury mechanisms as soon as possible. Once the child has been resuscitated and stabilized, a detailed examination of the head, face, neck, chest, abdomen, pelvis, spine and extremities should be performed using clinical signs and appropriate imaging techniques. A detailed record is kept of all these steps and the child is then referred and moved to the most appropriate clinical area.

LIFE-THREATENING INJURIES

It is important that life-threatening injuries are identified and treated as early as possible.

In the child with chest injuries, life-threatening situations include tension pneumothorax, massive haemopneumothorax, open pneumothorax, flail chest, cardiac tamponade, lung contusion, rupture of the trachea or a bronchus, disruption of great vessels and rupture of the diaphragm. The immediate treatment is to ensure a clear airway and give high flow oxygen. Patients may need chest drainage or aspiration, intubation and ventilation, needling and drainage of the pericardium and fluid resuscitation. Experienced anaesthetic and surgical help should be sought urgently.

For abdominal injuries, operation is indicated if there is a penetrating injury, signs of perforation of bowel or shock not responding to treatment. Sometimes a kidney is explored if it is traumatized. Clinical examination after the child has been resuscitated plus computed tomography (CT) scan and/or ultrasound of the abdomen are very useful while diagnostic peritoneal lavage usually is useless. Early expert surgical help is vital.

SPECIAL PROBLEMS OF HEAD INJURY IN CHILDREN

The head injury itself can cause damage to the child's brain but lack of adequate oxygen and/or bloodflow to the brain after the injury result in secondary damage. It is essential to maintain adequate brain oxygen and blood supplies to limit this secondary damage. To do this, the resuscitation priorities should be meticulously followed. In head injury this is particularly important because the pressure inside the skull cavity may rise rapidly if there is brain swelling or an expanding blood clot. Controlling the airway, ventilation and blood pressure all help to improve blood flow and oxygen supply to the brain. Ventilation to a normal or slightly low arterial CO_2 helps to reduce intracranial

pressure and diuretics such as frusemide and mannitol can assist in reducing brain swelling. Steroids are no longer used in head injury.

Serious head injury is indicated by the history of the injury, loss of consciousness, impaired consciousness or responsiveness, seizures, focal neurological signs, or if there is a penetrating injury. The rapid assessment of conscious level and pupils is supplemented by detailed examination of lacerations, bruises, skull vault fractures, skull base fractures and fundi. Conscious level, focal neurological signs and pupillary signs are examined in more detail also. Appropriate X-rays and scans are carried out.

Deterioration in conscious level, convulsions or pupillary signs indicate the need for urgent measures to control intracranial pressure and definitive surgical management. All patients with a Glasgow Coma Score <8 should be intubated and ventilated immediately. Others may need intubation and ventilation for transport, for adequate imaging or as indicated by other injuries. The transfer must be conducted in accordance with the principles outlined in Chapter 11 but speed is essential and may not allow time for a retrieval team from the tertiary centre to attend.

LEARNING POINTS

1. An alphabetical scheme for rapid assessment of injured children allows comprehensive evaluation in 60 s.

2. The cervical spine must be assumed to be injured and unstable until proven otherwise.

3. Early involvement of senior anaesthetic, surgical and trauma staff is vital for successful management of the injured child.

4. The head injured child presents particular problems and clear guidelines for intubation and ventilation, referral for imaging and/or neurosurgery and safe transport must be followed.

FURTHER READING

Advanced Life Support Group. *Advanced paediatric life support*. BMJ Publishing Group, London, 1993.
Gentleman D, Dearden M, Midgley S *et al*. Guidelines for resuscitation and transfer of patients with serious head injury. *British Medical Journal* 1993; **307**: 547–552.

5

Airway management

D.N. Robinson

Skilled management of the airway is a core skill requirement for paediatric intensive care. A number of neonates, infants, and children will require intensive care solely for the establishment and safe maintenance of an airway, and many patients will undergo endotracheal intubation and mechanical ventilation as part of their overall management. Concentrated practice in managing the airway can best be obtained by full-time supervised experience in the operating theatre or PICU with a paediatric anaesthetist or intensivist.

ANATOMY AND PHYSIOLOGY

There are important differences between the airway anatomy of the infant or child and that of the adult,[1,2] and these differences have important pathophysiological and practical implications.

In absolute terms, the airway is much smaller and, because resistance to breathing is related to the fourth power of the radius, relatively small amounts of oedema in the walls of the airway can greatly increase the resistance to breathing. This relationship holds when airflow is laminar—during turbulent airflow (such as might occur during crying) resistance becomes related to the fifth power of the radius. The infant has a relatively large tongue in relation to the oropharynx, making respiratory obstruction more likely should muscle tone be reduced or lost. The large tongue may also make direct larngoscopy more awkward than is the case with adults. In infants, the larynx is situated higher in the neck than in adults—at birth, the epiglottis is at the level of C1, falling to the level of C3 by 6 months. Thereafter, the larynx continues to descend to reach the adult level of C6 at around the time of puberty. This high position of the larynx decreases the angle between the base of the tongue and laryngeal inlet, creating the impression that the larynx is situated more anteriorly. The infant epiglottis is softer, shorter and floppier than in the adult. It is Ω-shaped and angled away from the long axis of the trachea. In adults, the larynx is shaped like a cylinder and the narrowest portion occurs at the level of vocal cords. In infants and prepubertal children the larynx is funnel-shaped and the narrowest portion is at the level of the cricoid ring.[3] This means that an endotracheal tube must be chosen based on the size of the

airway at the cricoid ring, and not on the size at the glottic opening. If too large an endotracheal tube is passed, subglottic oedema may occur causing post-extubation stridor, or in the longer term fibrotic changes leading to subglottic stenosis can occur. An airleak at 20–30 cmH$_2$O pressure should always be checked for following intubation.

BASIC AIRWAY MANAGEMENT

Oxygen administration

If the airway is adequate and the patient is breathing spontaneously, supplemental oxygen may be delivered by a variety of means. Oxygenation should be assessed by continuous pulse oximetry supplemented when indicated by arterial or capillary blood gas analysis.

Nasal cannulae

These are available in different sizes and provide a lightweight, easily tolerated method of administering supplemental oxygen. From the flowmeter, oxygen flows through a water bath and then to the patient via two short soft prongs which are inserted into the nares. The delivered oxygen concentration depends on the flow administered and the patient's peak inspiratory flow rate. It cannot be assessed accurately, and probably will not exceed 40%. The humidifying properties of the upper airway remain intact, but with fresh gas flows of greater than about 3 l/min there may be excessive mucosal drying.

Head box

Head box oxygen is suitable for use with infants, but is often poorly tolerated by toddlers or older children. It allows high concentrations of humidified oxygen to be given in a controlled manner. The inspired concentration of oxygen can be measured by an oxygen analyser in the box near to the infant's airway. Exhaled gases escape through the opening for the neck and relatively high flows of oxygen are required in order to flush carbon dioxide from the box.

Face masks

Face masks can be tolerated by older children, and different devices allow for the degree of sophistication required. Simple loose fitting masks can provide up to about 40% oxygen depending on the oxygen flow rate and peak inspiratory flow rate. When higher concentrations are required, a tightly fitting mask with reservoir bag, or alternatively a mask which incorporates a venturi device delivering a set concentration of oxygen can be used.

Mask and bag/valve assemblies

Proficiency in bag-mask ventilation is essential for emergency airway management and to provide optimal ventilation and oxygenation prior to endotracheal intubation.

Masks are available in a variety of materials and sizes. The black rubber Rendell-Baker Soucek face mask[4] provides a contoured fit to an infant's face and is designed to minimize airway deadspace. In practice it may be difficult to obtain an airtight seal using this face mask, and many prefer to use modern, plastic masks with a soft inflatable rim. As well as being easier to use, these masks have the advantage of being transparent, thus allowing observation of colour or the presence of vomit.

Self-inflating resuscitation bags are generally made in sizes to suit infants, children and adults. The widely available Laerdal bags are available with a 240 ml volume for infants up to about 18 months of age, a 500 ml volume for older children and a 1600 ml volume for adults. The infant and child bags have a pressure pop-off valve set at 45 cmH$_2$O to prevent inadvertent barotrauma. The patient end of the bag connects to a valve allowing positive pressure to be applied. Most, but not all bags will also allow spontaneous respiration through the valve, and this must always be checked for an individual bag/valve assembly. With an attached reservoir bag it is possible to provide close to 100% oxygen with a resuscitation bag; without a reservoir most bags will not provide more than 50% oxygen, due to the entrainment of atmospheric air. With skill and some practice in its use, a paediatric anaesthetic breathing system has much to commend it. 100% oxygen is reliably administered and a 'feel' is obtained for ventilation and the compliance of the lungs. Disposable systems are lightweight and inexpensive. The Jackson-Rees modification of the Ayres T-piece[5] consists of a T-piece to which an opened tailed bag has been added to allow positive pressure ventilation and the observation of spontaneous breaths. Positive pressure is applied by occluding the open tail of the bag using the palm of the hand, ring and little fingers while the bag is squeezed using the thumb and first two fingers. Such a system depends on a continuous supply of oxygen, and it is essential that a self-inflating bag is always available as a back-up.

Pharyngeal airways

Oropharyngeal airway

Guedel oropharyngeal airways are available in sizes from 000 (small neonate) to 4 (large adult). They consist of a curved airway with a flanged bite section and are designed to lie between the tongue and posterior pharyngeal wall. As a guide, when laid on the child's face, the correct size of airway will extend from the centre of the mouth to the angle of the jaw. If the gag reflex is present, insertion of an oropharyngeal airway is poorly tolerated and may provoke coughing, vomiting, or laryngospasm. In infants and smaller children,

the airway is inserted with the aid of a tongue depressor or laryngoscope blade 'right way up' after opening the airway using a chin lift. In older children, the airway can be inserted with its concave side facing the hard palate until the tip reaches the soft palate. It is then rotated through 180° and slid backwards over the tongue into its final position. It may be necessary to try different sizes of airway from the original estimate.

Nasopharyngeal airway

Small-sized nasopharyngeal airways are not readily available, and an appropriately sized endotracheal tube cut short can be substituted, the approximate length being from the nares to the tragus of the ear. In a semiconscious patient with intact gag reflex, a nasopharyngeal airway is better tolerated than an oral airway. Their use is contraindicated with basal skull fractures, and as bleeding is easily provoked, care should be taken with patients who have deranged coagulation. A well-lubricated tube is inserted by passing it directly backwards along the floor of the nose. Some gentle pressure and slight rotation will ease the tip of the tube past the turbinates, whereupon a definite give is felt. A safety pin, or the endotracheal tube connector should be inserted into the proximal end of the tube to prevent it falling into the nose. Flanged silastic nasopharyngeal airways are available which prevent ingress of the tube into the nose.

ENDOTRACHEAL INTUBATION

Equipment

The equipment that should be laid out prior to endotracheal intubation is shown in Table 5.1.

Table 5.1 Equipment for endotracheal intubation

Oxygen and ventilating mask and bag

Suction apparatus with Yankauer sucker

Selection of oropharyngeal airways

Laryngoscope and spare

Endotracheal tubes—one each of predicted size together with half sizes larger and smaller

Endotracheal tube stylet

Magill forceps

Gauze swabs

Lubricating jelly

Plaster remover and Tincture of Benzoin solution to clean and prepare skin for adhesive tape

Precut lengths of adhesive tape

Laryngoscopes

Straight and curved blade laryngoscopes are available in a range of sizes to suit infants and children. Up to the age of about 1 year a straight blade is usually preferred. The position of the epiglottis is high and anterior and because it is large and floppy the laryngeal inlet tends to be obscured. The straight blade is designed for the tip to be placed under the laryngeal surface of the epiglottis that is then lifted upwards to expose the glottis. Remember that this surface is innervated by the vagus nerve and a bradycardia can be induced. A variety of straight blade designs exist including Robertshaw, Wisconsin, Anderson-Magill, Oxford, Miller and Seward. The choice between these different designs is largely a matter of individual choice, and there is benefit to be gained from trying a variety of designs until preferences are formed for particular situations. Longer straight-blade laryngoscopes can also be used in older children, however from about 2 years onwards an ordinary size 3 adult Mackintosh curved blade can be used successfully in most patients. The tip of the curved blade is placed short of the epiglottis in the vallecula, and then lifting the laryngoscope tip upwards exposes the glottis because the epiglottis is lifted by the hyoepiglottic ligament. This area is innervated by the glossopharyngeal nerve and heart-rate changes are less likely to be induced.

Endotracheal tubes

In modern practice, the only endotracheal tubes used in the intensive care setting are non-reusable and made of PVC. The materials from which these tubes are made are non-irritant and non-toxic, having been implantation-tested in animals. This is indicated by the letters 'IT' on the tube. Non-cuffed tubes are used in children under 8 years of age. Below this age the narrowest section of the airway occurs at the level of the cricoid cartilage and because the larynx is funnel shaped a satisfactory fit can be obtained using a plain tube. A cuffed tube decreases the effective internal diameter of the tube. It is important to select a tube size that allows a leak pressure of less than about 25 cmH$_2$O to minimize the risk of postextubation laryngospasm or longer term subglottic stenosis.[6-8] The Cole tube, which has a shouldered tapered distal portion has been widely used in neonatal practice, but it has been shown that the shoulder increases airflow turbulence and resistance to breathing and this tube is also known to cause laryngeal injury,[9] and should no longer be used. In paediatric anaesthesia practice preformed north- or south-facing oral tubes are popular,[10] but because of the difficulty of passing a suction catheter down these tubes, they are best avoided for intensive care. Orotracheal intubation is suitable for short-term use but in the longer term nasotracheal intubation is more comfortable, gives rise to fewer complications and allows easier and more secure fixation of the tube.

A guide to endotracheal tube size and length is shown in Table 5.2. Various formulae also exist to help in estimating tube size and length:

- internal diameter (mm) = (age in years/4) + 4
- oral tube length (cm)   = (age in years/2) + 12
- nasal tube length (cm) = (age in years/2) + 15.

Another useful method of gauging the correct length of tube to insert is to have the distance from the tip of the tube in centimetres at the point where it passes between the cords to be the same as the internal diameter of the tube in millimetres. It should be remembered, however, that tables and formulae should only be used as a guide. The correct size of tube is one that passes easily, permits ventilation and allows a gas leak at less than about 25 cmH$_2$O. The correct length of tube is one whose tip is seen to lie in mid-trachea on an AP chest X-ray with the head in neutral position.

Drugs to facilitate intubation

Although in an emergency, endotracheal intubation can be achieved without the use of drugs, in most situations the judicious use of sedative and neuro-muscular blocking agents will greatly ease the process and limit any trauma or rise in intracranial pressure associated with the procedure. However, these drugs may be associated with life-threatening complications and it is imper-ative that their pharmacology is thoroughly understood. If there is any doubt about the ability to establish an airway and maintain ventilation, these drugs are contraindicated.

Intravenous anaesthetic and sedative agents
Included in this category are the intravenous anaesthetic induction agents, benzodiazepine sedative agents and opioid analgesics.

Thiopentone
In paediatric anaesthesia thiopentone remains the most commonly used intravenous induction agent, and is the agent against which all others must be judged. The 2.5% solution is highly alkaline, and may cause tissue necrosis if extravasation occurs. Accidental arterial administration may result in severe pain and arterial spasm leading to distal gangrene. Thiopentone is highly lipid soluble, its maximal concentration in brain being reached in one circulation time. Following bolus administration, its short duration of action is due to redistribution of drug. It is metabolized in the liver by oxidation to an inactive metabolite, its elimination half-life in infants and children following a single dose being around 6 h.[11] Thiopentone causes a dose-dependent reduction in myocardial contractility and a reduction in venous return. In healthy patients, this is seen as mild hypotension with a compensatory tachycardia. However,

Table 5.2 Endotracheal tube size and length

Age	Weight (kg)	Internal diameter (mm)	Length (orotracheal, cm)	Length (nasotracheal, cm)	Suction (French)
Birth	<1	2.5	5.5	7	6
Birth	1	3.0	6	7.5	7
Birth	2	3.0	7	9	7
Birth	3	3.0	8.5	10.5	7
Birth	3.5	3.5	9	11	8
3 months	6	3.5	10	12	8
1 year	10	4.0	11	14	8
2 years	12	4.5	12	15	8
3 years	14	4.5	13	16	8
4 years	16	5.0	14	17	10
6 years	20	5.5	15	19	10
8 years	24	6.0	16	20	10
10 years	30	6.5	17	21	12
12 years	38	7.0	18	22	12

in the presence of hypovolaemia or impaired cardiac function thiopentone given in normal doses may cause catastrophic cardiovascular decompensation. Thiopentone causes a fall in cerebral bloodflow and reduces cerebral oxygen consumption leading to a fall in intracranial pressure. Intraocular pressure is also reduced. Thiopentone is a potent anticonvulsant. In fit children who have received no premedication, a dose of 5–7 mg/kg of thiopentone is required. In the critically ill, dose should if possible be titrated to effect and as little as 1–2 mg/kg may suffice.

Ketamine
Ketamine is a phencyclidine derivative which produces a state of dissociative anaesthesia and analgesia. Compared to thiopentone its onset is slow, taking 1–2 min and its duration of action is longer, being in the region of 10–20 min. It is eliminated by hepatic metabolism and in children has an elimination half-life of about 1½ h.[12] Uniquely amongst the intravenous induction agents, ketamine causes cardiovascular stimulation with a rise in blood pressure and heart rate, and is therefore useful in the presence of cardiovascular compromise. It also is a potent bronchodilator, making it the agent of choice when intubation is required in severe acute asthma. However, ketamine is relatively contraindicated in the presence of raised intracranial pressure or raised intraocular pressure, both of which may be further increased. Ketamine causes an increase in salivation, making the concurrent use of an antisialogue advisable. In older children and adults, the occurrence of unpleasant dreams and hallucinations is a feature of ketamine anaesthesia. However, these phenomena are less common in younger children and infants and do not appear to pose a problem when subsequent sedation is given in the intensive care environment. Intravenous dosage of ketamine is 1–2 mg/kg, and it may also be given intramuscularly in a dose of 10 mg/kg.

Midazolam
Midazolam is a water-soluble benzodiazepine, with a relatively slow onset and intermediate duration of action. It is metabolized by oxidation in the liver and has an elimination half-life of about 1½ h in children.[13] It is most commonly used as a sedative agent either by intermittent bolus or continuous infusion, but is also a useful agent to facilitate endotracheal intubation, particularly when used in combination with short acting opiates. In fit children it has minimal cardiovascular effects, but hypotension may be precipitated in the presence of cardiovascular compromise. Like other benzodiazepines, midazolam has sedative, anxiolytic, hypnotic, amnesic and anticonvulsant effects. Dose is in the range 0.05–0.2 mg/kg.

Fentanyl/alfentanil
These opioids are useful adjuncts to other induction agents. Whilst having minimal cardiovascular effects, they blunt the haemodynamic response to

intubation and may help to limit rises in intracranial pressure. They may cause rigidity of the chest wall making ventilation difficult unless neuromuscular blocking drugs are also administered. In situations of cardiovascular compromise where the use of an intravenous induction agent is felt to be inadvisable, sedation may be achieved using a combination of benzodiazepine and opiate. Fentanyl is given in a dosage of 1–10 micrograms/kg, alfentanil 10–30 micrograms/kg.

Neuoromuscular blocking agents

Neuromuscular blocking agents cause a reversible chemical paralysis and are indicated to allow atraumatic laryngoscopy, intubation, and to facilitate subsequent mechanical ventilation. They render a patient apnoeic, and are contraindicated if there is any doubt on behalf of the operator of his ability to establish an artificial airway and maintain ventilation. Neuromuscular blocking agents belong to one of two types: depolarizing agents, and non-depolarizing agents which will be considered in turn.

Depolarizing neuromuscular blocking agents

Suxamethonium   Succinylcholine or suxamethonium is the only clinically available member of this group. Chemically, it consists of two linked molecules of acetylcholine and its mode of action is to bind to the nicotinic receptors on the postjunctional membrane at the neuromuscular junction. The membrane is maintained in a depolarized, non-responsive state until the drug diffuses away and is metabolized by plasma cholinesterase. Suxamethonium has a uniquely rapid onset of action, paralysis being complete in as little as 30 s following intravenous administration. It also has the shortest duration of action of the available neuromuscular blockers, this being in the order of 5 min. Side-effects seen with suxamethonium include sinus bradycardia and nodal beats. In adults, bradycardia occurs most commonly after the administration of a second dose,[14] but in children bradycardias may occur after a single dose.[15] It is therefore prudent to pretreat with a dose of atropine 0.01 mg/kg, or at least to have atropine ready for immediate administration. Patients with burns, muscular denervation and muscular dystrophies have the potential to develop rapid life-threatening hyperkalaemia following the administration of suxamethonium. This potential develops within 2 d of burn injury, and suxamethonium is contraindicated in these situations. Suxamethonium is know to increase intragastric pressure in adults, and this might lead to an increased likelihood of regurgitation of gastric contents. However, this rise in intragastric pressure was not seen in infants and children,[16] and subsequent work[17] has shown that suxamethonium as well as raising the intragastric pressure also raises the lower oesophageal pressure, and therefore the barrier pressure and hence the likelihood of regurgitation is unchanged. Suxamethonium also raises both the intraocular and intracranial pressure. It

must therefore be used with caution in situations where there is an open globe injury, or there is risk of increased intracranial pressure. The use of thiopentone is these situations will limit or even reduce pressure changes.[18] Infants require a larger dose of suxamethonium (2 mg/kg) than older children and adults (1 mg/kg). Suxamethonium may also be given by the intramuscular route (3–5 mg/kg), when it will have a slower onset and longer duration of action. Despite its potential for producing side-effects, suxamethonium remains unique in its ability to produce rapid, profound neuromuscular blockade, and it is the drug of choice for providing paralysis for emergency endotracheal intubation.

Non-depolarizing neuromuscular blocking agents

These agents produce a competitive block at the neuromuscular junction by binding to, but not activating acetylcholine receptors. Although modern drugs are notable for their lack of side-effects, all drugs in this group have a longer onset time and longer duration of action than suxamethonium. If bag-mask ventilation should prove difficult, or be inadvisable for example in patients with a full stomach, removal of the patient's ability to breathe spontaneously using one of these agents may lead to disaster. Vecuronium and atracurium are the most commonly used drugs to facilitate intubation. The role of the recently introduced agents mivacurium and rocuronium has yet to be defined in the area of paediatric intensive care. Satisfactory intubating conditions may be achieved more quickly using rocuronium than other available non-depolarizing agents.[19] In the infant, maturation of neuromuscular transmission does not occur until 2 months of age,[20] and these patients are therefore relatively sensitive to non-depolarizing agents.

Once partial spontaneous recovery of neuromuscular function has occurred, all non-depolarizing neuromuscular blocking agents may be reversed using neostigmine in combination with an anticholinergic agent (neostigmine 50 micrograms/kg, glycopyrrolate 10 micrograms/kg, or atropine 20 micrograms/kg).

Vecuronium   Vecuronium, like pancuronium, is a water-soluble steroid. It is excreted in the bile, and to a lesser extent unchanged in urine. It is remarkably free of side-effects, and the same dose may be used in infants as in adults,[21] although the duration of action will be longer in infants than in children. A dose of 0.1 mg/kg will produce satisfactory intubating conditions in about 90 s.

Atracurium   Atracurium, like vecuronium is a non-depolarizing neuromuscular blocking agent of intermediate duration of action.[22] It is eliminated by Hoffmann elimination and ester hydrolysis, and is therefore useful for use in renal hepatic failure. Although it may produce histamine release it is devoid of cardiovascular effects. Its onset of action is similar to vecuronium, and a dose of 0.5 mg/kg should produce satisfactory intubating conditions in about 90 s.

Other agents

Atropine

Vagal stimulation, drug effects and hypoxia may cause bradycardia during intubation. Atropine 20 micrograms/kg can be used to prevent or treat bradycardia due to the first two causes, but may mask bradycardia due to hypoxia. Atropine may be given prophylactically when emergency intubation using suxamethonium muscle paralysis or halothane inhalational anaesthesia is used. Otherwise, atropine should always be drawn up ready for administration.

Lignocaine

The use of lignocaine to limit rises in intracranial pressure due to endotracheal intubation is discussed in a later section. Suxamethonium and tracheal intubation related rises in intraocular pressure can be protected against by pretreatment with intravenous lignocaine 1.5 mg/kg without causing a significant decrease in arterial pressure.[23]

Technique of intubation

In order to visualize the laryngeal inlet, it is necessary for the axes of the mouth, pharynx and larynx to be aligned. In children older than 2 years of age, the classic 'sniffing the morning air position', where the head is extended on the neck and the occiput is raised, is best achieved by placing the head on a small pillow and lifting the chin into the sniffing position. Below 2 years of age, intubation is best achieved with the infant lying on a flat surface as the relatively large occiput of the infant produces the necessary anterior displacement of the neck.

Orotracheal intubation using a curved blade laryngoscope

Held in the left hand, the blade of the laryngoscope is introduced into the mouth to the right of the midline. It is advanced to the midline over the back of the tongue until the epiglottis is visualized. The tip of the blade comes to rest in the vallecula between the base of the tongue and the superior surface of the epiglottis. At this point, the laryngoscope is elevated upwards in the axis of the blade and because of its attachment via the hyoepiglottic ligament the epiglottis is elevated to reveal the laryngeal inlet (Fig. 5.1). It is important that the laryngoscope is lifted and not used a lever against the teeth or gums, as this hinders visualization of the larynx and may cause trauma. The endotracheal tube is introduced from the right side of the mouth, and can be seen as it passes through the glottis.

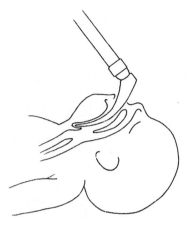

Fig. 5.1 Intubation using a curved blade laryngoscope.

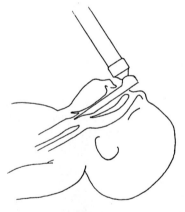

Fig. 5.2 Intubation using a straight blade laryngoscope.

Orotracheal intubation using a straight blade laryngoscope

Using a straight blade, the initial and final manoeuvres are the same as for the curved blade. However, the tip of the blade is passed under the epiglottis to lie against its inferior surface which is then lifted to reveal the laryngeal inlet (Fig. 5.2). Alternatively, the tip of the blade may be passed beyond the larynx and then carefully withdrawn to reveal the glottic opening.

Nasotracheal intubation

In nearly all situations, it is advisable to initially secure endotracheal intubation via the oral route. A nasal tube can then be exchanged for the oral one with minimal interruption of ventilation. An assistant holds the oral tube and assumes responsibility for ventilating the patient using a bag. The operator passes the precut nasal endotracheal tube into the pharynx by gently passing it directly along the floor of the nose. Laryngoscopy is then performed and the laryngeal inlet visualized with the oral tube *in situ*. Using Magill forceps held in the right hand, the tip of the nasal tube is picked up and aligned with the glottis anterior to the oral tube. The assistant is then asked to withdraw the oral tube and the operator replaces it with the nasal one, guiding it through the glottis with the forceps. Because of the greater curvature imposed on the nasotracheal tube and the high anterior position of the infant larynx, it is necessary to use forceps to lift the tip of the tube to the glottic opening. Occasionally, a tube passed via the nose will be difficult to advance into the trachea because it sticks against the anterior larynx. This may be overcome by rotating the proximal end of the tube through almost 180°, whereupon it will be felt to spring into the trachea. Alternatively, using the forceps to grip either side of the tube, downward pressure is exerted on the larynx to straighten the axis from the pharynx to the trachea and allow passage of the tube.

Securing the endotracheal tube

Both oral and nasal endotracheal tubes can be secured using adhesive tape. The skin is prepared by applying tincture of benzoin, and two lengths of tape are used. These are cut in half for about half of their length. For fixation of a nasal tube, the lower portion of the tape is applied to the upper lip and across the cheeks, and then the upper torn section is wrapped around the tube. This is repeated with the other tape. For fixation of an oral tube, it is the lower torn section of tape that is used to wrap around the tube. Commercial products may incorporate a device where the endotracheal tube adaptor grips the tube and provides sticky attachments to the face. The use of frames, such as those described by Tunstall or Birtles, to secure a nasotracheal tube may be useful in the more vigorous infant or child.

Special situations

Full stomach

The use of anaesthetic agents and neuromuscular blocking drugs to facilitate endotracheal intubation will abolish protective laryngeal reflexes, and in the presence of a full stomach risk the aspiration of gastric contents into the tracheobronchial tree should regurgitation occur. Some situations where a full stomach must be assumed are shown in Table 5.3.

Table 5.3 Risk of full stomach

Recent food intake	Drug-induced ileus
Peritonitis	Bowel obstruction
Postoperative ileus	Pyloric stenosis
Metabolic ileus	Hypoperfusion states
diabetic ketoacidois	Fear, pain or anxiety
hypokalaemia	Trauma
uraemia	Deep sedation

Elective fasting will rarely be a feasible option in intensive care, and besides, will do little to improve most of the situations listed in the table. Passage and aspiration of a nasogastric tube may be helpful in reducing the liquid content of the stomach, but is less effective in clearing food or blood. Gastric acidity can be reduced by giving antacids via a nasogastric tube, but only clear antacids, such as 0.3 M sodium citrate 10–30 ml, should be used as particulate antacids containing aluminium or magnesium may themselves cause a severe pneumonitis.[24] H_2 receptor antagonists are effective in reducing gastric acidity,[25] but require longer than an hour following administration. They will of course have no effect on existing gastric contents. In the presence of a full stomach, the period between the administration of sedative and neuro-muscular blocking drugs to the time that the airway is secured by an endo-tracheal tube must be managed so as to minimize the risk of regurgitation and aspiration.

Rapid sequence intravenous induction
This is the most commonly used technique in patients with a full stomach. The technique is summarized in Table 5.4. Following preoxygenation with 100% oxygen, anaesthesia and muscle paralysis are obtained by the rapid infusion of drugs. As soon as consciousness is lost, an assistant performs Sellick's manoeuvre.[26] The thumb and forefinger hold and firmly press the cricoid cartilage backwards, compressing the oesophagus between the cricoid cartilage and the vertebral column. As the cricoid cartilage forms a complete ring, the trachea is not distorted and visualization of the larynx is indeed often improved. It is vital that the assistant performing Sellick's manoeuvre correctly identifies the cricoid ring, as compression of the thyroid cartilage distorts the larynx and may make laryngoscopy difficult. It has been shown in infants that cricoid pressure is effective in occluding the oesophagus in the presence or absence of a nasogastric tube, and that a nasogastric tube can act as a blow off valve if intragastric pressure rises.[27] Cricoid pressure is maintained until the position of the endotracheal tube is confirmed—most reliably by the observation of the expired carbon dioxide trace, or at least by auscultation of both lungs and over the stomach. Before performing a rapid sequence intravenous induction, it is important to assess the airway and be sure that

Table 5.4 Rapid sequence intravenous induction

Check all equipment is working and drugs including atropine are prepared and ready for use.

Trained assistant is available to apply cricoid pressure and a second person available to help.

Suction with Yankauer is switched on and immediately to hand.

Position patient for intubation.

Preoxygenate with 100% oxygen, ideally for 3 min ensuring a tight seal with mask.

Give intravenous anaesthetic induction agent:

No cardiovascular compromise	Thiopentone	5 mg/kg
Possible cardiovascular compromise with head injury	Thiopentone	2 mg/kg
Consider alfentanil 15 micrograms/kg or lignocaine 1.5 mg/kg		
Possible cardiovascular compromise with no head injury	Ketamine	2 mg/kg
Severe cardiovascular compromise	Ketamine	1 mg/kg

   Or consider midazolam 0.05 mg/kg plus alfentanil 15 micrograms/kg

Cricoid pressure is applied as consciousness is lost.

Give neuromuscular blocking agent:

Suxamethonium	2 mg/kg for infants
	1 mg/kg for older children
Vecuronium	0.1 mg/kg
	Gentle bag/mast ventilation until paralysis complete

Intubate when paralysis is complete.

Maintain cricoid pressure until endotracheal tube position is confirmed.

---

intubation is not likely to be difficult. Because predetermined doses of drugs are usually given, dosage may be either excessive or inadequate resulting in circulatory instability. The usual drugs used are thiopentone and suxamethonium. If the patient is hypotensive, ketamine or etomidate may offer a more suitable alternative. This is discussed further in the next section. If suxamethonium cannot be used, then vecuronium or atracurium will provide adequate intubating conditions in 60–90 s. The relatively new drug, rocuronium may provide satisfactory intubating conditions in a shorter time than either of these two agents.[19]

Inhalational induction

If there is doubt about the ability to maintain the airway or it is thought that endotracheal intubation may be difficult, an inhalational induction using halothane in 100% oxygen may be used. Spontaneous respiration is maintained until the airway is secured. In paediatric intensive care, this situation most commonly occurs in patients with suspected epiglottitis or croup, and the management of these patients is discussed in a later section.

Cardiovascular instability

Cardiovascular instability may be due to hypovolaemia or impaired cardiac function. In the moribund child, endotracheal intubation may be accomplished without the use of sedative or neuromuscular blocking drugs. In the presence of hypovolaemia fluid resuscitation should begin along with establishment of an airway and maintenance of ventilation. To facilitate intubation minimal doses of sedative drugs should be given cautiously. If not otherwise contraindicated, for example traumatic hypovolaemia with head injury, ketamine 1–2 mg/kg may be the drug of choice.

Raised intracranial pressure

Neurological disease and injury are among the most common reasons for admission to the paediatric intensive care unit. Trauma, infection, intracerebral bleeding, hydrocephalus, and mass lesions may all produce or threaten an increase in intracranial pressure. Hypotension, hypoxia and hypercarbia will compromise cerebral perfusion. Endotracheal intubation and ventilation will secure the airway, optimize oxygenation and allow control of carbon dioxide levels. However, laryngoscopy and endotracheal intubation are intensely stimulating and even in the severely obtunded patient may cause an acute rise in intracranial pressure. Such a rise may reduce cerebral perfusion, causing brain ischaemia or herniation. If the patient is haemodynamically stable, the induction agent of choice is thiopentone (4–6 mg/kg), which will lower intracranial pressure.[28] If the operator is confident that the airway will not pose any problems, muscle paralysis may be achieved using a non-depolarizing agent. Hyperventilation with a bag and mask during the time drug effect takes place will lower carbon dioxide and reduce intracranial pressure. Where there is the possibility of a full stomach, suxamethonium should be used as part of a rapid sequence induction technique. In the presence of cardiovascular compromise, induction using a reduced dose of thiopentone, or a technique employing a benzodiazepine in combination with fentanyl or alfentanil can be used. Ketamine may cause a large rise in intracranial pressure[29] and its use is therefore contraindicated. Many techniques have been tried to prevent or limit the rise in intracranial pressure due to laryngoscopy and intubation. They include the use of a further dose of thiopentone,[30] the use of intravenous lignocaine (1.5 mg/kg)[31] and the use of various hypotensive agents. The possibility of a full stomach must be considered in all patients and in trauma patients cervical spine injury must also be considered.

Cervical spine instability

Cervical spine injury may be produced by trauma causing fractures of the spinal column, compression or ligamentous disruption. Compared to adults, the cervical spine in children is more mobile, and injuries of the cervical spine

are rare,[32] usually involving the upper three vertebrae. Because of the mobility of the spine, severe cord injury can result from stretching without fracture or disruption of ligaments. Atlantoaxial rotary subluxation, odontoid epiphyseal separation and ligament disruption are the most common injuries. All severely injured patients are assumed to have an unstable cervical spine until excluded clinically and on X-ray examination. In children and infants radiographs of the cervical spine can be extremely difficult to assess and computed tomography (CT) or magnetic resonance imaging (MRI) may be required. Often intubation will be required during resuscitation before cervical spine injury or instability can be excluded. In these cases, it is essential that manipulation of the head and neck during the process of intubation does not worsen the situation.

In adult practice much controversy exists over the best method to achieve endotracheal intubation in such situations. Previously, Advanced Trauma Life Support (ATLS) guidelines have recommended nasotracheal intubation as being the method of choice. However, the most recent guidelines[33] give equal emphasis to orotracheal and nasotracheal intubation, the choice being dependent on the experience of the operator. In one trauma centre, orotracheal intubation following rapid induction of anaesthesia with the application of cricoid pressure and manual in-line stabilization of the head and neck was shown to be a safe and effective method of securing the airway in patients with cervical spine injury.[34]

In paediatric practice, Pediatric Advanced Life Support guidelines[1] emphasize that spinal cord injury without radiographic abnormality occurs, and by definition cannot be excluded by X-ray examination and that cervical spinal cord injury must therefore be assumed in all children who have suffered severe trauma. The orotracheal route for endotracheal intubation is the preferred method in children under 8 years of age. During intubation the head must remain in a neutral position. Blind nasotracheal intubation in the child is difficult, and not recommended in the emergency situation. Conscious infants or children tolerate awake intubation poorly and a struggling child who moves risks further cord damage. In the unconscious child, intravenous anaesthesia and muscle relaxation are required to limit increases in intracranial pressure associated with endotracheal intubation. Therefore in the severely injured child at risk of having sustained cervical cord injury the method of choice for achieving endotracheal intubation is via the oral route following intravenous anaesthesia and muscle relaxation. The head is held in a neutral position without traction by an assistant who ensures that movement of the neck does not occur.

Upper airway obstruction

Upper airway obstruction is discussed at length in a later section.

Table 5.5 Conditions associated with difficult intubation

Micrognathia	Short thick neck
Hyperglossia	Airway tumours—intrinsic and extrinsic
Restricted mouth opening	Head and neck trauma
Restricted neck movement	

Difficult intubation

Some conditions associated with difficulty in performing direct laryngoscopy and intubation are listed in Table 5.5. However, it must be remembered that difficulty with intubation may occur in patients with no obvious abnormal anatomical features and again it is worth emphasizing the use of neuro-muscular blocking agents is contraindicated if there is doubt that an airway can be maintained and the patient's lungs ventilated using a bag and mask.

Aids to difficult intubation include the use of stylets and malleable light wands. A retrograde technique using a Seldinger wire has been described in a child of 30 months,[35] but the technique is not suitable for infants. The wide availability of the flexible fibreoptic laryngoscope has revolutionized the management of difficult or impossible intubation by conventional means.[36] The smallest available fibreoptic laryngoscope will pass through a 2.5 mm endotracheal tube, but does not have a directable tip nor a suction channel. The smallest available instrument incorporating both these features will pass through a 4.5 mm endotracheal tube.[37] The most important point to be remembered about all of these aids to difficult intubation is that they must be practised and mastered prior to encountering the real difficult intubation.

Complications

Immediate complications due to endotracheal intubation include cardiac arrhythmias, the pressor response to laryngoscopy, aspiration, and trauma to the structures of the airway. Failure to maintain oxygenation during the process of intubation may lead to hypoxaemia. Accidental extubation is a relatively common complication in the paediatric population, particularly in infants under 1 year and in association with inadequate sedation.[38] Partial or complete obstruction of the tube is also relatively common, and is most likely to occur in tubes of 4 mm internal diameter or less.[39] Factors that contribute to the development of tube obstruction include poor suctioning techniques, inadequate humidification and kinking of the endotracheal tube. Endo-bronchial intubation with associated atelectasis or collapse can be prevented by cutting the tube to a suitable length, and always ensuring that the tip of the tube lies in the mid-trachea on chest X-ray (see above). Aspiration or seepage may occur past non-cuffed endotracheal tubes, but a correctly sized tube will protect against clinically significant aspiration.[40] Although the use of cuffed

endotracheal tubes has been described in paediatric intensive care,[41] their use cannot be recommended. Later complications include ulceration of the nares and acquired subglottic stenosis.

Extubation

Extubation can be attempted when the indication for intubation has passed. Normally, a period of 12–24 h on continuous positive airway pressure (CPAP) is allowed when the child is observed for signs of developing respiratory distress. The inspired oxygen concentration should be 40% or less, and a set of satisfactory arterial blood gases obtained. Remember that small endotracheal tubes and their connectors are very hard to breathe through and impose an extra load on the child's work of breathing. If a very small tube has had to be used or in an infant, inspiratory assistance or a slow IMV rate may be preferable to CPAP. When the indication for intubation has been upper airway obstruction due to epiglottitis or croup, there should preferably be an audible gas leak from around the tube, although in some cases where swelling is severe, this is not possible. The child is fasted for 4–6 h prior to planned extubation, and for a further 4 h following extubation, lest reintubation should be required. Maintenance intravenous fluids are given during this period. Sedation can be reduced or withdrawn in the hours prior to extubation, in order to ensure the presence of protective airway reflexes. Equipment and drugs for reintubation should be available. Endotracheal and pharyngeal suctioning are performed, and following preoxygenation with 100% oxygen the tube is removed and humidified oxygen administered. Postextubation stridor may occur in 1–10% of patients,[7,8,42–44] the most important factor in its genesis probably being failure to ensure that the correct size of endotracheal tube is used.[8,45] Symptoms of respiratory distress, stridor and recession appear within 2 h. Initial treatment is humidified oxygen and nebulized adrenaline (0.5 ml/kg of 1:1000, maximum 5 ml).[46] Dexamethasone (0.5 mg/kg) may be of benefit,[7] and is often given prophylactically, although a double-blind study failed to show benefit from this practice.[47] If treatment is ineffective, reintubation with a smaller tube for 24–48 h may allow extubation subsequently. Repeated failure of extubation due to the development of stridor is an indication for laryngotracheobronchoscopy under general anaesthesia.

UPPER AIRWAY OBSTRUCTION

Acute airway obstruction is a common reason for admission to the paediatric intensive care unit. Partial obstruction causes noisy, stridorous breathing. When the site of airway obstruction is at or above the vocal cords, the stridor is heard during inspiration. Expiratory stridor occurs when the site of obstruction is below the cords. There are many causes of upper airway obstruction,

both congenital and acquired, and some of the more important are discussed below. Management of endotracheal intubation in the presence of airway obstruction is discussed in the section on acute epiglottitis.

Laryngomalacia

Laryngomalacia is the commonest congenital cause of upper airway obstruction. It is thought to be due to flaccidity of the laryngeal cartilage and presents with inspiratory stridor either at birth or in the first weeks of life. The diagnosis is made at direct laryngoscopy in the anaesthetized spontaneously breathing infant, when the laryngeal inlet is seen to collapse on inspiration. Treatment is most often expectant, as the condition resolves by about 2 years of age with growth. Laser treatment of the larynx may be of benefit and in a small number of infants long-term tracheostomy may be required.

Laryngeal web

Laryngeal webs will frequently cause symptoms which are noted at birth. Diagnosis is made at laryngoscopy under general anaesthesia when the web can be removed.

Tracheomalacia

Tracheomalacia results when the trachea lacks rigidity due to malformed cartilage rings. Stridor occurs during expiration. It is particularly common in infants who have had repair of a tracheoesophageal fistula or when there has been external compression of the trachea as occurs with external haemangiomas or vascular rings.

Acute epiglottitis

Acute epiglottitis is a common life threatening condition in preschool children, though any age group can be affected. The causative organism is usually *Haemophilus influenzae* type B, though *Streptococcus pneumonae*, *Staphylococcus aureus* and *Haemophilus parainfluenzae* may also be responsible. It is a non-suppurative inflammatory oedema of the supraglottic structures and epiglottis. In children, even small degrees of oedema may lead rapidly to complete obstruction, and experienced personnel are essential for management. It is also important to remember that sudden total obstruction can occur, and under no circumstances should the child be removed from close medical supervision and the facilities for immediate intubation. The history and clinical picture are usually diagnostic, with a short history of sore throat, fever, stridor and drooling. The child is usually very quiet and sits forward with the mouth open. Cough is not a feature and respirations are deliberately slow. Cyanosis,

pallor and bradycardia indicate an urgent need to establish a patent airway. If the diagnosis is in doubt, a lateral X-ray of the neck may show the enlarged epiglottis and surrounding oedema, but under no circumstances should the child be removed to the X-ray department for this investigation. No attempt should be made to visualize the pharynx or perform stressful procedures such as venous cannulation as obstruction may be precipitated.

The airway is secured under general anaesthesia by the most experienced anaesthetist available in the operating theatre or intensive care unit. All equipment should be to hand, and an ear, nose and throat (ENT) surgeon prepared to perform tracheostomy may be called in. The child is kept sitting and induced using halothane in 100% oxygen, delivered by a paediatric T-piece circuit, only being laid flat prior to intubation. Induction may be slow because of reduced alveolar ventilation, and patience is important—CPAP applied via the face mask and partial occlusion of the T-piece tail help to overcome obstruction as anaesthesia deepens. At laryngoscopy, the cherry red epiglottis is usually seen, and the airway secured initially with an oral endotracheal tube, before changing to a nasal one. The majority of cases can be extubated within 24 h after treatment with cefotaxime.

The introduction of widespread vaccination against *Haemophillus influenzae* in infancy has dramatically reduced the incidence of acute epiglottitis.

Croup

Laryngotracheobronchitis or croup commonly occurs at between 6 months and 2 years of age. The cause is usually viral, occurring in the winter months. The onset is gradual, preceded by the signs of an upper respiratory tract infection. Admission to hospital is not usually required, the child responding to humidification, oral fluids and paracetamol. The inspiratory and expiratory stridor, barking cough and signs of upper airway obstruction resolve over a period of hours. About 10% of children presenting to hospital will require admission—most of whom will be managed with only humidified oxygen and intravenous fluids. The use of a clinical croup score (Table 5.6)[48] may be useful in assessing the need for intervention in patients. A score of less than 4 indicates conservative management, a score of 7 or more despite full conservative management indicates the need for an artificial airway. Antibiotics are not given unless secondary bacterial infection is suspected. The use of steroids is now less controversial. An analysis of nine published trials supported their use, showing an improvement in clinical condition and a reduction in the need for intubation.[49] Nebulized budesonide is convenient and effective. If simple measures fail, then the child should be transferred to intensive care for monitoring and treatment. This should include continuous pulse oximetry and a chest X-ray. At this point, oxygen and racemic adrenaline and the mainstay of treatment. Racemic adrenaline is given as 0.5 ml of a 2.25% solution diluted to 5 ml with saline in 100% oxygen. If

Table 5.6 Downes and Raphaely clinical croup score

Signs/score	0	1	2
Inspiratory breath sounds	Normal	Harsh with rhonchi	Delayed
Stridor	None	Inspiratory	Inspiratory, and expiratory
Cough	None	Hoarse cry	Bark
Retractions	None	Flaring and suprasternal retractions	Flaring, suprasternal, subcostal and intercostal retractions
Cyanosis	None	In air	In 40% oxygen

racemic adrenaline is not available, then 0.5 ml/kg of ordinary 1:1000 adrenaline up to a maximum of 5 ml can be used instead. The electrocardiograph should be monitored and treatment stopped if the heart rate exceeds 200 or arrhythmias occur. The adrenaline can be repeated within 1 h if deterioration follows an initial improvement, or if the first dose is ineffective. If there is a lack of response to adrenaline, or if the child appears to be tiring, then an artificial airway should be established as for acute epiglottitis. Intubation is normally required for between 3 and 6 d.

Bacterial tracheitis

With the reduction in the incidence of epiglottitis, bacterial tracheitis is becoming relatively more common. It is usually caused by staphylococcal infection often after croup and is managed in many centres like severe croup. Flucloxacillin is given and prolonged intubation may be needed. Tube blockage with secretions and mucosal slough is often very troublesome.

Cervical fascial space infections

Infection may involve the submandibular space, the lateral pharyngeal space or the retropharyngeal/prevertebral space. Infection in any of these planes may spread to involve one or more other anatomical planes. Additionally, extension may occur to the mediastinum, carotid sheath or directly to intra-cranial structures.

Submandibular space—Ludwig's angina

This is rarely seen. It is a woody gangrenous cellulitis of the submandibular area which may spread to involve the small muscles around the larynx. Infection is usually from the 2nd or 3rd lower molar and due to *Staphylococcus*

or *Streptococcus*. Clinically, the patient is febrile, complains of pain and neck stiffness, drools and has dysphagia. The mouth is held open by swelling of the tongue. Lateral X-ray of the neck may show soft tissue swelling around the airway and submandibular gas. Treatment, in the first instance, involves close observation and intravenous antibiotic treatment with penicillin, cephalosporin, or metronidazole. If swelling continues to advance or respiratory difficulty develops, then an artificial airway should be established. This is best achieved by fiberoptic intubation with tracheostomy or cricothyroidotomy as a standby. Pus collections develop relatively late, and surgical decompression may be useful if the patient fails to respond adequately to antibiotics alone. Infected teeth are also extracted at this time.

Retropharyngeal/prevertebral space

These spaces lie between the deep cervical fascia surrounding the pharynx and oesophagus anteriorly and the vertebral spine posteriorly. The retropharyngeal space extends from the base of the skull to the level of the superior mediastinum. The prevertebral space extends from the base of the skull to coccyx. Infection may spread from one space to the other, and mediastinitis is a danger. In children, infection most frequently reaches the space by lymphatic spread from suppurative adenitis. There may be fever, drooling, and neck stiffness. Dysphagia and dysnoea may occur due to a mass effect or laryngeal swelling. Swelling of the posterior pharyngeal wall is usually seen. Dangers include airway obstruction and abscess rupture with aspiration. In adults, the most common route of infection is by penetrating trauma or instrumentation. X-rays show anterior displacement of the larynx and trachea. Treatment is by surgical exploration and drainage. The development of mediastinitis carries a mortality of 25%.

Suppurative parotitis

Acute bacterial parotitis affects primarily elderly malnourished, dehydrated, or postoperative patients. There is firm erythematous swelling in front of and behind the ear extending to the angle of the mandible. There is marked pain and tenderness, but no trismus. Systemic toxicity is usually present. Progression of the infection may lead to massive swelling of the neck and compromise of the airway. Treatment is by early surgical decompression.

Peritonsillar abscess

Quinsy is a complication of acute tonsillitis involving the peritonsillar space. There is fever, sore throat, trismus, and drooling. The abscess is usually unilateral and associated with cervical lymphadenopathy. Complications include aspiration of pus, airway compromise and spread of infection to the neck.

Treatment involves needle drainage, formal surgical exploration and antibiotic treatment with penicillin.

Diphtheria

Corynebacterium diphtheriae infection is now very rare. The grey shaggy membrane may be visible on the pharyngeal wall or tonsillar bed. Treatment is with antitoxin and penicillin or erythromycin.

TRACHEOSTOMY

In adult practice, it is common to perform surgical tracheostomy when 14–21 d of translaryngeal intubation have elapsed. In paediatric practice, much longer periods of oro- and particularly nasotracheal intubation are well tolerated, and with good care few complications occur.

Indications for tracheostomy include congenital airway obstruction, laryngeal trauma, facial burns, paralysis of the vocal cords and compromise of the airway as a result of translaryngeal intubation. A requirement for prolonged mechanical ventilation, possibly outside of an intensive care environment, will require tracheostomy. The occasions when tracheostomy is performed electively in the longer-term intensive care patient to provide a more comfortable airway and as an aid to weaning from ventilation will be much less frequent in paediatric than in adult practice.

At operation, when the trachea is identified two silk sutures are placed as far laterally as possible directly into the tracheal rings. Subsequently, these sutures will aid in replacing a tube that has become displaced—by pulling them apart towards the shoulders, the stoma will be opened and the trachea elevated towards the surface. No tracheal cartilage is removed as this may give rise to subsequent instability and tracheal collapse leading to failed decannulation.[50] Because the tracheostomy is sited below the cricoid ring, it can usually be 0.5 mm larger than the preceding endotracheal tube. A non-cuffed plastic tube is most commonly sited, and is firmly secured in place using tapes. After operation, a chest X-ray confirms the position of the tube, and a check is made for the appearance of any surgical air. In the first 2 d following tracheostomy, secretions will be increased, and frequent suctioning is necessary. Humidified oxygen must be provided to prevent the formation of inspissated secretions. Although many units perform the first tube change at 1 week, it is our practice to change the tube every 2 d, as blockage of the tube is the most frequent complication. The first change is done by the ENT surgeon who performed the tracheostomy, and when a tract is well formed at 1 week, the lateral retention sutures are removed.

Early complications of tracheostomy include bleeding, pneumothorax, pneumomediastinum and surgical emphysema. Obstruction or dislodgement

of the tracheostomy tube, and formation of false passage can occur at any time. Later complications include infection, skin breakdown due to the securing tapes, formation of tracheal granulations, tracheal strictures, and fistula formation.

Decannulation of the tracheostomy is achieved by using progressively smaller tracheostomy tubes to allow breathing through the larynx. When the smallest available tube is in place and respiration appears easy, the tube is removed and the stoma covered with a dressing. Frequently, following prolonged presence of a tracheostomy it is prudent to perform a laryngotracheobronchoscopy under general anaesthesia to exclude any of the longer term complications of tracheostomy.

CRICOTHYROTOMY

Given proper equipment and training in management of the airway, cricothyrotomy will be an extremely rare event,[1] but may be of use to allow oxygenation in the presence of complete upper airway obstruction due to foreign body, trauma, or infection.

A roll is placed under the shoulders and the cricothyroid membrane located between the thyroid and cricoid cartilages. A 20-gauge needle is used initially to locate and enter the trachea, which is confirmed by the aspiration of air. A 14-gauge cannula with attached syringe is then inserted through the cricothyroid membrane directed toward the midline caudally and posteriorly at a 45 ° angle. Aspiration of air confirms position in the trachea, after which the cannula is advanced over its needle which is then withdrawn. Air is again aspirated to check the final position of the cannula. A standard luer lock cannula can be connected to a 3 mm endotracheal tube connector to allow attachment to a ventilating device. Ventilation with a bag connected to the endotracheal tube connector may allow some oxygenation to take place, but carbon dioxide levels will rise. The use of jet ventilation as described in adults is very hazardous in children, with serious barotrauma in the presence of complete upper airway obstruction a major problem. Remember, the child must have a patent *expiratory* pathway as well as a means of delivering inspired oxygen.

LEARNING POINTS

1. The anatomy and size of the child's airway mean that airway maintenance skills must be taught and maintained regularly.

2. A wide range of sizes of airway equipment must be kept wherever children are managed.

3. Airway obstruction is common in children and the decision to intervene to secure the airway is usually based on clinical signs.

4. An inhalational induction with 100% oxygen and halothane with spontaneous respiration and CPAP is the favoured anaesthetic technique for securing the airway in the child with airway obstruction. This is a procedure for senior, experienced staff.

REFERENCES

1 American Heart Association, American Academy of Pediatrics. *Pediatric advanced life support manual.* American Association, Dallas, 1994.
2 Thompson AE. Pediatric airway management. In *Pediatric critical care* (ed. BP Fuhrman, JJ Zimmerman). Mosby, St Louis, 1992.
3 Eckenhoff J. Some anatomic considerations of the infant larynx, influencing endotracheal anesthesia. *Anesthesiology* 1951; 12: 401–410.
4 Rendell-Baker L, Soucek DM. New paediatric facemasks and anaesthetic equipment. *British Medical Journal* 1962; 1: 1960–1962.
5 Rees GJ. Anaesthesia in the newborn. *British Medical Journal* 1950; 2: 1419–1422.
6 Stocks J. Prolonged intubation and subglottic stenosis. *British Medical Journal* 1966; 2: 1199–1200.
7 Koka BV, Jeon IS, Andre JM *et al.* Postintubation croup in children. *Anesthesia and Analgesia* 1977; 56: 501–505.
8 Black AE, Hatch DJ, Nauth-Misir N. Complications of nasotracheal intubation in neonates, infants and children: A review of 4 years' experience in a children's hospital. *British Journal of Anaesthesia* 1990; 65: 461–467.
9 Quiney RE, Gould SJ. Subglottic stenosis, a clinico-pathological study. *Clinical Otolaryngology* 1985; 10: 315–327.
10 Ring WH, Adair JC, Elwyn RA. New pediatric endotracheal tube. *Anesthesia and Analgesia* 1975; 54: 273–274.
11 Sorbo S, Hudson RJ, Loomis JC. The pharmacokinetics of thiopental in pediatric surgical patients. *Anesthesiolology* 1984; 61: 666–670.
12 Grant IS, Nimmo WS, McNicol LR *et al.* Ketamine disposition in children and adults. *British Journal of Anaesthesia* 1983; 55: 1107–1111.
13 Salonen M, Kanto J, Iisalo E *et al.* Midazolam as an induction agent in children: a pharmacokinetic and clinical study. *Anesthesia and Analgesia* 1987; 66: 625–628.
14 Stoelting RK, Peterson C. Heart rate slowing and junctional rhythm following intravenous succinylcholine with and without preanesthetic medication. *Anesthesia and Analgesia* 1975; 5: 705–709.
15 Leigh MD, McCoy DD, Belton KM *et al.* Bradycardia following intravenous administration of succinylcholine chloride to infants and children. *Anesthesiology* 1957; 18: 698–702.
16 Salem MR, Wong AY, Lin YH. The effect of suxamethonium on the intragastric pressure in infants and children. *British Journal of Anaesthesia* 1972; 44: 166–170.
17 Smith G, Dalling R, Williams TIR. Gastro-oesophageal pressure gradient changes produced by induction of anaesthesia and suxamethonium. *British Journal of Anaesthesia* 1978; 50: 1137–1143.

18 Edmondson L, Lindsay SL, Lanigan LP *et al.* Intra-ocular pressure changes during rapid sequence induction of anaesthesia. A comparison between thiopentone and suxamethonium and thiopentone and atracurium. *Anaesthesia* 1988; **43**: 1005–1010.

19 Puhringer FK, Khuenl-Brady KS, Koller J *et al.* Evaluation of the endotracheal intubation conditions of rocuronium (ORG 9426) and succinylcholine in outpatient surgery. *Anesthesia and Analgesia* 1992; **75**: 37–40.

20 Goudsouzian NG. Maturation of neuromuscular transmission in the infant. *British Journal of Anaesthesia* 1980; **52**: 205–213.

21 Fisher DM, Millar RD. Neuromuscular effects of vecuronium (ORG NC45) in infants and children during N_2O, halothane anesthesia. *Anesthesia* 1983; **58**: 519–523.

22 Brandom BW, Rudd GD, Cook DR. Clinical pharmacology of atracurium in paediatric patients. *British Journal of Anaesthesia* 1983; **55**: 117S–121S.

23 Grover VK, Lata K, Sharma S *et al.* Efficacy of lignocaine in the suppression of the intra-ocular pressure response to suxamethonium and tracheal intubation. *Anaesthesia* 1989; **44**: 22–25.

24 Gibbs CP, Schwartz DJ, Wynne JW *et al.* Antacid pulmonary aspiration in the dog. *Anesthesiology* 1979; **51**: 380–385.

25 Guay J, Santerre L, Gaureault P *et al.* Effects of oral cimetidine and ranitidine on gastric pH and residual volume in children. *Anesthesiology* 1989; **71**: 547–549.

26 Sellick BA. Cricoid pressure to control regurgitation of stomach contents during induction of anaesthesia. *Lancet* 1961; **2**: 404–406.

27 Salem MR, Wong AY, Fizzotti GF. Efficacy of cricoid pressure in preventing aspiration of gastric contents in paediatric patients. *British Journal of Anaesthesia* 1972; **44**: 401–404.

28 Shapiro HM, Galindo A, Wyte SR *et al.* Rapid intraoperative reduction of intracranial pressure using thiopentone. *British Journal of Anaesthesia* 1973; **45**: 1057–1062.

29 Shapiro HM, Wyte SR, Harris AB. Ketamine anaesthesia in patients with intracranial pathology. *British Journal of Anaesthesia* 1972; **44**: 1200–1204.

30 Unni VKN, Johnston RA, Young HSA *et al.* Prevention of intracranial hypertension during laryngoscopy and endotracheal intubation. Use of a second dose of thiopentone. *British Journal of Anaesthesia* 1984; **56**: 1219–1223.

31 Hamill JF, Bedford RF, Weaver DC *et al.* Lidocaine before endotracheal intubation: intravenous or laryngotracheal? *Anesthesiology* 1981; **55**: 578–581.

32 Kewalramani LS, Kraus JF, Sterling HM. Acute spinal-cord lesions in pediatric population: epidemiological and clinical features. *Paraplegia* 1980; **18**: 206–219.

33 The American College of Surgeons Committee on Trauma. *Advanced trauma life support program for physicians: instructor manual.* American College of Surgeons, Chicago, 1993.

34 Criswell JC, Parr MJA, Nolan JP. Emergency airway management in patients with cervical spine injuries. *Anaesthesia* 1994; **49**: 900–903.

35 Borland LM, Swan DM, Leff S. Difficult pediatric endotracheal intubation: A new approach to the retrograde technique. *Anesthesiology* 1981; **55**: 577–578.

36 Rucker RW, Silva WJ, Worcester CC. Fiberoptic bronchoscopic nasotracheal intubation in children. *Chest* 1979; **76**: 56–58.

37 Fan LL, Sparks LM, Fix EJ. Flexible fiberoptic endoscopy for airway problems in a pediatric intensive care unit. *Chest* 1988; **93**: 556–560.

38 McCready M, Greenwald BM, Scolavino J. A prospective evaluation of unplanned endotracheal extubations in a paediatric intensive care unit (PICU). *Critical Care Medicine* 1994; **22**: A154.

39 Redding GJ, Fan L, Cotton EK *et al.* Partial obstruction of endotracheal tubes in children. *Critical Care Medicine* 1979; **7**: 227–231.
40 Goitein KJ, Rein AJ-JT, Gornstein A. Incidence of aspiration in endotracheally intubated infants and children. *Critical Care Medicine* 1984; **12**: 19–21.
41 Deakers TW, Reynolds G, Stretton M *et al.* Cuffed endotracheal tubes in pediatric intensive care. *Journal of Pediatrics* 1994; **125**: 57–62.
42 Orlowski JP, Ellis N, Amin NP *et al.* Complications of airway intrusion in 100 consecutive cases on a pediatric ICU. *Critical Care Medicine* 1980; **8**: 324–331.
43 Abbott TR. Complications of prolonged nasotracheal intubation in children. *British Journal of Anaesthesia* 1968; **40**: 347–353.
44 Battersby EF, Hatch DJ, Towey RM. The effects of prolonged naso-tracheal intubation in children. *Anaesthesia* 1977; **32**: 154–157.
45 Kemper KJ, Benson MS, Bishop MJ. Predictors of postextubation stridor in pediatric trauma patients. *Critical Care Medicine* 1991; **19**: 352.
46 Jordan WS, Graves CL, Elwyn RA. New therapy for postintubation laryngeal edema and tracheitis in children. *Journal of the American Medical Association* 1970; **212**: 585–588.
47 Tellez DW, Storgion SA, Galvis AG *et al.* Corticosteroids for prevention of post-extubation laryngeal edema: a double-blind study. *American Review of Respiratory Disease* 1987; **135**: 126A.
48 Downes JJ, Raphaely RC. Pediatric intensive care. *Anesthesiology* 1975; **43**: 238–250.
49 Kairys SW, Olmstead EM, O'Connor GT. Steroid treatment of laryngotracheitis: a meta-analysis of the evidence from randomized trials. *Paediatrics* 1989; **83**: 683–693.
50 Filston HC, Johnson DG, Crunrine RS. Infant tracheostomy. *American Journal of Diseases of Children* 1978; **132**: 1172–1176.

FURTHER READING

Baskett PJF, Dow A, Nolan J, Maull K. *Practical procedures in anesthesia and critical care.* Mosby, London, 1995.

6

Paediatric ventilatory care

M. Kerr

ANATOMY AND PHYSIOLOGY

The first breath marks the most radical change which will ever take place in the respiratory system. The adjustment from a fluid-filled to an air-filled lung is dramatic, but it is only the first of many adaptations which will take place as the lungs mature. The aetiology and clinical course of respiratory failure in infants and children is often quite unlike that seen in adults. The response to ventilatory support may also differ according to age. An understanding of the immature respiratory system can help explain these clinical differences and allow ventilatory management to be tailored to the needs of the patient.

Airway anatomy

Anatomical factors can make laryngoscopy and visualization of the vocal cords difficult in the infant. The larynx is more cephalad (C3–C4) and more anteriorly placed than in the adult. The epiglottis is long, floppy, and U-shaped, and lies at an angle of about 45° above the glottis. It may prove difficult to elevate the epiglottis in infants with a curved laryngoscope blade, and a straight bladed laryngoscope is often used to gain a better view.

The infant has a relatively large head and short neck, and it is easy for the head to become excessively flexed anteriorly. This, in conjunction with a relatively large tongue, creates a potential for respiratory obstruction. Infants are obligate nose-breathers. The nasal airways are, however, narrow and readily blocked by oedema and secretions, and it may prove difficult for the infant to convert to mouth breathing if the nose becomes obstructed.

The upper airway is narrowest at the cricoid ring in children, and oedema of this non-compliant region may develop due to trauma from too large a tracheal tube. Even 1 mm of circumferential swelling in the subglottic region can cause a substantial increase in resistance to breathing.[1] Great care is therefore needed in selecting the correct size of tube, and an audible leak present during positive pressure ventilation will indicate that the tube is not too large.

The trachea is short in children, and, because of this, inadvertent endobronchial intubation is more likely than in the adult. Firm and precise

fixation of the tracheal tube is essential once a satisfactory position has been confirmed. (See Chapter 5.)

The abdomen, diaphragm, and chest wall

There are various anatomical factors which reduce the efficiency of the infant's diaphragm as a respiratory pump. Despite this, respiration in this age group is almost completely diaphragmatic. Lung disease imposes a large additional workload on the diaphragm which can easily become too onerous. When this happens, respiratory failure develops.

In the infant and young child, the abdominal viscera are relatively bulky, and can exert considerable pressure on the thoracic contents, reducing functional residual capacity, and hampering diaphragmatic movement. These effects may be intensified if the gastrointestinal tract is distended.

The immature rib cage is cartilaginous and compliant. This makes breathing less efficient, as each time the diaphragm contracts, proportionately more force will go into deformation of the thoracic cage, and less into generation of a negative pressure in the thorax.

Even allowing for the anatomical difficulties described so far, diaphragmatic fatigue still occurs more easily in infants than in adults. It was thought that the muscle fibres in the infant's diaphragm were of a type more suited to rapid bursts of short-lived contraction rather than endurance. It now appears, however, that this lower threshold for fatigue is due to a decreased muscle mass.[2]

Metabolic factors

The high metabolic rate in infants and children necessitates a higher minute ventilation/body mass ratio. This means that if ventilation stops or becomes inadequate for any reason, oxygen reserves are used up quickly and there is a rapid fall in arterial oxygen saturation.

Control of breathing

In infants, during normal breathing, the intercostal muscles contract to reduce the compliance of the chest wall. In the very young, intercostal contraction is inhibited during rapid eye movement (REM) sleep, and the infant tends to compensate by increasing diaphragmatic activity. If there is coexistent lung disease, this work load may prove too heavy for the diaphragm, and respiratory failure develops. Sleep can therefore be a time when latent respiratory diseases present or when known pulmonary problems are exacerbated.

The Hering Breuer reflex is active in the newborn infant, but disappears in the early weeks. Head's paradoxical reflex is the stimulation of a large inspiration by a small lung inflation. It is active in the newborn, and remains present (especially under anaesthesia) through to adulthood.

The ventilatory responses to hypoxia and hypercarbia are essentially the same as in the adult. A notable exception to this is the apneoic and brady-cardic response to hypoxia in young infants. A vicious circle may develop whereby the infant is unable to sustain the normal hyperventilation response to hypoxia, and diaphragmatic fatigue develops. Periods of apnoea occur, wor-sening the oxygen deficit. Hypoxia leads to central nervous system depression which eventually overrides any stimulatory effects of oxygen lack.

Lung mechanics

Specific lung compliance (compliance/kg body mass) increases after birth to reach the adult value at 1 week of age. Compliance of the chest wall is, how-ever, very different from that in the adult. In the infant, the high compliance of the chest wall helps to determine the size of functional residual capacity. Functional residual capacity (FRC) is the volume of gas left in the lungs at the end of a normal expiration. It can be thought of as a point of balance between the outward elastic recoil of the thoracic cage and inward lung recoil. Because the chest wall is so compliant in infants the balance (FRC) is achieved at a lower lung volume.

In children, the relationship between FRC and closing volume plays an important part in lung physiology in health and disease. Closing volume is the lung volume at which small airways start to close and this impinges upon FRC in the infant and child (up to about age 6). This means that some airways close during normal tidal breathing, and that with each breath, some alveoli may end up being perfused but not ventilated. As a consequence, in children, more deoxygenated blood is 'shunted' across the pulmonary vascular bed into the systemic circulation.

Functional residual capacity is usually thought of as a 'buffer zone' against hypoxia, acting as a reservoir of oxygen if breathing stops for any reason. Be-cause of the regular airway closure during tidal breathing, the fast expenditure of any oxygen reserves, and the smaller size of the reservoir, FRC is less efficient at forestalling hypoxia in children than it is in adults.

In the infant, partial closure of the glottis during expiration provides approximately $3 \, cmH_2O$ of positive end expiratory pressure (PEEP). This distending pressure keeps FRC dynamically raised, so that fewer airways will close with each breath and shunt is minimized. Lung disease worsens the encroachment of closing volume on FRC, and the 'grunt' often heard in resp-iratory failure is an attempt to keep airway pressure as high as possible for as long as possible.

Other factors

The pores of Kohn are small fenestrations which allow communication between alveoli. These pores are less well developed in the immature lung,

allowing for less collateral ventilation if airway blockage occurs. If pressure builds up in one alveolus, it is not so easy for this pressure to vent into an adjacent alveolar sac. This increases the likelihood of alveolar rupture and escape of gas into the interstitium or the structures surrounding the lung. It is important to be aware of this increased susceptibility to barotrauma when mechanical ventilation is used in infants.

Immunological differences in children may render them more susceptible to certain respiratory infections than adults. The peak incidence of respiratory syncytial virus (RSV) bronchiolitis and pneumonia, for example, is in the age group under 6 months.

INDICATIONS FOR VENTILATORY SUPPORT

Artificial ventilatory support may be needed in respiratory failure to improve arterial oxygenation and CO_2 elimination, and to allow respite from fatigue. It is also an essential part of the treatment strategy in raised intracranial pressure, severe head injury and status epilepticus. Mechanical ventilation also has a role in reducing cardiac work, and is often employed pre- and postoperatively in congenital heart disease. In the child who has undergone thoracic or abdominal surgery, a period of ventilation may be necessary to facilitate good postoperative oxygenation and analgesia.

RESPIRATORY FAILURE

Pathophysiology

Respiratory failure can be defined as an inability of the respiratory system to maintain normal gas exchange: this may be due to 'lung failure' or 'pump failure' (Fig. 6.1). Conventionally, it is said to occur when arterial PCO_2 is greater than 50 mmHg (6.5 kPa) and arterial PO_2 is less than 50 mmHg (6.5 kPa) when breathing air. In practice, when considering whether to give ventilatory support, this rigid definition is not particularly useful. The decision to ventilate must be taken in light of the aetiology of respiratory failure and the severity of the underlying disease.

Evaluation of the child in respiratory distress

Useful information about the severity and cause of respiratory distress can be gained from clinical examination, and this should be directed towards assessing the features listed below.

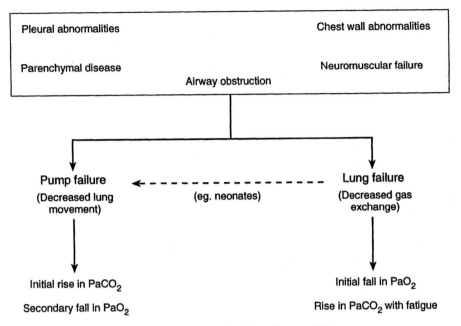

Fig. 6.1 Pathogenesis of respiratory failure.

Respiratory rate and tidal volume

Encephalopathy or metabolic acidosis often lead to hyperventilation with an increased respiratory rate and tidal volume. Decreased compliance (e.g. in pulmonary oedema or pneumonia) produces rapid and shallow respirations. In conditions where airway resistance is increased (e.g. asthma or bronchiolitis), respirations tend to be slower and deeper.

Inspiratory retractions—intercostal or suprasternal

Inspiratory retractions occur when high negative intrathoracic pressure is generated during inspiration. This high pressure is needed to shift gas into the lungs in the face of airway obstruction or poor compliance. Retractions are especially marked in the presence of extrathoracic obstruction.

Stridor

Inspiratory stridor is a feature of extrathoracic airway obstruction. Stridor is produced when a negative airway pressure during inspiration causes further narrowing at the site of obstruction. During expiration, the high positive pressure below the obstruction distends the airway and stridor is not heard in expiration as the obstructed area widens.

Expiratory stridor occurs when there is an intrathoracic cause of airway obstruction such as a tumour pressing on the trachea, a foreign body in the trachea or bronchi or when the tracheal or bronchial cartilages are eroded, softened, or incomplete (tracheomalacia, bronchomalacia). During inspiration, gas usually flows as the negative intrathoracic pressure opens up the large airways but on expiration, the airways tend to collapse inwards thus trapping gas in the smaller airways. Over time this may lead to rupture of the lung tissue, air leaks and critical respiratory failure.

Wheezing

Wheezing can occur in any disease where there is intrathoracic airway obstruction, and gas flows through narrowed airways.

Grunting

A grunt is produced by expiration through a partially closed glottis. As explained earlier, this manoeuvre improves oxygenation by keeping FRC and airway pressure raised during expiration. It is therefore most beneficial in small airway disease (bronchiolitis) and in alveolar diseases which produce widespread loss of FRC (pulmonary oedema or diffuse pneumonia).

Tachycardia

Hypoxia, hypercapnia, and anxiety are common features of respiratory failure which increase sympathetic drive and contribute to the development of tachycardia. Increased metabolic work of breathing and sometimes dehydration accompany respiratory failure, and these, too, produce an increase in resting heart rate.

Dehydration

The child who presents to the accident and emergency (A&E) department in respiratory failure may be dehydrated, and careful attention to fluid balance is essential in subsequent management.

Nasal flaring and use of accessory muscles

Nasal flaring occurs in an attempt to reduce upper airway resistance. Accessory muscles (mainly pectoralis minor, the scalene muscles, and serratus anterior) are brought into play to help overcome the increased work of breathing in respiratory failure.

Mental effects

Hypercapnia and hypoxia may contribute to a spectrum of mental changes ranging from anxiety and irritability to somnolence and obtundation.

If the heart rate or respiratory rate is increasing, if vital capacity is less than 15 ml/kg, or if conscious level is reduced, mechanical ventilatory support should be considered. Use of accessory muscles, a fall in PaO_2 despite increasing inspired oxygen (F_iO_2), or a rising $PaCO_2$ despite treatment are also indications for ventilatory support.

Restlessness, decreased conscious level, cyanosis and extreme pallor are ominous signs indicating an urgent need for respiratory support. Decreased respiratory effort, or a reduction in stridor or breath sounds may indicate imminent respiratory arrest.

Causes of respiratory failure

Chest wall, abdominal, and diaphragmatic abnormalities

Aetiology

The pain and physical restriction associated with chest wall trauma or surgery may hamper respiratory movements. Intra-abdominal pathology such as ascites, tumours, organomegaly, peritonitis or postoperative pain may also limit respiratory movements. Congenital defects, including abdominal wall defects (gastroschisis or omphalocele), narrow thorax and congenital diaphragmatic hernia not only produce mechanical respiratory problems, but may also be associated with pulmonary hypoplasia. Scoliosis is an unusual cause of respiratory compromise, but if the spinal angle is less than 50°, lung volume may be decreased significantly.

Clinical features

The underlying defect may be obvious on examination. Air entry is often reduced, and there may be tachypnoea and other signs of respiratory failure. In congenital diaphragmatic hernia, diaphragmatic excursion and muscle activity are reduced on the side of the hernia.

Chest X-ray

Anatomical abnormalities may be seen. Respiratory muscle weakness can lead to a visible decrease in lung volume and a high domed diaphragm. Abdominal abnormalities may result in a reduced lung volume on chest X-ray.

Management

Mechanical ventilation may be necessary to deal with the respiratory embarrassment caused by postoperative pain or trauma. Infants born with gastroschisis or a small omphalocele usually do well with a few days of postoperative ventilation. However, the infant with a giant omphalocele has a worse prognosis. Narrow thorax may, if it is an isolated defect, improve with pulmonary growth. In congenital diaphragmatic hernia, the degree of pulmonary hypoplasia determines survival. Preoperative ventilation may be necessary for these patients, and various ventilatory strategies, including high-frequency ventilation,

extracorporeal membrane oxygenation, and use of inhaled nitric oxide have been used in an attempt to improve arterial oxygenation in severe congenital diaphragmatic hernia.

Pleural abnormalities

Pneumothorax

Aetiology   Pneumothorax can be defined as gas in the pleural space.

Primary spontaneous pneumothorax arises in the absence of underlying lung disease. It is often caused by rupture of a bleb near the apex of the lung.

Secondary spontaneous pneumothorax is caused by underlying lung disease such as bronchopulmonary dysplasia, asthma, or cystic fibrosis. These diseases lead to hyperinflation of the alveolar sacs. In the infant with lung disease, pathological overdistension of alveoli is complicated by underdevelopment of the pores of Kohn. These pores usually provide collateral ventilation, and act as a 'safety valve' between alveoli. If this safety mechanism is absent, a leak is more likely to develop and eventually reach the pleural space or mediastinum.

Iatrogenic causes of pneumothorax include central venous catheter placement and bronchoscopy. Mechanical ventilation can also lead to pneumothorax, especially in the presence of excessive inflation pressures (e.g. in right main bronchus intubation), low lung compliance or intrinsic PEEP (if the respiratory rate is too fast).

Clinical features   A sudden onset of pain and dyspnoea may be accompanied by decreased chest wall motion, and bulging of the chest wall. Breath sounds are commonly decreased, and there may be a drop in blood pressure, heart rate, and pulse pressure. These signs are, however, not reliable indicators of pneumothorax, as they may be obscured by other lung disease, and transmitted breath sounds may be heard on the collapsed side. Tension pneumothorax produces a dramatic clinical picture with progressive dyspnoea, central cyanosis, and distended neck veins.

Chest X-ray   This will often provide the diagnosis, although a cross table lateral may be necessary to delineate collections of air around the heart, and in the supine patient.

Treatment   If the patient's respiration is severely compromised, and pneumothorax is suspected, especially in the case of tension pneumothorax, the delay involved in getting a chest X-ray may be fatal and emergency thoracocentesis followed by insertion of a chest drain is essential.

Therapeutic or diagnostic centesis is performed in the second or third intercostal space in the midclavicular line. It is often necessary to follow this with insertion of a chest drain, however, a primary spontaneous pneumothorax

may be resolved by thoracocentesis alone. Secondary pneumothorax usually requires a chest drain with suction.

Complications Bronchopleural fistula is a very troublesome complication, especially in mechanically ventilated patients. Attempts to improve ventilation by increasing tidal volume often only achieve more gas flow through the fistula. High-frequency ventilation may succeed where other ventilatory methods have failed. The fistula may persist for a long time, and if it persists after extubation, surgical closure may be required.

Treatment of pneumomediastinum rarely requires placement of a mediastinal drain and usually no action is required other than careful observation. In the case of pneumopericardium, pericardiocentesis is only warranted if there is haemodynamic compromise. Centesis of a pneumoperitoneum is indicated if it is causing respiratory difficulties and this is rarely the case. The partial pressure of oxygen in a pneumoperitoneum is the same as inspired: the partial pressure of oxygen in a perforated viscus is that of room air. Subcutaneous emphysema which develops from a pneumothorax needs no treatment.

Pleural effusion

Aetiology Pleural effusion is usually caused by a local increase in capillary hydrostatic pressure. An example of this is the parapneumonic effusion in pulmonary infection. Bacteriological culture of these effusions is initially negative, but such an effusion may at a later stage develop into an empyema (pus in the pleural space).

Fluid may accumulate in the pleural space in subdiaphragmatic conditions such as pancreatitis, or in systemic disease, e.g. connective tissue disorders. Pleural effusion may also be caused by an increase in lung water or a decrease in lymphatic outflow (e.g. mediastinal lymphadenopathy or disruption of the thoracic duct).

Clinical features Features of pleural effusion or empyema include fever, pain and breathlessness, and an ipsilateral decrease in chest wall mobility. Breath sounds are diminished, and the area is dull to percussion. A pleural rub is heard in 10% of children with empyema.

Investigations Diagnosis is by chest X-ray or ultrasound. Thoracocentesis may help to elucidate the cause.

Treatment If an effusion is causing significant respiratory distress, thoracocentesis should be performed. Antibiotics and placement of a chest drain (to help prevent subsequent fibrothorax) are the treatments of choice in empyema.

Haemothorax
The diagnosis of blood in the pleural space is made when there is a history of trauma and evidence of a pleural effusion. Bleeding is usually from low-pressure vessels, and often stops when the lung is re-expanded. Evidence of an underlying pneumothorax should be sought. Treatment is with a posteriorly placed chest drain. Haemothorax carries a risk of subsequent fibrothorax.

Neuromuscular disorders

Aetiology
Neuromuscular causes of respiratory failure can be classified as follows:

- **pharmacological** (e.g. salicylate overdose, aminoglycosides, suxamethonium apnoea, opioids, anaesthetic agents and prolonged action of non-depolarizing muscle relaxants)

- **endocrine and metabolic** (e.g. diabetic ketoacidosis, hyperthyroidism, hypocalcaemia, hypophosphataemia, hypokalaemia (rare), acidosis, hypoxaemia, and hypercapnia)

- **infectious** (e.g. encephalitis, sepsis, viral illness, tetanus and Guillain Barre)

- **intracranial lesions** (e.g. tumours or haematoma)

- **spinal lesions** (e.g. tumours, trauma or abscess).

Clinical features
Neurological causes of respiratory failure tend to be associated with irregular breathing and/or ineffective tidal ventilation. Hyperventilation without respiratory tract lesions may occur in encephalopathy or metabolic acidosis. Neuromuscular weakness is often associated with atelectasis, and this leads to ventilation perfusion mismatch and shunting and hypoxaemia. Involvement of the pharyngeal muscles can cause snoring, respiratory obstruction and aspiration of foodstuffs. Arterial PCO_2 may be normal initially, but will rise when respiratory failure supervenes. Neurological causes of respiratory failure are commonly associated with change in mental status, blood pressure or heart rate. These changes may be primary due to the cause, or secondary due to hypoxia or hypercapnia. Chest X-ray is usually normal except in the case of neurogenic pulmonary oedema.

Management
Noisy snoring inspiratory sounds, an impaired gag reflex and difficulty in swallowing indicate an urgent need to establish a patent airway. The patient's ability to cough and to breathe deeply should be evaluated. Mechanical ventilation should be considered if the patient is distressed, or has decreased pharyngeal muscle function, rapidly worsening vital capacity or evidence

Table 6.1 Causes of bacterial pneumonia

Neonates	4–10 years
Group B Streptococcus	*Streptococcus pneumoniae*
Gram negative bacilli	*(Haemophilus influenzae)*
Chlamydia trachomatis	
Listeria monocytogenes	Adolescents
	Mycoplasma
Infants and toddlers	*Streptococcus pneumoniae*
Haemophilus influenzae	
Streptococcus pneumoniae	All ages
	Staphylococcus aureus
	Klebsiella

of atelectasis on chest X-ray. An inspiratory muscle strength of less than 30 cmH$_2$O (measured as a forceful inspiration against a closed airway) also indicates a need for ventilatory support. Controlled mechanical ventilation is the mode usually chosen in patients with neuromuscular failure. A test period of 30–60 min spontaneous breathing with the tracheal tube in place will help decide whether or not weaning is feasible. If respiration is regular and comfortable for the patient, without periods of apnoea, and if the arterial PCO$_2$ is less than 45 mmHg (6 kPa) (with a pH of over 7.35), extubation should be successful.

Disorders of the lung parenchyma

Bacterial pneumonia

Aetiology The aetiological agent varies with age (Table 6.1).

Clinical features There is usually a prodromal phase with mild upper respiratory tract infection and pyrexia. This is superseded by a pattern of respiratory distress with inefficient tachypnoea and, especially in infants, grunting. The typical findings on auscultation are decreased breath sounds and crepitations, but these may be absent in infants.

Staphylococcal pneumonia can follow a rapid course in adolescents, and may be fulminant, with rapid development of shock and severe respiratory failure. Initially, the picture is similar to that seen in other pneumonias, but consolidation, pneumatocele, empyema and spontaneous pneumothorax may follow within a few hours.

Investigations Chest X-ray shows patchy lesions or lobar consolidation. Pneumatocele and empyema may also be seen.

Sputum is often difficult to obtain especially in infants and younger children. Bacteraemia is frequent in *Strep. pneumoniae* and *H. influenzae* infections and blood culture may be a useful aid to diagnosis in these circumstances.

Treatment   Ventilatory support may be needed during treatment of bacterial pneumonia. Care should be taken to avoid high airway pressures during mechanical ventilation if possible, as there is a significant risk of barotrauma. Antibiotic therapy should be given in light of the results of bacterial culture. If the organism is not known, a 'best guess' therapy may be directed towards the most commonly occurring organisms in the child's age group.

Viral pneumonia

Aetiology   Viral pneumonia in infants is usually due to RSV, but can also be caused by parainfluenza, adenovirus, and influenza A and B. Herpes simplex and cytomegalovirus should be considered in neonates and in the immunocompromised.

In RSV bronchiolitis and pneumonia, oedema, mucus and debris block the small airways, causing gas trapping and atelectasis. Airway reactivity may be increased, causing bronchospasm.

Clinical features   Respiratory syncytial virus infection occurs in yearly winter epidemics. The usual presentation is with an upper respiratory tract infection and cough. Some infants may present with apnoea. The chest appears hyperinflated, and expiratory wheezes are heard on auscultation. Tachypnoea, intercostal and subcostal recession indicate respiratory failure, and a decrease in breath sounds is an ominous sign of severe respiratory obstruction.

Diagnosis   Chest X-ray may show bilateral streaky infiltrates with hyperinflation of the lungs and a flattened diaphragm. Laboratory diagnosis is by tissue culture or immunofluorescence of nasopharyngeal secretions.

Treatment   Treatment is directed towards providing adequate humidity, oxygen and pulmonary toilet. A recent study[3] demonstrated the efficacy of continuous positive airways pressure (CPAP) via nasal cannulae in avoiding the need for intubation. However, if there is evidence of respiratory fatigue with hypercapnia and respiratory acidosis, intubation and ventilatory support with judicious use of CPAP and PEEP will be necessary. Up to 3% of hospitalized infants with RSV infection may require mechanical ventilation. The use of salbutamol in infants with RSV infection is controversial.

Pneumocystis pneumonia

Aetiology   *Pneumocystis carinii* causes an opportunistic infection in immunocompromised patients. Patients with acquired immune deficiency syndrome (AIDS), malignancy or congenital immune problems are susceptible to this pathogen.

Clinical features   Hypoxaemia is a prominent feature. Tachypnoea develops early with intercostal recession. Grunting and cyanosis may also be present.

Chest X-ray Chest X-ray shows diffuse bilateral interstitial and alveolar infiltration. Diagnosis is by finding *Pneumocystis carinii* in lung biopsy or bronchoalveolar lavage fluid. In infants, the artificial airways may be too narrow to permit standard bronchoscopy. In these circumstances, non-bronchoscopic bronchoalveolar lavage, using a fine suction catheter has been successfully used to obtain lavage fluid for diagnosis.[4]

Treatment Cotrimoxazole is the antibiotic therapy of choice. Oxygen administration should be guided by pulse oximetry and arterial blood gases. Assisted ventilation may be needed.

Legionella pneumonia

Aetiology *Legionella pneumophila* is the causative agent. This is usually a disease of older people, but can occur in children. Risk factors in the paediatric patient are asthma, renal failure or immunosuppressive use after transplantation.

Clinical features A 24-h flu-like illness is followed by a productive cough, nausea, vomiting, diarrhoea, and fever. This may progress to encephalopathy with lethargy, unsteadiness, and delirium. On examination, the patient appears toxic and in respiratory distress. Rhonchi are heard early before signs of lobar consolidation develop. There may be inappropriate anti-diuretic hormone secretion, and urine abnormalities vary from proteinuria to renal failure.

Diagnosis The chest X-ray reveals patchy rounded opacities throughout both lung fields. Often this progresses to lobar consolidation. A fourfold increase in serum antibody titre is diagnostic.

Treatment Erythromycin is the antibiotic of choice. Supplemental oxygen should be administered as required. Mechanical ventilation may be necessary.

Hydrocarbon pneumonia

Aetiology Hydrocarbons are most commonly encountered in the home as cigarette lighter fuels. Inhaled hydrocarbons may penetrate to the most distal airways and vaporize, leading to hypoxia. They may also destroy surfactant, damage the alveolar epithelium and cause atelectasis.

Clinical features The initial picture of coughing, gagging, choking, and cyanosis is followed by a non-productive cough. During the first 24 h, signs of increasing respiratory distress appear. In severe cases, there is pulmonary oedema, haemoptysis, pneumothorax and subcutaneous emphysema.

Chest X-ray No abnormalities may be seen initially, but usually changes appear within 12 h. These take the form of bilateral streaky and mottled

densities in the perihilar region, extending to the peripheries. Pneumothorax may be present.

Treatment   Treatment is essentially supportive. There is no evidence for the benefit of antibiotics or corticosteroids. Care must be taken with the use of high airway pressures in mechanical ventilation due to the risk of barotrauma. Even the most severely affected patient will usually, however, survive with minimal residual pulmonary damage.

Atelectasis

Aetiology   Atelectasis may be described as a collapsed normal lung parenchyma. It occurs due to hypoventilation, e.g. secondary to surgery and anaesthesia, weak respiratory muscles or complete airway obstruction. Alternatively, it may occur if the lung is abnormally compressed by heart, vessels or lymph nodes. A search should therefore always be made for potential causes as atelectasis may be misdiagnosed as pneumonia and inappropriate treatment given. The underlying physiological abnormalities include a reduced functional residual capacity, an increased closing volume and airway resistance. Hypoxaemia may be avoided in lobar atelectasis as vessels in the affected area constrict in response to alveolar hypoxia.

Clinical features   The features of atelectasis are those of respiratory distress. Breath sounds are decreased or absent, the affected lung is dull to percussion and the heart and trachea may be shifted to the affected side. Signs of large airway obstruction, e.g. endotracheal tube malposition, foreign body or mucus plug should be sought. Atelectasis in small infants often presents as an acute respiratory illness.

Chest X-ray   Chest X-ray may reveal multiple focal areas of opacity. The presence of an air bronchogram can be a prognostic sign. If present, it is likely to signify an intrabronchial obstruction which can be cleared, allowing recovery to occur more quickly.

Treatment   If atelectasis causes respiratory failure, a period of intubation and mechanical ventilation will be needed. Treatment is directed towards the initial cause and consists of physiotherapy, suction, 'bagging', percussion and repositioning at regular intervals. Flexible fibreoptic bronchoscopy is indicated if atelectasis is refractory after 3–4 days of intensive physiotherapy.

Pulmonary oedema may occur following re-expansion of the collapsed lung. The onset of this may be rapid (immediate to a few hours) with tachypnoea, intercostal recession, tachycardia, and cyanosis.

Pulmonary oedema

Aetiology   There are many causes of pulmonary oedema:

- increased microvascular pressure

- decreased interstitial pressure

- increased colloid osmotic pressure

- defective lymphatic drainage

- neurogenic oedema.

Clinical features   The patient with pulmonary oedema shows signs of respiratory distress, with crepitations and frothy pink sputum. Wheezing and hyperexpansion may occur early on.

Chest X-ray   Early changes are non-specific, with hyperexpansion due to gas trapping. Perivascular cuffing with Kerley A B & C lines (thickening of the interlobular septa) and evidence of pleural fluid may be present. When alveolar filling occurs, patchy densities in both lung fields give a 'butterfly' appearance with relatively clear peripheral fields. If there is associated left ventricular dysfunction, cardiomegaly and prominent pulmonary vasculature will also be seen.

Treatment   Treatment is aimed at reversing hypoxia and dealing with the cause. Ventilatory support may be necessary. Depending on the cause, diuretics, inotropes, and afterload reduction may be useful.

Acute respiratory distress syndrome

Aetiology   Acute respiratory distress syndrome (ARDS) is the result of acute damage to the alveolar epithelium and pulmonary capillary endothelium. A wide variety of agents may cause this damage. The pathogenesis of ARDS is complex, and is not yet fully understood. The end result can be summarized as a state of respiratory distress characterized by low compliance and reduced lung volumes, due to increased alveolar fluid and progressive atelectasis. Intrapulmonary shunting leads to severe hypoxia.

Clinical features   The predisposing illness or injury may be followed by a period of apparent clinical recovery (the latent period). Even at this stage, there are subtle changes in pulmonary haemodynamics in the child at risk of developing ARDS. The features of acute respiratory failure develop suddenly in these patients, and are associated with recalcitrant and progressive hypoxaemia. Respiratory distress worsens, hypercapnia develops, and the need for

mechanical ventilation becomes inevitable. The situation often becomes irretrievable with the development of multiorgan failure, frequently exacerbated by the underlying disease or by secondary infection.

Chest X-ray   The chest X-ray shows diffuse, bilateral infiltrates which worsen as the disease progresses. A complete 'whiteout' of both lung fields may develop. Cardiac size is normal.

Treatment   Although a few patients may manage with PEEP and supplemental oxygen, most require mechanical ventilation. It is important that the tidal volume delivered is not too high, as there is a real risk of pneumothorax in poorly compliant lungs. A tidal volume of 10–15 ml/kg and a respiratory rate of 30–40/min has been suggested.[5] Other modes of respiratory support, e.g. inverse ratio ventilation,[5] high-frequency ventilation and extracorporeal membrane oxygenation[6] have been used with some success. Pharmacological strategies which have been used in recent years include inhaled nitric oxide, exogenous surfactant, vasodilators, e.g. PGE$_1$, non-steroidal anti-inflammatory drugs, pentoxifylline, and antibodies against inflammatory mediators. Although many of these show considerable promise, their benefits are as yet unproven.

Smoke inhalation injury

Aetiology   Smoke inhalation injury describes a broad range of insults which can result from inhaling products of combustion. **Carbon monoxide (CO)** readily binds to haemoglobin, and reduces oxygen delivery to the tissues. As well as causing organ failure due to tissue hypoxia, and central nervous system (CNS) effects, CO is a direct myocardial depressant. **Cyanide** is produced from combustion of plastics etc., and also contributes to tissue hypoxia. A wide variety of other toxic products arise from combustion of synthetic materials found in the home. These are responsible for varying degrees of upper and lower airway inflammation and lung parenchymal damage. The effects of **heat** on the mucosa may produce airway obstruction, developing over a few hours. Bronchospasm and lower airway damage can arise from the irritant effects of inhaled **particulate matter**. ARDS and bacterial pneumonia are secondary effects which may develop after smoke inhalation injury.

Clinical features   It should be borne in mind that the child who comes to the A&E department with smoke inhalation injury may have other injuries (e.g. burns, soft-tissue injuries, cervical spine and other fractures). The patient may be obtunded or confused. Obvious respiratory distress or airway obstruction may be present and auscultation of the chest may reveal wheeze or crepitations. There are often signs of heat and soot exposure in the nares and mouth.

Investigations   Chest X-ray is often negative initially. Flexible fibre-optic bronchoscopy may be diagnostic or therapeutic. Carboxyhaemoglobin levels and arterial blood gases should be monitored.

Treatment   Humidified oxygen should be administered to displace carbon monoxide, to reverse hypoxaemia and to minimize airway oedema. Mechanical ventilation, often with PEEP may be necessary in respiratory obstruction or pulmonary damage. High-frequency ventilation may be of use in these patients.[7] Bronchodilators and antibiotics are used as required and a cyanide antidote is available for use in children at high risk of cyanide toxicity.[8] Excessive secretions should be removed by careful tracheal suction and bronchoscopy if necessary. Exogenous administration of surfactant is as yet an unevaluated treatment, which may prove promising.

Upper airways (see also Chapter 5)
Viral croup (acute laryngotracheobronchitis)

Aetiology   Viral croup is usually caused by parainfluenza virus types I and II. Occasionally, RSV or influenza viruses may be the causative organism. Infection leads to oedema and exudation in the subglottic region. Lower airway disease may occur secondary to distal spread of viral infection, and secretions produced can cause mucus plugging and atelectasis. Children in the age group 6 months to 3 years are predominantly affected.

Clinical features   There is usually a short history of upper respiratory tract infection with a harsh cough and hoarseness. Pyrexia, stridor, inspiratory flaring, retractions, and táchypnoea are common features found on examination. Hypoxaemia, hypercapnia and cyanosis are late features, and may reflect a near complete airway obstruction.

X-ray   Lateral neck radiographs may show narrowing of the subglottic region, and a widened hypopharynx. An anterio-posterior neck X-ray will show subglottic narrowing (the 'steeple sign'). This narrowing is characteristically exacerbated by inspiration.

Treatment   Treatment is aimed at loosening secretions and decreasing airway oedema. The benefits of humidifying inspired air in croup may not be as indisputable as once maintained.[9] This is, however, at present a widely used therapy, and further investigation is necessary before its usefulness can be discounted. Nebulized racemic adrenaline is an important component of therapy for croup which may forestall the need for intubation. Care should be taken to monitor the child's symptoms carefully, and to give a repeat dose if required, as the duration of action is about 2 h. Early administration of corticosteroids may also reduce the need to intubate. There are, however,

some children in whom these measures fail to provide adequate relief. This group show signs of respiratory failure including a PaO_2 of less than 50 mmHg on 50% oxygen, a $PaCO_2$ greater than 55 mmHg, and pH less than 7.35. There is often evidence of fatigue or somnolence. In these patients, the trachea should be intubated with gradual introduction of halothane in oxygen in controlled circumstances with the child breathing spontaneously. While intubated, the child should be allowed to breathe humidified oxygen, and the trachea gently suctioned periodically. Adequate intravenous hydration is important. Criteria for extubation include resolution of fever and of excessive tracheal secretions in conjunction with the development of a leak around the tracheal tube.

Bacterial tracheitis (membranous laryngotracheobronchitis)

Aetiology   Bacterial tracheitis is probably caused by viral infection with superimposed bacterial infection (usually *Staphylococcus aureus* or *Haemophilus influenzae*). The main pathological feature is subglottic oedema.

Clinical features   The presenting features are similar to those seen in the child with viral croup, although the child with bacterial tracheitis may appear more toxic with a high fever. There is a gradual onset of the signs of airway obstruction (cyanosis, hypoxia, hypercapnia, nasal flaring, and retraction). The white cell count is often raised.

X-rays   X-rays of the airway may show irregular radiopacities in the trachea, and narrowing of the subglottic region.

Treatment   Bacterial tracheitis is associated with the presence of copious thick, tenacious secretions in the trachea. These secretions may cause life-threatening airway obstruction, and it is often advisable to insert a tracheal tube. This allows clearance of the secretions by suction, however, rigid bronchoscopy may be needed to remove particularly tenacious material. The decision to extubate should be made after flexible bronchoscopy has revealed a decrease in secretions. Appropriate intravenous fluids and antibiotics should be given throughout the course of the illness.

Epiglottitis

Aetiology   About 85% of cases of acute epiglottitis are caused by *Haemophilus influenzae* type B. The small cross-sectional diameter of the airway, the anatomical relationship of the epiglottis to the glottis, and the abundance of loose connective tissue in the epiglottic region are factors which determine the development and obstructive effects of epiglottitis in the 2–5 year age group.

Clinical features A history of sore throat, worsening in severity, precedes dysphagia, dyspnoea and increasing anxiety. This is followed, within 4–6 h by the development of a high pyrexia, tachypnoea, drooling, and marked inspiratory stridor. At this stage, the child often sits with neck extended, supporting him or herself with straight arms, and moving as little as possible. This is the position in which, by this time, there is least resistance to breathing. These signs imply imminent respiratory obstruction.

Treatment If this diagnosis is truly suspected, X-ray of the airway is an unjustifiable delay. Examination of the airway with a tongue depressor may precipitate complete respiratory obstruction. Someone experienced in paediatric airway management should be summoned and a selection of tracheal tubes prepared. While preparation is being made to intubate, the child must not be left alone. The patient should be given 100% oxygen to breathe, and halothane introduced gradually to allow intubation while breathing spontaneously. If complete obstruction occurs before intubation, positive pressure ventilation can be given with a bag and mask. It has been documented recently that the best guide to extubation is return of a normal appearance on direct laryngoscopy.[10] Appropriate parenteral antibiotics are indicated throughout the course of the illness. Until sensitivities are known, cefotaxime may be used.[9]

Anomalies of the great vessels

Aetiology Congenital anomalies of the aorta, innominate, left common carotid, left pulmonary artery or right subclavian may compress the trachea, and cause respiratory difficulties. The oesophagus may also be compressed, leading to feeding problems.

Clinical features The symptoms and signs usually start early in life, and include feeding and breathing difficulties, the latter worsening in the presence of respiratory infection. Expiratory rhonchi and inspiratory stridor are heard.

Investigation Barium swallow is usually diagnostic.

Treatment Treatment is surgical, and is usually associated with a good outcome, except in the case of complete tracheal rings and distal tracheal stenosis.

Retropharyngeal infections

Aetiology Retropharyngeal infections may arise from lymphatic spread of infection from the nasopharynx, oropharynx, or external auditory meatus. A foreign body penetrating the posterior wall of the pharynx may also set up an

infective focus. The most common organisms involved are group A *Strepto-coccus* and *Staphylococcus aureus*.

Clinical features   The onset of fever is often sudden, and is accompanied by neck stiffness, drooling, dyspnoea, and a sore throat.

Treatment   Palpation may rupture the abscess, and lead to aspiration of pus. If the history is suspicious of retropharyngeal abscess, palpation should be avoided. If there is a significant degree of airway obstruction, orotracheal intubation should be performed with due care not to rupture the abscess. The definitive treatment is surgical drainage.

Tonsillar obstruction

Aetiology   Marked tonsillar enlargement may occur secondary to acute bacterial infection (usually with group A *Streptococcus*), peritonsillar abscess or glandular fever.

Treatment   A nasopharyngeal airway is usually sufficient to maintain airway patency. Surgery may be performed after treatment with antibiotics and resolution of the acute episode.

Other causes of upper airway obstruction

These are relatively rare, and include vocal cord paralysis, trauma, laryngo-tracheomalacia, mediastinal tumours, laryngeal papillomata, and congenital causes (Pierre Robin, Treacher Collins, and choanal atresia). Upper airway burns and inhalation injury can cause oedema and airway obstruction.

Lower airways

Status asthmaticus

Aetiology   Bronchospasm, mucosal oedema, and increased mucus secretion cause trapping of gas or alveolar collapse behind narrowed airways. Work of breathing increases and a ventilation–perfusion mismatch develops.

Clinical features

An acute episode of asthma may progress very rapidly to respiratory failure, and this should always be borne in mind. The patient with a severe asthma episode uses accessory muscles of respiration, and is obviously distressed. There may be expiratory wheezes. Cyanosis, reduced breath sounds and a normal or high PCO_2 are ominous signs.

Investigations   Chest X-ray may show infiltrates, atelectasis, pneumome-diastinum, or pneumothorax. Arterial blood gases should be taken, and pulse oximetry instituted.

Treatment   Nebulized beta agonists, intravenous aminophylline, and corticosteroids are the pharmacological mainstays of treatment. If severe respiratory failure supervenes despite this therapy, and arterial oxygenation cannot be maintained despite giving humidified oxygen, mechanical ventilation will be needed to provide support until the airway obstruction is resolved. There are various approaches to mechanical ventilation in status asthmaticus. Two recent studies[11,12] have emphasized the importance of limiting the peak airway pressure e.g. to 45 cmH$_2$O. Slow ventilatory rates (12 bpm) and a tidal volume of 10–12 l/min are chosen to allow for optimal alveolar filling and emptying. Although this results in a degree of hypercapnia, this appears to be a safe trade-off to avoid complications of overpressure such as pneumothorax. Correction of acidosis with bicarbonate may lead to hyponatraemia and hyperosmolarity, and is not advisable. It appears to be safer to tolerate hypercapnia and acidosis than to try to correct them. Dworkin and Kattan[11] instituted PEEP of 4–7 cmH$_2$O after severe bronchoconstriction had been reversed, and recovery had started. It may be that this is a useful strategy which guards against the later development of atelectasis in areas which are becoming well perfused again. Theoretically, this approach should help to avoid hypoxia caused by shunting, although its efficacy has not yet been formally evaluated.

Foreign body inhalation

Aetiology   All manner of foreign bodies are commonly inhaled by accident. Peanuts and sunflower seeds account for over 50% of all aspirated objects. Aspirated material most frequently lodges in the right main bronchus.

Clinical features   The initial inhalation episode is often associated with a sudden onset of coughing, hypoxia and gagging. Airway obstruction may be complete, needing urgent cardiopulmonary resuscitation and removal of the offending object, either under direct vision, or by external manoeuvres, e.g. Heimlich. If obstruction is incomplete, it may cause inspiratory stridor (trachea or hypopharynx) or expiratory wheezing (main bronchus). Presentation is not always immediate, and aspiration of a foreign body should be considered in all children with respiratory distress. Breath sounds may be decreased, but this is not a reliable sign in all cases. Oesophageal foreign bodies may also cause stridor or wheeze due to secondary airway compression.

Investigation and treatment   The request for a chest or upper airway X-ray should include a description of the foreign body. The object itself may be seen on X-ray, or the effects it produces, e.g. atelectasis or hyperinflation distal to the blockage. Inspiratory and expiratory films may be of use in demonstrating a 'ball-valve' effect. Occasionally, endoscopy (flexible or rigid bronchoscopy) is needed to identify the foreign body, as well as to remove it.

If the patient is well, this need not be done as an emergency. If secondary infection develops, antibiotics are indicated.

VENTILATION OF THE CHILD WITH A HEAD INJURY

Indications for intubation

The child who has sustained a head injury should be intubated if the airway needs to be protected from aspiration of blood or stomach contents, or if the patient cannot maintain a reliable airway themselves. Intubation is also indicated if mechanical ventilation is required. When considering intubation in the head injured patient, it should always be borne in mind that the patient may also have a cervical spine injury, and appropriate measures should be taken to prevent further injury.

Indications for ventilation

Ventilatory support in the head injured patient will be needed if spontaneous ventilation is inadequate, for example, if the PaO_2 is less than 75 mmHg or $PaCO_2$ greater than 40 mmHg while breathing 60% oxygen. Head injury patients may also hyperventilate, and mechanical ventilation is recommended if the $PaCO_2$ is less than 25 mmHg. Mechanical ventilation is also indicated if conscious level is deteriorating or depressed (less than 8 on the Glasgow Coma Scale), if there are refractory convulsions, if analgesia is required for other injuries, or if intracranial pressure is raised.

Aims of ventilation

Ventilation in the management of head injury is directed towards optimizing the balance between cerebral oxygen delivery and oxygen consumption. Oxygen delivery to the brain can be kept at a satisfactory level by providing adequate oxygenation, avoiding hypercapnia and maintaining normal arterial pressure. Careful attention to fluid balance and avoidance of anaemia also help to optimize cerebral oxygen delivery. Adequate sedation and analgesia will minimize rises in arterial and venous pressure, and consequently help keep intracranial pressure within safe limits. Intracranial pressure may be reduced by ventilating to a moderately reduced $PaCO_2$. Hyperpyrexia and convulsions should be avoided as they increase cerebral oxygen consumption.

Controlled mechanical ventilation with morphine/midazolam sedation and often with vecuronium as a muscle relaxant is the usual ventilatory strategy employed. In some centres, the patient is nursed in a 15° head-up posture. Physiotherapy should be performed with great care, with supplemental sedatives if necessary to avoid sudden rises in intracranial pressure. Weaning from

ventilation should be started when the patient is neurologically stable and after consultation with the neurosurgeons. To permit spontaneous breathing $PaCO_2$ should be gradually allowed to increase to 40 mmHg and sedation gradually stopped.

VENTILATION IN CARDIAC DISEASE

Mechanical ventilation may be needed in children with congenital heart disease, especially in the perioperative period. The requirement for mechanical ventilatory support after cardiac surgery is fairly common, although the incidence of postoperative ventilation seems to have diminished in recent years.[13]

Respiratory failure may develop for a number of reasons in the child who has had cardiac surgery. Increased lung water and pulmonary bloodflow decrease pulmonary compliance and increase airway resistance. The effects of cardiopulmonary bypass on the inflammatory response and the surfactant system exacerbate these changes in lung mechanics. In addition, sedative and analgesic drugs which have been given during surgery may decrease respiratory drive in the immediate postoperative period.

Controlled mechanical ventilation is often used after cardiac surgery. Positive end expiratory pressure may be used to combat atelectasis, but PEEP can impair venous return and increase pulmonary vascular resistance (PVR), and this is usually a disadvantage in the postoperative cardiac patient. As pulmonary vascular resistance rises, the right ventricle becomes distended, displacing the interventricular septum and reducing left ventricular compliance. A high PVR is particularly disadvantageous after a Fontan or Glenn procedure, where pulmonary blood flow is not subject to ventricular pumping, but occurs passively. Occasionally, PEEP may be beneficial in that it may be used to improve oxygenation, and offset hypoxic vasoconstriction. It is also thought that PEEP may help to staunch high levels of postoperative bleeding.

Pulmonary vascular resistance may be very high or labile in the child with congenital heart disease. Avoidance of hypoxia and hypercapnia, and maintenance of a near normal FRC can offset this tendency somewhat. Inhaled nitric oxide is now being tested as a promising strategy to reduce PVR when needed.

It appears that in right ventricular dysfunction, ventilation may be used to augment the output of the failing right ventricle. Overinflation of the lungs flattens small vessels in the pulmonary bed: expiration then allows refilling of these vessels, generating a 'pumping' effect. Intermittent positive pressure ventilation with high pressures and high volumes has been showed to be beneficial in children with right heart failure.[14] Inflation volumes can be reduced as right ventricular function improves.

Pressure support ventilation has also been shown to benefit some post-operative cardiac surgery patients.[15] It can also be used in combination with synchronized intermittent mandatory ventilation.

VENTILATORS

Characteristics of a ventilator for paediatric intensive care

The ideal paediatric ventilator for use in intensive care should be lightweight, compact, and easy to understand with clearly marked controls and parts which are easy to clean and replace. Alarms should include warnings of high pressure, low pressure (disconnect) and incorrect inspired oxygen concentration. The ventilator should be versatile, allowing ventilation in different modes, with a wide range of possible respiratory rates and volumes. Adequate ventilation should be possible in the face of changing lung mechanics, and a direct readout of circuit pressure, respiratory frequency and inspiratory times is desirable. A facility to interchange between pressure and flow generation is useful. The resistance and compressible volume of the circuit should be low and the response times rapid.

Classification of ventilators

Mechanical ventilators may be classified according to how they provide gas flow in the inspiratory phase, and to how they change from inspiration to expiration (cycling).

The inspiratory phase

Pressure generators
In a pressure generator, a certain preset peak pressure of gas is delivered to the patient. The flow rate may be constant or non-constant. The pressure delivered by this type of ventilator is not affected by respiratory system compliance or resistance. However, gas *flow* is affected by lung mechanics. Flow decreases as airway resistance increases, and tidal volume decreases as compliance decreases.

It is possible to compensate for leaks in the circuit, and around the tube with this type of ventilator and to provide a more reliable tidal volume in the presence of a leak. For this reason, pressure generators are often used in infants and children under 10 kg who are almost invariably ventilated with a tube leak. Pressure generators also have a rapid response time and can be used at the high respiratory rates needed in small children. Their major disadvantage is an inability to provide reliable ventilation in the face of changing lung mechanics.

Flow generators

Flow generators are more commonly used in the older child. A predetermined tidal volume is set, and the ventilator generates either a constant or non-constant flow. Whether or not these different patterns of inspiratory flow have any benefit in improving oxygenation is controversial.

The airflow produced by a flow generator is not influenced by pulmonary mechanics. The pressure produced is, however, dependent on pulmonary mechanics. If compliance decreases, alveolar pressure increases. If resistance increases, the rate of rise in alveolar pressure decreases, and the pressure gradient between the mouth and the alveoli increases.

In infants and young children, the compliance of the ventilator tubing may absorb all of a preset tidal volume. As the child gets larger, however, the ratio of compressed to delivered volume favours delivered volume, and flow generators can be used satisfactorily in the older age group.

Microprocessor controlled ventilators

These recently developed ventilators are very versatile, offering a wide range of ventilatory modes, waveforms and cycling mechanisms. They incorporate sophisticated safety check mechanisms and allow real-time monitoring of ventilatory parameters, and often lung mechanics. These parameters can be stored in memory and retrieved to show trends. Two types of control mechanism are used in these ventilators: open loop or closed loop. In open loop control, no account of measured data is taken. In closed loop ventilation, theoretically changes in lung mechanics and compliance of tubing may be taken into account and used to correct ventilatory parameters. In practice, however, response times may not be fast enough and compensation for changing lung mechanics or tubing compliance may not be complete.

Cycling from inspiration to expiration

Volume cycling

In this mode, the ventilator cycles into expiration once a preset tidal volume has been delivered. Peak inspiratory pressure varies, depending on lung mechanics. If compliance is very low or resistance is very high, there will be a considerable increase in pressure. As a safety mechanism, excess pressure may be vented through a safety valve or the ventilator may automatically terminate inspiration once a set pressure has been reached. The volume of gas actually delivered to the patient depends on the compressibility of the ventilator circuit, and on lung mechanics. It may be impossible for a volume cycled ventilator to deliver a constant tidal volume in the face of changing lung mechanics, as excess gas may be vented if airway pressure rises too much. However, the use of low compliance ventilator tubing improves the accuracy of the volume delivered.

An end inspiratory pause may be incorporated with volume cycled ventilation. The theory behind this is that time is allowed for gas to redistribute

to compartments with longer time constants, thus producing more even ventilation. In practice, however, the improvement in ventilation may be a non-specific one arising from an increased mean airway pressure.

Time cycling

This type of ventilator cycles from inspiration to expiration after a preset time. The cycling mechanism may be pneumatic or electronic. If time cycling occurs in a flow generator, it is equivalent to volume cycling as time × flow = volume.

The inspiratory time and the expiratory time controls determine the ratio of inspiration to expiration. The tidal volume delivered is a product of inspiratory time and inspiratory flow. All of this volume is not, however, delivered to the patient, as some of it may be absorbed by the compliance of the ventilator tubing.

In time cycled ventilation, the duration of the inspiratory phase is preset, and is independent of peak inspiratory pressure or lung mechanics. Inspiratory flow, tidal volume and peak pressure, however, are affected by changing lung mechanics. In the face of decreased compliance or increased resistance, increasing the inspiratory time will allow a larger tidal volume to be delivered. Peak airway pressure should be carefully monitored in low compliance or high resistance states as high pressures may be reached, with the attendant risk of barotrauma.

Pressure limited ventilation can be used in the time cycled mode. In pressure limited ventilation, when a preset airway pressure is reached, the breath is not terminated (as in pressure cycled ventilation), but the preset pressure is sustained as a plateau throughout the set inspiratory time. This can be achieved by the incorporation of a pressure relief valve into the circuit, allowing gas to vent, and to continue venting once the set pressure has been reached. Gas continues to flow from the ventilator to the patient and the venting mechanism during the plateau.

This mode of ventilation may help gas to be delivered more evenly to areas of lung with different time constants as alveoli are stented open for longer, allowing improved gas distribution. Pressure limited ventilation is also useful when there is a risk of barotrauma from high airway pressures.

It is important to note that a pressure limited ventilator cannot detect tube kinking. If the ventilator tubing becomes obstructed, the ventilator will just continue ventilating and venting gas once plateau pressure has been reached. The use of a capnometer is therefore recommended to detect tube kinking and blockage.

Pressure cycling

In pressure cycling, the ventilator cycles into expiration when a preset pressure is reached within the ventilator circuit, irrespective of tidal volume delivered. This mode allows a large peak flow to be delivered. Pressure cycling

can compensate well for tube leakage, provided the requisite pressure can be reached, and the leak is not large enough to prevent cycling altogether.

If respiratory compliance falls or resistance rises, the delivered tidal volume will decrease. Delivered tidal volume can be increased by increasing the set pressure however, care must be taken when the compliance improves, as the same pressure may then result in overdistension. Problems may also occur if compliance decreases, or secretions block the airway, as the preset pressure will be reached quickly, and underventilation can occur. If, on the other hand, there is a tubing disconnect, the ventilator will never reach the preset pressure, and will not cycle. Tidal volume lost in compliant ventilator tubing may result in delays in cycling.

Flow cycling

When flow has fallen to a certain critical level, inspiration is halted. Flow cycling may be used in microprocessor controlled ventilators in the pressure support mode. Inspiration is terminated once the flow has fallen to a certain percentage of peak inspiratory flow rate.

The inspiratory:expiratory ratio

Expiration is a purely passive process, therefore, to allow adequate emptying of the lung, the expiratory time needs to be longer than the inspiratory time. Usually , the inspiratory:expiratory (I:E) ratio is set at 1:2. This ratio should, however be adjusted according to the patient's respiratory problem and consequent changes in lung mechanics. In diseases where compliance is low and the lungs empty rapidly, the expiratory time may be decreased. In diseases where resistance is high, and the lungs empty slowly, expiratory time may need to be lengthened.

VENTILATORY STRATEGIES

Controlled mechanical ventilation

In controlled mechanical ventilation (CMV), there is no continuous gas flow through the circuit, and the patient cannot breathe spontaneously. The machine delivers repeated mandatory breaths of a rate and volume determined by the operator. There is no synchronization with the patient's own ventilatory efforts.

Controlled mechanical ventilation may be the only option in severe cardio-vascular or respiratory compromise. It is also especially useful in neuromuscular causes of respiratory failure, status epilepticus, and ventilation to reduce intracranial pressure.

Because the patient on CMV is unable to make any spontaneous respiratory efforts, the presence of a disconnect alarm is essential.

Intermittent mandatory ventilation

In intermittent mandatory ventilation (IMV), the ventilator delivers a predetermined number of breaths per minute, while the patient breathes spontaneously in between breaths.

The main disadvantage of this system is that the patient may not receive his or her full required minute volume. If the total volume to be delivered by IMV breaths is set at less than the required minute volume, underventilation may occur if the patient does not generate enough spontaneous breaths in between mandatory breaths to make up the balance. Asynchrony between the patient and the ventilator may also cause underventilation, for example if the patient breathes out while the ventilator is in the inspiratory phase.

Provision for spontaneous breathing requires a large fresh gas flow equal to or greater than the patient's peak inspiratory flow rate. The presence of a reservoir in the circuit is often employed to allow spontaneous breathing. A continuous flow system with or without a reservoir bag works well in children.

Synchronous intermittent mandatory ventilation (SIMV) was developed in an attempt to overcome the problems of asynchrony encountered with IMV. In this system, the patient can breathe spontaneously and initiate ventilator-delivered breaths via a demand valve. Actuation of the demand valve requires the patient to generate a negative pressure in the circuit. This is a major disadvantage in infants and children in whom the work of breathing is already high. The effort required to trigger the ventilator may raise the workload to an intolerable level. In tachypnoea, inadequate sensing may lead to asynchrony between the patient and the ventilator. More rapid sensing in conjunction with the Siemens Servo 900C ventilator for example has been achieved by using less complaint, paediatric ventilator tubing, and a more proximally placed airway pressure monitor.[16]

Advantages put forward for IMV and SIMV include possible reduction of respiratory alkalosis (although the evidence for this is controversial), decreased need for sedation or muscle relaxation, a lower mean airway pressure (and a reduced risk of barotrauma) and less haemodynamic effects than CMV. Reduction of mean airway pressure allows a higher level of PEEP or CPAP to be used. It also appears that FRC and ventilation perfusion ratio are less disrupted by IMV/SIMV than with controlled mechanical ventilation. SIMV is very widely used to facilitate weaning from ventilatory support.

Mandatory minute ventilation

Mandatory minute ventilation (MMV) ensures the delivery of a preset minute volume either by spontaneous or mandatory breaths. A constant gas flow (equal to a preset minute volume) is delivered to a reservoir maintained at constant pressure. The patient breathes spontaneously from the reservoir, and any remaining flow is collected in a bellows. Once the bellows contains a

preset amount, this gas is delivered as a ventilator breath. Selection of the correct minute volume is difficult. If it is too high, the patient may become apnoeic due to hypocapnia and if too low, the patient may be underventilated. As minute volume is determined by both respiratory rate and tidal volume, the patient may increase respiratory rate but not breathe an adequate tidal volume. This is especially a problem in children where ventilatory failure is met initially with an increase in respiratory rate rather than tidal volume. In these circumstances, ventilation may become extremely inefficient. All currently available ventilators with MMV also have pressure support which should help to overcome this problem by increasing the tidal volume of each spontaneous breath.

Pressure support ventilation

In pressure support ventilation (PSV), the patient makes an inspiratory effort which triggers the ventilator to deliver a flow which raises the airway pressure until a certain preset level is reached. This pressure is maintained until inspiratory flow stops. Pressure support can usually be varied from 0 to 30 cmH$_2$O.

Use of this mode poses problems in paediatric critical care as the fast respiratory rates in children may not be compatible with sensing and delivery systems which have a phase lag. As a result, asynchrony between the patient and the ventilator can develop. A pressure support ventilator in children should have a very sensitive means of detecting inspiration, and should be capable of a fast response over a broad range of gas flows. Usually a decrease to 25–50% of peak flow can be used as an indication to terminate inspiratory pressure. In infants and children, however, inspiratory times are faster, making the termination point more difficult to determine.

In lungs with low compliance, initial filling may occur at a fast flow rate, therefore termination of pressure support may be premature and complete filling may not take place. On the other hand, air leakage around a tube or high compliance may cause a slow decrease in pressure, and cause inspiratory pressure support to be sustained for a long time.

Pressure support ventilation has been studied in children aged 3–5 years.[15] It was found that as pressure support increased, minute ventilation did not change, but tidal volume increased, respiratory rate decreased, and work of breathing decreased. It should be noted, however, that in this study, PSV was used as a weaning mode in postoperative cardiac surgery patients, and this may not be representative of the situation in respiratory failure.

Pressure support ventilation allows the patient to set their own respiratory rate, tidal volume and gas flow. This is advantageous, as it allows feedback mechanisms to operate from mechanoreceptors in the chest wall and helps in the establishment of a regular, controlled pattern of breathing. The degree of autonomous respiratory control allowed by PSV also increases patient comfort. Pressure support ventilation may be used at low levels in the

spontaneously breathing patient to overcome the additional work of breathing imposed by a narrow tracheal tube. Alternatively, it may be used at a maximum level (10–12 ml/kg tidal volume) to provide full ventilation and then be gradually reduced during weaning. It may also be used as a weaning mode following controlled mechanical ventilation.

Pressure support ventilation is only of use in patients with a good respiratory drive and well established pattern of ventilation. If a reliable respiratory drive is not present, there is a real risk of apnoea. Pressure support should not be used in patients with varying lung mechanics, as potentially high and unpredictable airway pressures may be generated.

Volume support

In this mode, the ventilator assists the child's inspiratory effort just enough to achieve a target, preset tidal volume. The advantage of this mode of ventilation is that the amount of support is automatically adjusted breath-by-breath. If the child's efforts decrease, a minimum safe backup ventilatory support is delivered.

Positive end expiratory pressure

Positive end expiratory pressure is, as the name implies, application of a positive distending pressure to the lungs at the end of every inspiration when mechanical ventilation is used. PEEP improves arterial oxygenation by increasing FRC and ensuring that more alveoli are stented open at end expiration. This decreases shunting of deoxygenated blood across the lungs, and airway resistance is reduced as lung volume increases.

There are, however, some negative effects associated with PEEP. Cardiac output is reduced by higher levels of PEEP. This probably occurs by two mechanisms. First, right ventricular filling is reduced by increasing intrathoracic pressure. Secondly, pulmonary vascular resistance is increased, raising right ventricular afterload, shifting the intraventricular septum, and reducing left ventricular compliance. Pulmonary vascular resistance is minimal at normal FRC, therefore titration of PEEP should be aimed towards normalizing FRC.

It must be borne in mind that with the application of PEEP, all alveoli do not expand equally, and that some areas with high compliance will be distended more than others. At higher levels of PEEP, this can lead to overventilation and underperfusion, potentially increasing shunt fraction as bloodflow is diverted to underventilated regions of the lung. PEEP also reduces glomerular filtration rate and increases antidiuretic hormone secretion, leading to sodium and water retention.

A balance must be struck between the positive and negative effects of PEEP, and 'optimal PEEP' is the aim of therapy. This is a level of PEEP

which maximizes oxygenation without introducing deleterious cardiovascular effects. The best way to ascertain optimal PEEP is to optimize oxygen delivery. This, however, requires placement of a pulmonary artery catheter, and is not routinely done in paediatric intensive care units. Clinical parameters such as heart rate, blood pressure and oxygenation are relied upon. Optimal PEEP is often said to coincide with the best obtainable respiratory system compliance. However, it was recently demonstrated[17] that in paediatric patients, heart rate and blood pressure did not reflect the cardiovascular depression which occurred at higher levels of PEEP. It was also found that neither compliance nor PaO_2 predicted optimal oxygen delivery. The best approach in practice is to aim for a non-toxic level of inspired oxygen with an acceptable PaO_2 and to provide pharmacological support for the cardiovascular system if needed.

Application of PEEP, especially in children, carries an ever-present risk of barotrauma. Increased intrathoracic pressure may lead to an increase in intracranial pressure, and care should be taken in light of this when ventilating head injured patients. In general, the deleterious effects of PEEP are less with intermittent mandatory ventilation.

Continuous positive airway pressure

This is the equivalent of PEEP in the spontaneously breathing patient. CPAP is a continuously applied distending pressure which works in the same manner as PEEP to improve oxygenation. Gas is delivered through a high flow system with a reservoir bag. CPAP may be applied via a tracheal tube, via nasal cannulae or via a face mask in small newborn infants. It should be noted that application of CPAP by face mask has been associated with gastric distension and aspiration of gastric contents and that CPAP via nasal cannulae has been associated with an increased risk of intraventricular haemorrhage. Nasal cannulae may also increase the work of breathing. The preferred system for delivery of CPAP is by the tracheal tube. Overall, CPAP has less effect on the haemodynamics than mechanical ventilation.

This ventilatory strategy is useful to support spontaneous breathing (e.g. at a level of 2–3 cmH$_2$O) in children who have atelectasis. It may also have a beneficial effect, by increasing pulmonary vascular resistance in patients with left ventricular overload due to increased pulmonary bloodflow. CPAP is also employed during weaning from mechanical ventilation.

Airway pressure release ventilation (APRV, BIPAP)

In airway pressure release ventilation (APRV, BIPAP), a constant distending pressure is applied to the lung. When the ventilator cycles (according to a preset I:E ratio), a valve opens to release the distending pressure, and to allow gas flow out of the lung. The valve then closes, and the pressure is rapidly

restored. This type of ventilation may cause less trauma to the alveoli and oxygenation may be achieved at lower pressures.

Airway pressure release ventilation allows spontaneous breathing with the application of CPAP. It is useful in low compliance states, as the lung can empty easily and distension of uncompliant alveolar walls is limited. It is of little use, however, in high airway resistance, where gas flow out of the lung is slow when the pressure is released.

A CPAP circuit in which the flow is greater than or equal to peak inspiratory flow rate with a rapid response pressure release valve in the expiratory limb is needed for APRV. Low resistance tubing is also necessary to provide a rapid drop in airway pressure to allow CO_2 elimination. I:E ratios commonly used are 3:1–5:1. Settings include peak inspiratory pressure, inspiratory time, expiratory time and PEEP.

APRV is at present under investigation in patients with normal or reduced lung compliance. When airway pressure release ventilation was compared with SIMV and PSV it was found that APRV provided a lower peak inspiratory pressure, but less patient comfort and more asynchrony.[18] Davis and co-workers[19] used APRV in patients with ARDS, and found that they could achieve an adequate level of oxygenation with reduced peak inspiratory pressures and PEEP, although they demonstrated no advantageous cardiovascular effects from this. It is not certain whether alveolar damage is lessened by APRV.

Inverse ratio ventilation (IRV)

Inverse ratio ventilation can be achieved by three methods. Slowing of the inspiratory flow rate or inclusion of an end inspiratory hold will prolong inspiratory time. Thirdly, pressure controlled inverse ratio ventilation (PCIRV) uses a rapid initial flow, followed by a decelerating flow to maintain a plateau of pressure at a preset level. Each new breath starts just before expiratory flow has fallen to zero; this causes a PEEP like effect to occur, allowing gas distribution to lung units that would not otherwise be ventilated. The effect of this improved gas distribution is a reduction in shunt and improved CO_2 elimination. Pressure controlled inverse ratio ventilation may also reduce trauma to alveoli by holding open alveolar sacs and preventing them from repeatedly snapping open and shut.

Complete neuromuscular relaxation is needed if PCIRV is to be used. An initial drop in PaO_2 may be seen when the transition to PCIRV is made, and this can be offset by increasing the inspired oxygen concentration. Although the peak pressure with PCIRV may be reduced to half of the pressure which was needed on CMV, this pressure is applied for a longer time, and therefore the mean pressure may be actually higher. Familiarity with the equipment used and close monitoring of haemodynamic and respiratory parameters is essential. The cardiovascular effects of inverse ratio ventilation are similar to those of PEEP.

Pressure controlled inverse ratio ventilation may be useful in patients ventilated with PEEP who are needing higher and higher inspiratory pressures to maintain adequate ventilation. When adult patients with ARDS or pneumonia were studied, it was found that PCIRV reduced peak airway pressure and PEEP.[20] Ventilation and arterial oxygenation improved at the cost of a raised mean airway pressure.

High-frequency ventilation

High-frequency ventilation can be arbitrarily defined as ventilation at a respiratory rate of over 60 bpm. These high respiratory rates may be delivered by various methods. **High-frequency positive pressure ventilation (HFPPV)** employs a high pressure flow generating ventilator coupled with a flow interruptor. **High-frequency jet ventilation (HFJV)** makes use of a high pressure gas source connected to a small cannula and a flow interruptor. Ventilating gases are entrained by the venturi effect. Interruptors may be electromagnetic, solenoid, rotating fenestrated sphere or fluidic. In both HFPPV and HFJV, expiration is passive. Gas trapping and air leaks are potential problems with HFJV in children. **High-frequency oscillation (HFO)** produces to and fro gas waves in the airway by movement of a piston pump or a loudspeaker. Frequencies used in HFO are higher (up to 40 Hz) and, as expiration is active, the removal or clearance of CO_2 is very efficient.

There are various theories which explain how gas exchange occurs during HFV. If the tidal volume is large enough, direct ventilation of proximal alveoli may occur. At airway bifurcations, gas flow is not uniform, and may stream in the centre to travel further. Gas may mix between alveoli with different time constants (Pendelluft) and diffusion and cardiogenic mixing may also occur.

High-frequency ventilation can be superimposed on CMV at a low rate. This has the effect of 'sighing' the airways open to overcome alveolar opening pressure, and then dropping the pressure to above closing pressure. This may reduce the damage caused by alveoli snapping open and closed.

Positive end expiratory pressure can be produced in conjunction with HFV, and oxygenation and CO_2 removal may be increased by increasing the driving pressure and inspiratory time. Use of HFO allows adequate humidification to be delivered and allows spontaneous ventilation. During spontaneous breathing, it has a similar effect to CPAP on oxygenation which can be improved by increasing mean airway pressure. The amplitude of oscillation can be adjusted by subjective assessment of chest vibration and by $PaCO_2$ levels.

It is essential that staff are familiar with the device delivering HFV before this mode is used. Hypotension has been reported in association with HFV, but reduction of cardiac output can be avoided if the lungs are not over-inflated during ventilation. There are conflicting reports as to whether or not HFV increases the risk of intraventricular haemorrhage. Necrotizing tracheobronchitis was reported in the early days of high-frequency jet ventilation,

however, poor humidification of inspired gas may have played a considerable part in this.

HFO is increasingly common with the availability of reliable, easy to use machines which can be used in neonates and children up to 20 kg. Oxygenation is controlled by manipulating FIO_2 and mean airway pressure while CO_2 removal is controlled by circuit flow, amplitude of the oscillation waveform and I:E ratio.

HFO shows great promise in bilateral confluent lung disorders and is being used in association with surfactant therapy and nitric oxide to salvage babies who would otherwise need EMCO support.

Extracorporeal membrane oxygenation (see also Chapter 7)

Extracorporeal membrane oxygenation (ECMO) developed in the wake of cardiopulmonary bypass. There are two forms of ECMO: venoarterial and venovenous. In venoarterial ECMO, blood is drained from the right atrium via a large catheter in the internal jugular vein. It is then pumped through a collapsible bladder (the venous return monitor) linked to an alarm which sounds if the bladder becomes empty. The blood then passes to a membrane oxygenator, where gas exchange occurs, and a heat exchanger, to return to the systemic circulation via a catheter with its tip at the junction of the innominate artery and the aortic arch.

Venovenous ECMO can be performed via two catheters, with the outflow catheter inserted in the right atrium via a great vein, and the inflow catheter inserted in the femoral vein. Single catheter venovenous ECMO utilizes a catheter in the right atrium. The proximal lumen is used for outflow, and the distal lumen for return. In venovenous ECMO, the oxygen saturations obtained are lower than those in venoarterial. There is no pump to support the circulation, therefore, if perfusion becomes persistently poor, it may be necessary to convert to venoarterial ECMO.

During ECMO, the lungs do not participate in gas exchange, and are ventilated with an inspired oxygen concentration of at or near room air, and a low respiratory rate. Arterial oxygen concentration is controlled by the flow rate of blood through the circuit.

ECMO has been widely used to support infants with meconium aspiration or congential diaphragmatic hernia. Venoarterial ECMO can also be used to provide cardiovascular support for children with remediable causes of cardiac failure, or as a bridge to transplantation; for example, in myocarditis, cardiomyopathy, or congenital heart disease. ECMO has been successfully used in respiratory failure. Moler *et al.*[21] in a recent study documented 25 non-neonatal patients who received ECMO for acute respiratory failure. 88% survived to be discharged home.

Criteria for institution of ECMO usually include an oxygenation index of about 0.4–0.55. Oxygenation index appears to be the most reproducible

predictor of mortality between centres.[22] Extracorporeal membrane oxygenation does not cure lung disease: it rests the cardiovascular and respiratory systems. Therefore it should be offered to patients who have a high risk of dying from a potentially recoverable lung disease.

Risks of ECMO are related to large vessel cannulation, return of unfiltered blood products to the aorta, heparinization, technical accidents, and being ill enough to require ECMO in the first place. Heparinization to an activated clotting time of about 200 s is required during ECMO. Bleeding is a worrying complication and intracranial bleeding can spell disaster.

Extracorporeal carbon dioxide removal

In extracorporeal CO_2 removal, the lungs provide oxygenation, while an extracorporeal circuit provides CO_2 removal via a single or double venous catheter. This avoids the entry to the arterial system, but cannot be used in severe lung disease where pulmonary oxygenation is not possible.

Intravascular oxygenation

Intravascular oxygenation (IVOX) involves placement of a bundle of hollow fibres in the inferior vena cava. These hollow fibres which act as a membrane oxygenator are introduced in compacted form via the femoral vein, and unfurl when they reach the inferior vena cava. Oxygen passes in through the inflow limb, and is sucked out through the outflow limb. The oxygenator surface area is the most important factor in determining the degree of oxygenation which can be obtained. IVOX cannot completely take over from mechanical ventilation, but it can provide a useful adjunct to oxygen and carbon dioxide exchange. Heptic, renal and thrombotic complications have been reported.[23]

Differential lung ventilation

Differential lung ventilation may be useful in severe unilateral lung pathology e.g. bronchopleural fistula, aspiration pneumonia, lobar pneumonia, atelectasis, or chest trauma, where the ventilatory requirements of both lungs vary. It allows a different ventilatory strategy to be applied to each lung. It does, however, pose considerable problems in the paediatric population, where, due to the increase in total tube-wall thickness, airflow resistance will be higher. Two ventilators or circuits are also needed, and this can cause logistic problems. Various strategies have been employed, including differential CPAP (although, in children this may be associated with an intolerable increase in work of breathing), high-frequency ventilation on one side and conventional ventilation on the other or so-called selective PEEP. Recent evidence has shown that synchronization of the two sides is probably unimportant. Migration of the tracheal tube may be a problem, and it is important to monitor

inspiratory and expiratory tidal volumes and inflation pressures on both sides. Bronchoscopic guidance can be used to ensure accurate placement of the tube. The tidal volume is usually set at about 6 ml/kg per lung.

Postural changes

Ventilation in the prone position may augment functional residual capacity and diaphragmatic movement, and improve ventilation of dorsal areas of the lung.

VENTILATORY SUPPORT AND PHYSIOLOGY

Mechanical ventilation produces physiological effects which encompass virtually all bodily systems.

Respiratory system effects

Functional residual capacity and respiratory system compliance fall. There tends to be a more uneven distribution of ventilation, dead space and shunting increase, and as a consequence, arterial alveolar oxygen difference becomes greater. Mucociliary clearance and lung water clearance are also altered.

Intrinsic PEEP

If, for any reason, expiratory time is not long enough to allow full expiration (e.g. due to increased airway resistance, or a short expiratory time set on the ventilator), airway pressure may be positive at the end of expiration. This phenomenon is called intrinsic PEEP, and will have the same physiological effects as a similar level of applied PEEP. Intrinsic PEEP can be detected by occluding the expiratory port of the ventilator immediately before inspiration, and reading the pressure on the ventilator manometer. Development of intrinsic PEEP can be offset by the use of bronchodilators to reduce airway resistance in bronchospasm, or by lengthening the expiratory time.

Cardiovascular effects

Intermittent positive pressure ventilation causes a reduction in cardiac output. This is probably due not only to reduced venous return and increased pulmonary vascular resistance (especially in lung disease) but also to decreased left ventricular compliance. In all forms of mechanical ventilation, the degree of cardiovascular depression is dependent on the peak airway pressure. Intermittent mandatory ventilation generally has a less depressive effect on the cardiovascular system than for example controlled mechanical ventilation.

This is partly due to the decreased number of mechanical breaths provided, but also increased work of breathing against a demand valve may cause catecholamine secretion, increased cardiac work, and a positive inotropic effect.

Renal effects

Renal vein pressure increases, and renal artery pressure decreases with intermittent positive pressure ventilation. Cardiac output also decreases. These factors together lower renal perfusion pressure and lead to decreased glomerular filtration rate and urine output. An additional hazard occurs with the use of ultrasonic nebulizers where fluid retention and hyponatraemia may occur due to absorption of large amounts of hypotonic fluid.

Intracranial pressure

During mechanical ventilation, intracranial pressure may rise due to reduced venous return initially, but this is often followed by a fall due to reduction in CO_2.

Endocrine effects

Secretion of atrial natriuretic factor is decreased by mechanical ventilation. Renin and aldosterone increase and there are variable effects on antidiuretic hormone. The net effect of this is that sodium retention is increased.

Gastrointestinal tract

Paralytic ileus may occur for 24–72 h after mechanical ventilation is commenced. Decreased hepatic bloodflow may lead to altered metabolism of drugs and other compounds. It is possible that changes in gastrointestinal haemodynamics are responsible for the increased incidence of gastrointestinal bleeding seen in ventilated patients.

STARTING VENTILATION

Once the decision to ventilate has been made, initial ventilatory parameters need to be chosen. From this starting point, ventilation can be tailored to the patient's individual needs, and to their response to ventilation. In controlled mechanical ventilation, the tidal volume is usually set at 10–15 ml/kg and the respiratory rate is adjusted to deliver a total minute volume of 150–200 ml/kg/min. Adequacy of ventilation can be assessed by observing chest expansion, air entry, and airway pressure and by monitoring arterial oxygen saturation (SaO_2), PaO_2 and $PaCO_2$. With normal resistance and compliance,

a tidal volume of 10–15 ml/kg, a peak flow of 30–40 ml/min and an I:E ratio of 1:2, peak inspiratory pressure should be between 20 and 30 cmH$_2$O. If compliance is decreased or resistance increased, peak inspiratory pressure increases. Peak inspiratory pressure can be reduced by decreasing peak flow, prolonging inspiratory time or reducing tidal volume and increasing respiratory rate. If airway pressure is still unacceptably high, another method of ventilation may be indicated.

When controlled mechanical ventilation is started, an inspired oxygen concentration of 60% is often selected. Alternatively, ventilation may be started with 100% oxygen, and the fraction decreased until it is as low as possible with an acceptable oxygen saturation.

Tidal ventilation should be adjusted in light of the airway pressure, arterial blood gases, and pH to match metabolic needs and to overcome dead space ventilation and tubing compliance.

The I:E ratio is usually set at 1:2. It should be borne in mind that if the airway resistance is high, a short inspiratory time will not allow ventilation with an adequate tidal volume. If the I:E ratio is too high—greater than 1:1—gas trapping may result.

PHYSIOTHERAPY AND AIRWAY CARE

Techniques

Chest physiotherapy can be defined as those techniques which loosen airway secretions and expand closed lung units, thus improving distribution of ventilation, and improving lung mechanics. These objectives can be achieved by postural drainage (placing the affected part uppermost to allow drainage of secretions by gravity), percussion of the chest with a cupped hand and vibration. Chest physiotherapy is not necessarily appropriate in all ICU patients. Indications include acute atelactasis, pneumonia, foreign body aspiration, and conditions producing copious secretions including cystic fibrosis, bronchiectasis, and lung abscess. Caution is required in conditions where there is a risk of bleeding, e.g. clotting disorders, active tuberculosis, haemoptysis and during the first 24 h after tracheostomy. Chest physiotherapy may be hazardous in lung damage, fractured ribs, brittle bones, untreated pneumothorax, and raised intracranial pressure.

When chest physiotherapy is being performed in the ventilated patient, a second person is often needed to safeguard the position of lines and tubes and to help position and restrain the child. Often an anaesthesia bag is used to inflate the lungs in between suctioning episodes. Each suction time should be short (5–10 s). A small volume of normal saline may be used to facilitate loosening of secretions. Suctioning of secretions is usually performed when a tracheal tube is in place, but it may be performed in the non-intubated patient if secretions are excessive.

Complications

Hypoxaemia may occur during suctioning as gas is sucked out along with secretions. This complication can be minimized by limiting suctioning to a short time. Hypoxia may also occur as PEEP is temporarily removed for suction. This can be offset by use of adaptors which maintain PEEP during the procedure. If the external diameter of the catheter is no greater than half that of the tube, the inward flow of gas replaces the gas lost in suction. Atelectasis can occur if the catheter obstructs an airway while a negative pressure is being applied. Atelectatic areas can be re-expanded by 'bagging', and it is advisable to hand ventilate with 100% oxygen prior to suctioning.

The risk of accidental extubation or decannulation can be minimized if two people are present during physiotherapy.

Damage to tracheal tissue is a hazard during suctioning, worsened by the use of uninterrupted suction or high pressure. A soft flexible catheter with a rounded tip, and an end hole rather than a side hole causes least trauma. Negative pressure should only be applied while the catheter is being withdrawn.

Other complications of chest physiotherapy include pneumothorax, raised intracranial pressure and transient bacteraemia. Bradycardia and other arrhythmias may occur: this is probably due to hypoxaemia. If this happens, suction should be temporarily stopped, and ventilation with 100% oxygen commenced.

Humidification

In infants and children, the small diameter endotracheal tube is very prone to blockage by secretions. Medical gases are supplied in dry form, and the presence of a tracheal tube bypasses the normal humidifying mechanisms of the upper airways and humidity must be supplied from an external source. Various types of humidifier are available, but not all are suitable for use in the paediatric intensive care unit. Heat and moisture exchanger humidifiers can cause problems in children, as they increase resistance to breathing and increase dead space. If humidification of inspired gas is too enthusiastic water can condense, and large quantities may be absorbed. For this reason, in the paediatric intensive care unit a nebulizer is of little use for humidification. A heated water bath (at about 40 °C) is a suitable method, but it should be noted that there is a danger of overheating, and appropriate alarms should be used.

WEANING FROM MECHANICAL VENTILATORY SUPPORT

Weaning is the controlled withdrawal of ventilatory support. Timing is all important, and weaning should not be considered if there is persistent hypoxia, organ dysfunction, mental confusion, or agitation.

Table 6.2 Signs of unsatisfactory weaning

Anxiety	Decreasing spontaneous tidal volume
Hypercapnia	Hypertension
Hypoxia	Hypotension
Tachypnoea	Sweating
Dyspnoea	Pallor

Measures of arterial oxygenation may be used along with other parameters to assess the feasibility of weaning from mechanical ventilation. An alveolar arterial oxygen difference of less than 300 mmHg on 100% inspired oxygen, and a PaO_2 over 60 mm Hg or SaO_2 greater than 92% on 40% inspired oxygen may indicate that the patient is ready to wean. A tidal volume on spontaneous ventilation greater than 3 ml/kg will allow adequate elimination of CO_2. Vital capacity should be greater than 10 ml/kg and there should be effective respiratory muscle strength, cough, and secretion clearing. A spontaneous ventilatory rate less than 60 breaths/min in neonates and less than 45 breaths/min in older children may be compatible with controlled withdrawal of ventilatory support. There should be reasonable evidence of a well-established respiratory pattern. Nitrogen balance should be positive, and the patient should be haemodynamically stable. It is difficult to state absolute criteria accurately.

When it has been decided to cut back ventilatory support, sedation is reduced, and muscle relaxants discontinued. There is no one weaning strategy which will work infallibly, and no evidence points to any one method being superior to others.

Intermittent mandatory ventilation may be started, and the rate gradually reduced. Alternatively, pressure support may be started at a level of full ventilatory support and gradually reduced. Mandatory minute ventilation may be used as a weaning mode in conjunction with pressure support. Once it has been established that spontaneous ventilation is possible, introduction of CPAP is a useful strategy to combat atelectasis.

Weaning programmes should be commenced early on in the day. A careful vigil is kept for indications that weaning is not progressing satisfactorily (Table 6.2).

SEQUELAE OF VENTILATION

Sequelae of intubation

Acutely, intubation can result in trauma to the larynx, pharynx, trachea and teeth. Subglottic and laryngeal oedema may develop, especially if too large a

tube is used. The tracheal tube may introduce infected secretions from the pharynx and nasal cavity into the trachea, and crusting in the airways is a hazard of non-humidified gases. Disconnection or plumbing errors and accidental self-extubation can be immediately life threatening.

Delayed complications include vocal cord granulomata and scarring, tracheomalacia, tracheal stenosis, arytenoid ulceration, and sinusitis. The last is a complication of nasal intubation.

Complications of tracheostomy

Complications which may occur acutely during and subacutely after the placement of a tracheostomy include pneumomediastinum, pneumothorax, and bleeding. Infection and mucus plugging may be troublesome while the patient with a tracheostomy is in the intensive care unit. Tracheal and subglottic stenosis and tracheomalacia are late complications.

Barotrauma and 'volutrauma'

Mechanical ventilation of lungs which are poorly compliant, and/or have a high airway resistance can lead to a group of effects known collectively as barotrauma. The gross manifestations of this damage are pneumothorax, pneumomediastinum, pneumoperitoneum and surgical emphysema.

Although barotrauma literally means 'damage due to increased pressure', it has recently been suggested that the cellular effects seen in mechanical ventilation are due to overdistension of alveoli rather than overpressure, and the term 'volutrauma' has been coined.[24] The cellular effects of volutrauma include desquamation, epithelial damage and a leak of protein into the alveoli.

Oxygen toxicity

It is difficult to tell how great a problem oxygen toxicity poses in the ventilated intensive care patient. Certainly, human volunteers spontaneously breathing 90–95% oxygen in the first 24 h get mild chest pain, decreased tracheal mucus velocity, tracheobronchitis, and increased alveolar permeability. After 24–48 h, vital capacity, compliance and diffusing capacity decrease, and dead space and shunt increase. Animal experiments have shown that the effects of 100% oxygen over a number of days may be lethal. There is, therefore, good reason to suspect that high oxygen concentrations for prolonged periods of time may be damaging to the lung. The generally accepted wisdom at present is that 100% oxygen is safe to be used for up to 24 h, and 40% oxygen is considered safe to use indefinitely.

Infection

Gram-negative organisms are most frequent culprits in nosocomial infection in the intensive care unit. Handwashing with a bactericidal agent, strict aseptic technique when handling the airway and limited examination of patient by people not involved in their care have been put forward as strategies for prevention of infection.

LEARNING POINTS

1. Meticulous care of the paediatric airway is fundamental to ventilatory care.
2. New ventilation modes and technologies have allowed improvements in synchronized support of spontaneous ventilatory efforts.
3. The roles of high frequency ventilation and extracorporeal life support are becoming clearer when applied to children.

REFERENCES

1   Eckenhoff JE. Some anatomic considerations of the infant larynx influencing endotracheal anesthesia. *Anesthesiology* 1951; **12**: 401–410
2   Robotham JL, Martin LD, Wetzel RC *et al.* Maturation of the respiratory system. In *Textbook of pediatric critical care* (ed. PR Holbrook). WB Saunders, Philadelphia, 1993.
3   Soong WJ, Huang B, Tang RB. Continuous positive airways pressure by nasal prongs in bronchiolitis. *Pediatric Pulmonology* 1993; **16**: 163–166.
4   Ashton MR. 'Blind' bronchoalveolar lavage. *Lancet* 1992; **340**: 1104.
5   Greaves TH, Cramolini GM, Walker DH *et al.* Inverse ratio ventilation in a 6 year old with severe post traumatic adult respiratory distress syndrome. *Critical Care Medicine* 1989; **17**: 588.
6   Sarnaik A, Lieh-Lai M. Adult respiratory distress syndrome in children. *Pediatric Clinics of North America* 1994; **41**: 377–363.
7   Ruddy RM. Smoke inhalation injury. *Pediatric Clinics of North America* 1994; **41**: 317–336.
8   Hall AH, Rumack B. Clinical toxicology of cyanide. *Annals of Emergency Medicine* 1986; **15**: 1067–1074.
9   Cressman WR, Myer CM III. Diagnosis and management of croup and epiglottitis. *Pediatric Clinics of North America* 1994; **41**: 265–276.
10 Gonzalez C, Reilly JS, Kenna MA *et al.* Duration of intubation in children with acute epiglottitis. *Otolaryngology, Head and Neck Surgery* 1986; **95**: 477–481.
11 Dworkin G, Kattan M. Mechanical ventilation for status asthmaticus in children. *Journal of Pediatrics* 1989; **114**: 545–549.
12 Cox RG, Barker GA, Bohn DJ. Efficacy, results and complications of mechanical ventilation in children with status asthmaticus. *Pediatric Pulmonology* 1991; **11**: 120–126.

13 DiCarlo JV, Steven JM. Respiratory failure in congenital heart disease. *Pediatric Clinics of North America* 1994; **41**: 525–542.

14 Pinsky MR, Marquez J, Martin D *et al*. Ventricular assist by cardiac cycle-specific increases in intrathoracic pressure. *Chest* 1987; **91**: 709.

15 Tokioka H, Kinjo M, Hirakawa M. The effectiveness of pressure support ventilation for mechanical ventilatory support in children. *Anesthesiology* 1993; **78**: 880–884.

16 Martin LD, Rafferty JF, Wetzell RC *et al*. Inspiratory work and response times of a modified pediatric volume ventilator during synchronised intermittent mandatory ventilation and pressure support ventilation. *Anesthesiology* 1989; **71**: 977–981.

17 Witte MK, Galli SA, Chatburn RL *et al*. Optimal positive end expiratory pressure therapy in infants and children with acute respiratory failure. *Pediatric Research* 1988; **24**: 217–221.

18 Chiang AA, Steinfield A, Gropper C *et al*. Demand flow airway pressure release ventilation as a partial ventilatory support mode: comparison with synchronised intermittent mandatory ventilation and pressure support ventilation. *Critical Care Medicine* 1994; **22**: 1431–1437.

19 Davis K, Johnson DJ, Branson RD *et al*. Airway pressure release ventilation. *Archives of Surgery* 1993; **128**: 1348–1352.

20 Lain DC, DiBenedetto R, Morris SL *et al*. Pressure controlled inverse ratio ventilation as a method to reduce peak inspiratory pressure and provide adequate ventilation and oxygenation. *Chest* 1989; **95**(5): 1081–1088.

21 Moler FW, Custer JR, Bartlett RH *et al*. Extracorporeal life support for severe pediatric respiratory failure: an updated experience 1991–1993. *Journal of Pediatrics* 1994; **124**: 875–880.

22 Klein MD, Whittlesey GC. Extracorporeal membrane oxygenation. *Pediatric Clinics of North America* 1994; **41**: 365–384.

23 Gasche Y, Romand JA, Pretre R *et al*. IVOX in ARDS: Respiratory effects and serious complications. *European Respiratory Journal* 1994; **7**: 821–823.

24 Dreyfus D, Saumon G. Role of tidal volume FRC and end-inspiratory volumes in development of pulmonary edema following mechanical ventilation. *American Review of Respiratory Diseases* 1993; **148**: 1194–1203.

7

Circulatory support

K.J. Millar

Restoration or maintenance of a normal circulation is one of the cornerstones of intensive care. The circulatory system exists primarily to carry oxygen and nutrients to the tissues and to carry carbon dioxide and products of metabolism to their sites of excretion. Efficient functioning of this system depends on:

- adequate circulatory volume (and composition)

- adequate pump function

- appropriate vessel resistance and capacitance.

Oxygen delivery to the tissues is the product of blood oxygen concentration and cardiac output. Efforts to support a failing circulation are directed towards maintaining cardiac output, usually in the face of increased demand due to illness.

THE DEFICIENT OR IMBALANCED CIRCULATION[1-4]

Hypovolaemic shock

An inadequate circulating volume may be due to bleeding, fluid loss (e.g. gastroenteritis, burns, diabetic ketoacidosis), or insufficient fluid intake or administration. The child is well able to compensate for losses of 10–15% of circulating blood volume. Initial compensatory mechanisms include peripheral vasoconstriction and an increase in heart rate to maintain perfusion of vital organs. With ongoing hypovolaemia, poor tissue and organ perfusion leads to anaerobic metabolism and a build-up of lactic acid. Ensuing cellular damage provokes harmful activation of clotting and kinin pathways.

The first signs of hypovolaemia are tachycardia and poor peripheral perfusion. Hypotension is a late sign in hypovolaemic shock, indicating a loss of more than 25% of circulating volume and failure of compensatory mechanisms. Agitation progressing to obtundation reflects insufficient cerebral oxygenation. With loss of more than 40% of circulating volume the child becomes ashen and unresponsive, with bradycardia and an unrecordable blood pressure. Acidosis and anuria or oliguria will be present. This is a grave clinical picture, and even aggressive resuscitation may not save the child at this point.

Septic shock

Septic shock is a circulatory maldistribution produced by an exaggerated inflammatory response to invasive infection. Invading bacteria produce toxins that activate the host's normally protective immune mechanisms. Unchecked, however, this complex cascade results in a harmful excess of cytokines which disrupt cardiovascular homeostasis and normal cellular metabolism. Vasomotor paralysis with vascular pooling and increased capillary permeability contribute to an effective hypovolaemic state. Myocardial contractility is often directly impaired, further reducing tissue oxygen delivery. At a cellular level, decreased oxygen availability and deficient oxygen utilization in the face of an increased metabolic demand lead to lactic acidosis.

In the early stages, clinical signs can be difficult to distinguish from common infection, with fever, tachycardia and warm peripheries. This high output phase gives way to poor peripheral perfusion, decreased urine output and, finally, hypotension. The development of confusion or somnolence at any stage is an important warning sign of worsening shock.

Cardiac failure and cardiogenic shock

In cardiac failure the abnormal or stressed heart can only maintain an adequate output by employing various compensatory mechanisms. Cardiogenic shock occurs when these are overwhelmed and the heart is no longer able to provide enough forward flow to meet tissue metabolic requirements.

Cardiac output is governed by four major variables.

1. Preload dictates ventric ular filling and is therefore affected by both venous return and ventricular compliance. Ventricular filling will directly determine intraventricular pressure and end diastolic volume.

2. Afterload reflects the direct resistance to ventricular output, which, in turn, affects the systolic loading state of that ventricle.

3. Inotropism is the ability of the myocardium to generate an efficient muscular contraction for ventricular emptying. This is affected by the intrinsic anatomic and physiological state of the heart, along with potent nurohormonal influences.

4. Heart rate directly determines cardiac output as well as the time for diastolic ventricular filling and coronary perfusion.

The heart of the young child, in particular the newborn infant, has a limited ability to cope with a demand for an increase in cardiac output for several reasons:

1. It contains more non-contractile elements.

2. It functions at a higher end diastolic volume (higher preload).

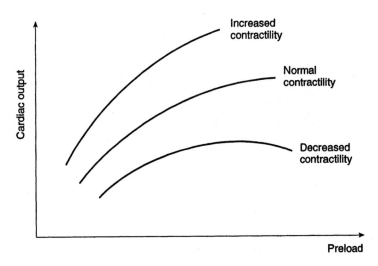

Fig. 7.1 The Frank–Starling curve.

3. It functions at a faster rate.

4. It is poorly able to develop increased tension in response to increased afterload.

The Frank–Starling curve represents the relationship between cardiac output and preload. An increase in stroke volume (cardiac output) is produced by increasing ventricular preload up to an optimum value. Beyond this level output will diminish. The inotropic state of the heart will alter the relationship as shown below (Fig. 7.1).

Cardiac output depends on heart rate and stroke volume (CO = HR × SV).

The child has a relative inability to increase stroke volume. Improving cardiac output is therefore heavily reliant on increasing heart rate.

The failing ventricle will dilate, increasing end diastolic volume. End diastolic pressure rises concomitantly, leading to back pressure and venous congestion. Atrial and venous distension, along with arterial hypotension produce an increase in sympathetic tone via stretch and baroreceptors. Alpha adrenergic stimulation causes peripheral, renal, and gastrointestinal vasoconstriction. Beta stimulation causes tachycardia and increased contractility, and cholinergic stimulation is responsible for the characteristic increased sweating.

Hypoperfusion of the juxtaglomerular apparatus leads to renin secretion with a consequent increase in angiotensin and aldosterone levels. These will directly and indirectly cause salt and water retention.

Pure left ventricular failure produces an increase in pressure in the pulmonary vascular bed. The lungs become less compliant and transudated fluid decreases the efficiency of gas exchange.

Right ventricular failure causes systemic venous congestion with enlargement of the liver and, in older children, peripheral oedema and visible distension of neck veins.

In cardiogenic shock the above measure to maintain cardiac output and tissue perfusion are insufficient to cope with ongoing demands and output becomes markedly diminished. Peripheral vasoconstriction raises systemic vascular resistance, and this increased afterload further impairs ventricular output. As tissue oxygen delivery falls off anaerobic metabolism and lactic acidosis ensue.

There are numerous causes of cardiac failure, but they can be broadly categorized into conditions that place either an increased pressure or volume load on the ventricle, and conditions that affect myocardial efficiency.

The infant with cardiac failure is tachypnoeic and sweats visibly. This sweating is frequently most visible on the forehead and is more pronounced during feeding and exertion. Ongoing cardiac failure increases metabolic demands sufficiently to cause failure to thrive. On examination, tachycardia is usually associated with a triple rhythm. Wheezes or crackles may be audible on auscultation, and hepatomegaly is a reliable sign. In older children, peripheral oedema and jugular venous distension are more easily visible.

In cardiogenic shock, the child will be extremely unwell, vasoconstricted and hypotensive with a poor urine output. Tachycardia progresses to bradycardia with worsening shock, and severe metabolic acidosis is present.

Pulmonary hypertension

Pulmonary arterial hypertension is usually a result of chronic exposure to excessive pulmonary bloodflow in children with large left to right shunts at aortopulmonary or ventricular level. The normal drop in pulmonary vascular resistance after birth is delayed and the real value of the nadir reached is higher than in normal children. Thereafter, ongoing exposure to the shearing forces of high bloodflow through the lungs leads to intimal proliferation, hyalinization and fibrosis. Irreversible obstructive pulmonary vascular disease may occur in children as young as 12–18 months of age. At this stage operative correction of the defect will not alleviate pulmonary hypertension.

Acute postoperative pulmonary hypertensive crisis is an occasional but life-threatening phenomenon in children following repair of high-flow left to right shunt lesions. Increased pulmonary vascular resistance impairs pulmonary bloodflow. The consequent hypoxia exaggerates pulmonary vasoconstriction, further elevating the pulmonary artery pressure. Diminished left atrial return produces a drop in cardiac output, reflected by a fall in systemic arterial pressure.

Treatment of postoperative pulmonary hypertension consists of ensuring adequate sedation and paralysis, hyperventilation with a high F_IO_2, and the administration of drugs aimed at producing pulmonary vasodilation.

The duct-dependent circulation

The ductus arteriosus is the channel by which blood bypasses the pulmonary circulation and enters the systemic circulation during fetal life. The muscular element of the ductal media and its constrictive response to oxygen increase towards term. In the fetus, patency is maintained by placental, ductal and umbilical vessel PGE_2. After birth, exposure to an increased arterial PaO_2 and removal of placental PGE_2 result in muscular contraction of the media. Normally, functional closure is attained within 24 h in the term baby.[5]

In some types of congenital heart disease the ductus is essential in maintaining an adequate circulation, and closure results in catastrophic shutdown of either the pulmonary or systemic circulation. In hypoplastic or atretic lesions of the left side of the heart (e.g. hypoplastic left heart, aortic interruption, critical aortic stenosis), distal systemic perfusion depends on right to left bloodflow through the ductus. Acute circulatory collapse and profound metabolic acidosis follow its closure. In hypoplastic or atretic right-sided lesions (e.g. tricuspid or pulmonary atresia), ductal closure interrupts pulmonary bloodflow producing marked cyanosis. In cases where the systemic and pulmonary circulations are working in parallel (e.g. transposition of the great arteries), the ductus may provide critical mixing. Usually there is also some circulatory mixing at atrial or ventricular level.

The administration of drugs to reopen the ductus and to maintain its patency in these cases is a temporary measure which will buy time until further shunting procedures can be undertaken.

GENERAL MEASURES

It is important to consider the child's immediate environment within the intensive care unit. The child should be appropriately warmed so that vital energy is not wasted in attempts to conserve heat. Special consideration should be given to the small newborn infant with its relative inability to thermoregulate.

Major metabolic disturbances (e.g. hypoglycaemia, hypocalcaemia, hyperkalaemia) must be dealt with, as these can be directly harmful as well as detrimental to further attempts to improve the child's circulation. Mild metabolic acidosis will often correct with warming and volume expansion and require no further treatment. Severe or persistent acidosis is, however, detrimental to cardiac function and correction with bicarbonate is warranted.

OPTIMIZATION OF CIRCULATING VOLUME

A reduction in circulating blood volume, for whatever reason, will reduce pre-load and ventricular filling. This, in accordance with the Frank–Starling relationship, will decrease the cardiac output. Increasing preload by volume expansion is a simple and commonly used first-line measure in situations where circulation seems inadequate.

There has been lengthy debate about the type of fluid to use as an initial volume expander, focusing mainly on whether crystalloid (electrolyte containing) or colloid (protein and electrolyte containing) solutions are most appropriate. The proteins in colloid solutions are retained more easily in the intravascular space and maintain the oncotic pressure of the intravascular fluid. If, however, colloids leak into the interstitial space, they may increase the oncotic pressure in this compartment, encouraging further loss of intravascular fluid. Crystalloid solutions will rapidly distribute themselves into the intravascular and interstitial compartments, both of which are likely to be depleted. The development of pulmonary interstitial oedema, however, appears to be a largely theoretical concern. Intravascular volume replacement using crystalloid solutions will require a greater volume of fluid than if colloid solutions are being used.

The usual practice in the United Kingdom is to use a colloid solution in the first instance, as the initial aim is to increase intravascular volume.

Volume expansion—practicalities (Table 7.1)

Circulating blood volume

- 100 ml/kg at birth

- 80 ml/kg at 1 year.

Table 7.1 Solutions used in volume expansion

	Na (mmol/l)	K (mmol/l)	Cl (mmol/l)	Protein	Other (mmol/l)
Crystalloid					
0.9% saline	150		150		
5% dextrose, 0.45% saline	75		75		Glucose 50 g/l
Hartmanns solution	131	5	111		Lactate 29 Ca 2
Colloid					
Plasma protein solution	130–150	1	125–135	4.5% albumin	
Haemaccel	145	5	145	3.5% polygelin	Ca 6

Dose of volume expander

Give an initial dose of 20 ml/kg of colloid solution as a rapid intravenous infusion. Double this dose can be given if using a crystalloid solution. Repeat this dose if there is still evidence of diminished circulating volume. Large volumes of fluid may be needed to restore the circulation in septic shock. Children with meningococcal septicaemia can require more than 100 ml/kg of fluid during initial resuscitation, and need ongoing volume replacement.

When to stop

Central venous pressure (CVP) monitoring is the most frequently used means of assessing the response to volume expansion. If the CVP is rising, or greater than 10, and there is no improvement in perfusion, then there is probably little to be gained by further fluid administration. It must be remembered that the CVP gives little information about left ventricular function. If more detailed assessment of this is required, pulmonary capillary wedge pressure provides valuable additional information.

Haemorrhage

If inadequate circulating volume is due to ongoing blood loss, the most appropriate volume expander is blood, whenever it becomes available.

PHARMACOLOGICAL CIRCULATORY SUPPORT (TABLE 7.2)

Even after optimization of intravascular volume, the sick child often needs further and ongoing circulatory support. The drugs used to augment the failing circulation generally act on several receptors at different sites.[6] Their physiological effects can, therefore, be unpredictable, particularly given the diversity of complex clinical situations in which they are used. It is essential that adequate cardiovascular monitoring is established before treatment is instituted.

Adrenoreceptor activating drugs

Sympathomimetic drugs are commonly used in critically ill children.[7-9] These endogenous and synthetic compounds are all catecholamine derivatives which exert their effects by interacting with specific tissue adrenoreceptors.

Adrenoreceptor subtypes and major distributions are shown in Table 7.3, while the relative effects of sympathomimetic drugs on these various receptor groups are summarized in Table 7.4.

Table 7.2 Commonly used cardiovascular support drug infusions

Drug	Dose (μg/kg/min)	Diluent	Compatible	Incompatible	Comments
Adrenaline	0.05–2	0.9% NaCl 5, 10% D	Noradrenaline Dopamine Dobutamine Vecuronium Heparin, KCl	$NaHCO_3$ Ca gluconate Frusemide	
Noradrenaline	0.1–2	0.9% NaCl 5, 10% D	Adrenaline Dopamine Dobutamine Isoprenaline Ca gluconate Heparin	$NaHCO_3$ Frusemide	
Dopamine	2–15	0.9% NaCl 5, 10% D	Adrenaline Noradrenaline Dobutamine Isoprenaline GTN/SNP Morphine Vecuronium Heparin KCl Ca gluconate	$NaHCO_3$ Frusemide	See text for dose-receptor effects
Dobutamine	5–20	0.9% NaCl 5, 10% D	Adrenaline Noradrenaline Dopamine Isoprenaline GTN/SNP Vecuronium	$NaHCO_3$ Ca gluconate KCl Frusemide	
Isoprenaline	0.05–1	0.9% NaCl 5, 10% D	Adrenaline Noradrenaline Dopamine Dobutamine Ca gluconate KCl, heparin Vecuronium	$NaHCO_3$ Frusemide	
Enoximone	5–20 Loading: 90 for 10–30 min	0.9% NaCl	Dedicated line		
SNP	0.5–10 (see text)	0.9% NaCl 5% D	Depamine Dobutamine GTN Vecuronium	Frusemide	Protect from light

Table 7.2 (*cont.*)

Drug	Dose (µg/kg/min)	Diluent	Compatible	Incompatible	Comments
GTN	1–10	0.9% NaCl 5% D	Dopamine Dobutamine SNP, heparin Vecuronium	Frusemide	Absorbed onto PVC
Prostacyclin	0.01	0.9% NaCl	Dedicated line		
Tolazoline	2–6 Loading: 1 mg/kg over 60 min	0.9% NaCl 30–5% D	Dopamine Dobutamine Frusemide		
PGE$_1$	0.01–0.1	0.9% NaCl 5% D	Dedicated line		
PGE$_2$	0.01–0.1	0.9% NaCl 5% D	Dedicated line		

Table 7.3 Adrenoreceptor subtypes and major distributions

α_1	Heart	Increased contractility
	Vascular smooth muscle	Constriction
α_2	Gastrointestinal smooth muscle	Relaxation
	(Vascular smooth muscle)	Constriction
β_1	Heart	Increased rate + contractility
β_2	Bronchial, gastrointestinal, genitourinary, smooth muscle	Relaxation
	Skeletal smooth muscle	Relaxation, K uptake
DA$_1$	Liver	Glycogenolysis
	Renal, mesenteric, coronary vascular smooth muscle	Relaxation
DA$_2$	Adrenergic nerves of renal + mesenteric vascular bed	Decreased sympathetic discharge—vasodilation

Stimulation of adrenoreceptors leads to activation of an intracellular G protein, through which the receptor is coupled to its effector protein. α_1 stimulation ultimately results in an increase in intracellular inositol triphosphate and calcium concentrations. β_1, β_2, and DA, receptor stimulation increase intracellular cyclic AMP concentrations by activating adenylate cyclase.

Downregulation is the phenomenon where prolonged exposure to an agonist drug results in a decreased number of receptors being expressed on the target tissue. This can be a problem with β agonists, resulting in a

Table 7.4 Relative receptor effects of sympathomimetic drugs

Drug	α_1	β_1	β_2	DA_1
Adrenaline	++	++	++	−
Noradrenaline	+++	+	−	−
Dopamine	+	+	+	+
Dobutamine	+	++	−	−
Isoprenaline	−	+++	++	−

decreased response to a static drug dose. Formation of normal numbers of fresh receptors occurs only after withdrawal of the drug.

Adrenaline

Adrenaline is an endogenous catecholamine produced by the adrenal medulla. Administration at low doses (<0.2 microgram/kg/min) initially stimulates β_1 receptors, increasing heart rate and contractility. β_2 receptors are also stimulated, causing some peripheral vasodilation and a drop in diastolic arterial blood pressure, with subsequent reflex tachycardia. At higher doses (>0.5 microgram/kg/min), α agonism predominates and peripheral vasoconstriction occurs, elevating systemic arterial pressure.

Adrenaline is useful in situations where a poorly functioning myocardium is associated with hypotension, e.g. cardiogenic shock, septic shock, post-cardiac arrest. Infusion rates from 0.1 to 2 micrograms/kg/min are employed and the chronotropic and pressor responses are dose-related.

At high doses intense peripheral vasoconstriction is observed, and poor peripheral perfusion with diminishing urine output occurs. The tachycardia seen with these doses increases myocardial oxygen consumption and can lead to ischaemia. Extrasystoles and ventricular arrhythmias may occur. Adrenaline also promotes intracellular pumping of potassium by stimulation of skeletal muscle β_1 receptors and inhibits insulin release, causing hyperglycaemia.

Noradrenaline

Noradrenaline is an endogenous catecholamine secreted by the adrenal medulla and found in sympathetic nerve endings throughout the body. Administration of noradrenaline stimulates peripheral α_1 receptors producing a brisk rise in both systolic and diastolic arterial pressures. Unlike adrenaline, noradrenaline produces no β_2 stimulation to counteract this effect. β_1 stimulation tends to increase heart rate and contractility, but vagal reflexes overcome the chronotropic effect. The inotropic effect, however, remains.

Noradrenaline is used in situations where hypotension exists with relatively well preserved cardiac function. It can be a useful pressor in septic shock after adequate volume loading.

The dose used is 0.1–2 micrograms/kg/min, and should be titrated against desired clinical effect.

The decrease in heart rate seen with noradrenaline means that myocardial oxygen demand is not significantly increased. Arrhythmias are exceedingly rare. Intense peripheral vasoconstriction can decrease perfusion of skin and vital organs, and pulmonary vasoconstriction increases pulmonary vascular resistance.

Dopamine

Dopamine is the endogenous precursor of noradrenaline and is found in neural tissue throughout the body. Of all the drugs used for circulatory support, the effects of dopamine are the most dose-dependent.

At low doses (<5 micrograms/kg/min), stimulation of DA_1 and DA_2 receptors in renal and splanchnic blood vessels produces vasodilation and increased flow through these vascular beds. Coronary bloodflow is also increased. As well as improving renal bloodflow, dopamine also promotes natriuresis and diuresis through DA_1-mediated effects on renal tubular cells. At moderate doses (5–10 micrograms/kg/min) $β_1$ effects are more marked and there is an increases in cardiac rate and contractility. At high doses (>10 micrograms/kg/min) $α_1$ stimulation predominates, resulting in peripheral vasoconstriction and a rise in systemic vascular resistance. This separation into discrete dose receptor response categories is an oversimplification, and it is reasonable to expect mixed receptor responses at any dose.[10,11] There may also be considerable variation in dose response between different age groups, and between similar patients. Neonates and infants may have decreased sensitivity to dopamine as well as accelerated plasma clearance.[12]

Dopamine also has important effects on endocrine function, including enhancement of renin production and inhibition of prolactin, growth hormone, thyrotrophin, and gonadotrophin secretion.

Dopamine is frequently used to improve renal perfusion and as a modest inotrope post-cardiac surgery, or in septic shock where marked hypotension is not a feature. Starting 'renal' doses of 2–5 micrograms/kg/min are used, with increasing inotropic effect up to 10 micrograms/kg/min. At doses above this peripheral vasoconstriction limits use.

Myocardial oxygen consumption rises with heart rate and afterload at high doses, where extrasystoles and tachyarrythmias may also be encountered. Renal perfusion is impaired with increasing vasoconstriction. There have been reports of unpredictable digital, limb, and gut ischaemia even at low infusion rates of dopamine.

Dobutamine

Dobutamine is a synthetic catecholamine with predominantly β_1 agonist effects. Stimulation of β_1 receptors increases cardiac contractility. There is some β_2-mediated vasodilation, but only a minimal rise in heart rate is usually observed. The amount of α stimulation produced by dobutamine is insufficient to produce a rise in systemic vascular resistance.

Dobutamine is useful as an almost pure inotropic agent in situations where a pressor effect is not required, e.g. congestive heart failure and cardiomyopathy. A fall in systemic blood pressure will occur in patients with inadequate circulating volume.

Doses of 5–20 micrograms/kg/min should produce an increase in stroke volume and cardiac output, and should be titrated against haemodynamic effect.

Myocardial oxygen consumption is increased by dobutamine, and this is exacerbated in those few patients who do become significantly tachycardic. Extrasystoles and arrhythmias are extremely rare.

Isoprenaline

Isoprenaline is a synthetic sympathomimetic amine with specific β agonist properties. β_1 agonism results in increased cardiac rate and contractility. β_2 receptor stimulation produces peripheral vasodilation and further, reflex tachycardia. Mean and diastolic arterial pressure falls, and systolic pressure may fall or rise slightly. Some pulmonary vasodilation is usually also produced.

Isoprenaline is used in situations where atropine resistant bradycardia is producing haemodynamic compromise.

Doses of 0.05–1 microgram/kg/min will produce an elevation in heart rate and cardiac output. Infusion rates are titrated against heart rate.

Extreme tachycardia can occur and can be complicated by tachyarrhythmias. The increased work of the myocardium raises its oxygen consumption, while the shortened diastolic time associated with a higher heart-rate decreases myocardial oxygen delivery. Myocardial ischaemia and infarction are recognized complications. Care must be taken to ensure adequate volume loading prior to starting isoprenaline, if hypotension secondary to peripheral vasodilation is to be avoided.

Phosphodiesterase inhibitors

The phosphodiesterases are widespread intracellular enzymes that hydrolyse the cyclic nucleotides cAMP and cGMP. Cyclic AMP and GMP are important secondary messengers promoting intracellular enzyme phosphorylation. There are at least five different phosphodiesterase isoenzymes that differ in their distribution and affinities for cAMP and cGMP. Phosphodiesterase

(PDE) III is found in myocardial and vascular smooth muscle cells and reacts with both cAMP and cGMP. Phosphodiesterase III inhibitors competitively inhibit this isoenzyme, leading to elevated intracellular levels of cAMP and cGMP.

In the myocardium, high levels of cAMP increase the phosphorylation of several protein kinases, the ultimate effect of which is to increase the availability of calcium at the myofilaments, enhancing contraction. In vascular smooth muscle cells, phosphorylation of myosin light chain kinase produces relaxation and vasodilation. A similar sequence of phosphorylation of cGMP dependency proteins causes myosin light chain dephosphorylation and vasodilation in response to elevated levels of cGMP.[13,14]

Enoximone

Enoximone is a synthetic midazolone that specifically inhibits PDE III. This has a positive inotropic effect, increasing stroke volume and cardiac output, with minimal, if any, effect on heart rate. There is also marked peripheral (and probably pulmonary) vasodilation, lowering systemic vascular resistance.

Enoximone is ideal in situations where both augmentation of myocardial performance and reduction in afterload are required. It is frequently used in congestive cardiac failure, cardiogenic shock, and following cardiac surgery.

The dose ranges from 5 to 20 micrograms/kg/min, using the minimum infusion rate necessary for the desired clinical effect. If a rapid effect is required, a loading dose can be given. An infusion running at 90 micrograms/kg/min is administered for 10–30 min, after which time the infusion is reduced to the usual rate.

Although increased contractility might be expected to increase myocardial oxygen demand, this is more than offset by the reduction in afterload and improvement in coronary perfusion that enoximone produces. Myocardial oxygen extraction is, in fact, reduced. Tachycardia is rarely seen, although increased arterio-venous conduction may lead to elevated ventricular rates in patients with rapid atrial arrhythmias.

Enoximone is excreted 80% unchanged by the kidneys and a lower infusion rate may be required in children with impaired renal function. Elevation of renal cAMP levels might theoretically produce a decrease in renal bloodflow. However, this does not appear to be a problem clinically, perhaps due to the increase in cardiac output.

Milrinone

Milrinone is a bipyridine that also competitively inhibits PDE III. It has similar inotropic and vasodilatory effects to enoximone, but experience in children is limited. Recommended doses are 0.375–0.75 microgram/kg/min.

Vasodilators

In situations where cardiac output remains poor despite inotropic therapy, peripheral vasodilation can be a useful manoeuvre. Arterial dilators will reduce afterload, whilst venous dilators reduce preload and filling pressures. Both of the commonly used vasodilators act by generating nitric oxide that stimulates intracellular guanylate cyclase mediated cGMP production. Phosphorylation of cGMP dependent kinases results in vascular smooth muscle relaxation.

Sodium nitroprusside

Sodium nitroprusside (SNP) reacts very rapidly with erythrocyte oxyhaemoglobin to produce cyanide, cyanomethaemoglobin and nitric oxide (NO). The ensuing NO-mediated vasodilation is rapid and dramatic. Roughly equivalent effects are seen in venous and arterial vessels.

The clinical effect achieved by this drop in systemic vascular resistance depends on the haemodynamic state of the patient. If the myocardium is functioning adequately and blood pressure is normal, there is a marked fall in systemic and pulmonary arterial pressure, reflex tachycardia, and no real increase in cardiac output. If myocardial dysfunction exists, however, the afterload reduction will increase stroke volume and cardiac output. There will be a minimal effect on heart rate and systemic arterial pressure will be maintained.

Sodium nitroprusside is used in situations where poor cardiac contractility is associated with systemic vasoconstriction, e.g. congestive cardiac failure, late septic shock. It is also used to reduce acutely an abnormally elevated blood pressure and as a pulmonary vasodilator.

Infusion rates used range from 0.5 to 10 micrograms/kg/min. Infusion rates of >4 micrograms/kg/min should not be used for longer than 24 h.

Cyanide is released slowly from erythrocytes and is metabolized to thiocyanate in the liver by rhodanase, in the presence of thiosulphate. Cyanide toxicity is rarely a problem if thiosulphate levels are normal, but when seen produces sweating, tachycardia, and arrhythmias. A rising serum lactate is an early sign of cyanide toxicity, and this should be monitored in prolonged exposure. The antidote to cyanide toxicity is an infusion of either sodium thiosulphate or dicobalt edetate.

Thiocyanate has a half-life of approximately 3 d due to repeated enterohepatic circulation prior to renal excretion. Thiocyanate accumulation occurs in renal impairment and produces signs of central nervous system (CNS) stimulation. Thiocyanate levels should be checked in children with poor renal function, or who are exposed to SNP for long periods (>4 d). Recipients of prolonged infusions should also have serum methaemoglobin monitored as this intermediary metabolite of nitroprusside may accumulate.

Sodium nitroprusside is light-sensitive, and the infusion should be covered with an opaque wrapper.

Glyceryl trinitrate

Glyceryl trinitrate (GTN) also functions as a nitric oxide donating peripheral vasodilator. The rise in cGMP and vascular relaxation occurs primarily in venous smooth muscle. Some arterial vasodilation does occur, particularly at high doses. With reduction in venous tone there is a fall in central venous and left atrial pressures. This improves output in a ventricle that has been subjected to excessive preload. A drop in systemic vascular resistance occurs as the dose is increased.

Glyceryl trinitrate is a useful drug in congestive cardiac failure and pulmonary oedema where elevated left ventricular filling pressures are present. It is also occasionally used as a pulmonary vasodilator.

The usual infusion rate is 0.5 microgram/kg/min, increasing in increments of 0.2 microgram/kg/min to achieve the desired effect. Glyceryl trinitrate is absorbed by polyvinyl chloride plastics. A polyethylene infusion set should therefore be used.

The most common side-effects of GTN infusion are hypotension and tachycardia. These will resolve on reduction in rate or, if necessary, cessation of infusion.

Tachyphylaxis can be a problem in patients receiving infusions for long periods.

Pulmonary vasodilators

Postoperative pulmonary hypertension is the most common situation requiring acute reduction in pulmonary artery pressure in paediatric intensive care. Persistent pulmonary hypertension of the newborn infant demands a similar strategy. Other diseases may have an element of symptomatic pulmonary hypertension, for example acute respiratory distress syndrome (ARDS).

Systemic administration of vasodilators such as SNP, GTN, tolazoline, and prostacyclin will have some effect on lowering pulmonary artery pressure, but systemic arterial hypotension is a common and limiting problem. This unwanted effect may be minimized by the administration of low doses of vasodilators into central venous lines as close as possible to the pulmonary artery. Inhaled NO is a new therapy which appears to produce pulmonary vasodilation without affecting systemic arterial pressure.

For sodium nitroprusside and glyceryl trinitrate, see above.

Epoprostenol (prostacyclin, PGI₂)

Prostacyclin is a naturally occurring eicosanoid produced in the intima of blood vessels. It is an extremely potent vasodilator that seems to be important

in the usual reduction in pulmonary vascular resistance which occurs after birth. Prostacyclin is used to lower acutely pulmonary arterial pressure at a starting dose of 0.01 microgram/kg/min. This is increased in increments of 0.01 microgram/kg/min depending on clinical effect and patient tolerance.

The most common side-effect experienced is systemic hypotension, usually accompanied by tachycardia. Facial flushing is often observed. Prostacyclin inhibits platelet aggregation by elevating platelet cAMP. Care must be taken, therefore, in the thrombocytopenic or haemorrhagic patient. The antiplatelet and hypotensive effects disappear within 30 min of cessation of infusion.

Tolazoline

Tolazoline has both H_2 agonist and α adrenergic antagonist properties. It produces profound vasodilation and has traditionally been used to treat persistent pulmonary hypertension of the newborn (PPHN). A limited number of newborn infants with PPHN appear to benefit from the drug. This, along with its significant side-effects, means that tolazoline enjoys varying degrees of favour in different neonatal units.[15,16]

A loading dose of 1 mg/kg is infused over a 30–60 min period as close as possible to the pulmonary circulation, i.e. into a right atrial or central venous line draining into the superior vena cava (blood from the inferior vena cava is more prone to right to left shunting through a patent foramen ovale). Response to this dose is assessed by measuring the PaO_2 in postductal arterial blood. If an improvement is seen, an infusion at 2–6 micrograms/kg/min is commenced.

The most limiting side-effect of tolazoline infusion is systemic hypotension, and this frequent occurrence should be treated initially with volume expansion. Dopamine is often given concurrently to achieve some peripheral vasoconstriction. The histaminic action of tolazoline promotes gastric acid secretion, and prophylactic administration of gastric protectants is essential.

Tolazoline has a very large volume of distribution and is excreted unchanged by a saturable renal tubular active transport system. The half-life varies inversely with renal bloodflow, and drug accumulation is a potential danger. In neonates the infusion rate should be reduced if there is diminished urine production, or there is tubular dysfunction or immaturity.

Nitric oxide

Nitric oxide is an endogenous gaseous free radical. Its importance as a widespread biological mediator is beginning to be recognized.[17-20] In endothelial cells NO is produced from arginine by nitric oxide synthase. Nitric oxide then activates guanylate cyclase, increasing levels of intracellular cGMP that result in vascular smooth muscle relaxation. In the pulmonary and systemic circulations, basal vasodilator tone is maintained by the continuous, controlled production of NO in arterial and arteriolar endothelial cells. Hypoxic

pulmonary vasoconstriction may be partly mediated by diminished NO production.

The administration of inhaled NO is a new and attractive therapy in the treatment of pulmonary hypertension. The gas is delivered directly to all ventilated areas, reaching parts of the lung that are poorly perfused. It acts locally to produce vasodilation, thereby improving ventilation/perfusion matching. There is minimal, if any, distant systemic effect because, once in the circulation, NO reacts rapidly with haemoglobin to form methaemoglobin.

This form of treatment has been used successfully in PPHN, acute postoperative pulmonary hypertension and ARDS.

The minimum effective dose is still unclear, but is certainly lower than previously thought. Current practice is to start at a dose of 2–10 ppm. If there is no improvement, the concentration is increased slowly to a maximum of 20 ppm. If there is still no improvement, the patient is unlikely to respond to NO.

The gas can be administered into the inspiratory limb of a continuous flow ventilator circuit, but needs to be mixed with the gases within an intermittent flow ventilator if unpredictable variations in concentration are to be avoided.

Concentrations of NO and its cytotoxic metabolite, nitrogen dioxide, must be measured continuously at the patient. Nitrogen dioxide concentrations should not be allowed to rise above 2 ppm. Methaemoglobin should be measured every 12–24 h and not be allowed to rise above 2%.

This treatment is still at an early stage of development, and precise details of dosage, method of administration, monitoring and duration of therapy have yet to be standardized. It is, however, an exciting prospect, and one of great potential use in the treatment of pulmonary hypertension.

Drugs used to maintain patency of the arterial duct

As discussed previously, certain neonatal circulations are critically dependent on flow through the ductus arteriosus. Drug treatment aimed at keeping open or reopening the ductus should be considered in the following situations:

(1) a cyanosed newborn infant with no evidence of respiratory disease;

(2) a baby developing cyanosis in the first few weeks of life with no evidence of respiratory disease;

(3) a baby collapsing in the first few weeks of life with poor peripheral perfusion, cardiac failure, and acidosis.

There is often no time to wait for echocardiographic diagnosis before starting therapy.

Prostaglandin E₁ (PGE₁, alprostadil, Prostin)

PGE_1 relaxes the smooth muscle of the ductal intima.

0.01 microgram/kg/min is the usual starting dose, and is generally enough to keep the ductus open. If this is not achieved, the dose may be increased up to a maximum of 0.1 microgram/kg/min.

The most common adverse effect of PGE_1 is apnoea. Often babies in which it is used will be in poor condition and already intubated and ventilated. If, however, the baby is breathing spontaneously, apnoea occurs in 10–12% of cases and should be anticipated.

Pyrexia, flushing, tachycardia, bradycardia, diarrhoea, and seizures are all recognized side-effects. Prolonged administration has been associated with weakening of the ductal wall, gastric outlet obstruction and long bone cortical proliferation.

Prostaglandin E₂ (PGE₂, dinoprostone)

PGE_2 is also effective at relaxing ductal smooth muscle.

Doses from 0.01 to 0.1 microgram/kg/min are used, with the infusion rate kept to the minimum necessary to maintain ductal patency.

Side-effects experienced with PGE_2 infusion are similar to those described above for PGE_1.

Pharmacological circulatory support—practicalities

Monitoring

All the drugs discussed in this section have major haemodynamic effects. Appropriate cardiovascular monitoring should be in place to assess clinical response to treatment. In practical terms this means a minimum of an electro-cardiograph, pulse oximeter, central venous pressure line and arterial line.

Administration

All these drugs should be infused through a catheter in a large central vein. This is particularly true of drugs acting on adrenoreceptors which can cause tissue necrosis and scarring if extravasated. Only in extreme circumstances should any of these drugs be administered through a peripheral line. Extravasation of adrenaline, noradrenaline or dopamine should be treated promptly with local phentolamine—an α antagonist.

Prescribing and making up infusions

Doses of drugs cited cover a wide range, and mistakes are easily made in the calculation of infusion concentrations and rates. It is best to get used to

working with a limited number of concentrations, and to stick to them. Always double-check calculations:

- 15 mg/kg in 50 ml at 1 ml/h = 5 micrograms/kg/min
- 3 mg/kg in 50 ml at 1 ml/h = 1 micrograms/kg/min
- 1.5 mg/kg in 50 ml at 1 ml/h = 0.5 micrograms/kg/min
- 0.15 mg/kg in 50 ml at 1 ml/h = 0.05 microgram/kg/min (50 ng/kg/min).

Compatibilities

It is ideal but not always possible to use a separate line or lumen for each drug. Compatibilities and incompatibilities have been given where information is available. These are for guidance only, and lines should always be checked for clouding or discoloration. Fresh infusions should be routinely made up every 24 h.[21-23]

MECHANICAL CIRCULATORY SUPPORT

In some patients with severe circulatory or respiratory failure, maximal conventional care with drug therapy and mechanical ventilation will be insufficient to support them through their illness. Mechanical circulatory assistance can be used as a short-term measure to augment the efforts of, or provide a period of rest for, the acutely sick heart, circulation or lungs.[24-30]

Extracorporeal membrane oxygenation (ECMO)

The extension of cardiopulmonary bypass to a mode of support for the critically ill infant was first done successfully in the mid-1970s. With increasing experience and refinement, the technique has gained acceptance as a valuable means of circulatory assistance in neonatal and paediatric intensive care.

The majority of patients undergoing ECMO have been neonates with respiratory failure, with more than 8000 treated world-wide. More recently, however, paediatric ECMO has been increasingly used in a variety of diseases.

The basic principle of ECMO is to remove a proportion of the patient's venous blood and mechanically pump it through an extracorporeal oxygenator before returning it to the patient's circulation. It must be appreciated that this is a means of support only and not a disease-specific treatment. The underlying acute disease process must be recoverable within the period of rest provided by ECMO.

Significant complications can arise from systemic heparinization and the cannulation and ligation of major vessels in these extremely sick children. Absolute dependence on the extracorporeal circuit also places the child at risk of complications secondary to technical circuit faults. Rigorous patient

selection is therefore essential to avoid applying this invasive, expensive and potentially dangerous technique in inappropriate cases.

Patient selection

Patient selection criteria are aimed at identifying a group of patients with reversible disease, a high predicted mortality and in whom the risk of major complications is not unacceptably high.

Current neonatal ECMO criteria (UK Collaborative ECMO Trial) comprise:

- birthweight >2000 g

- gestation >34 weeks

- predicted mortality >80% (oxygenation index >40).

Exclusion criteria are:

- unrecoverable/irreversible disease

- high-pressure ventilation >7 d

- major congenital, chromosomal, or neurological abnormality

- necrotizing enterocolitis

- intraventricular haemorrhage >grade 1

- major pulmonary haemorrhage.

Paediatric selection criteria are less well defined, not least because of the much more heterogeneous group of patients and diseases considered. The basic aim of identifying salvageable patients early in their disease is the same, however.

Diseases treated

Extracorporeal life support has been most successful in newborn infants, with the overall survival being 81%. The most common primary diseases in this population are meconium aspiration (93% survival), congenital diaphragmatic hernia (58% survival), pneumonia (76% survival), PPHN (83% survival), and respiratory distress syndrome (84% survival).

In the paediatric population, ECMO support has been used in cardiac disease (e.g. postcardiac surgery low output state, cardiogenic shock, myocarditis), lung disease (e.g. ARDS, pneumonia, aspirtion), and a mixture of other diseases causing circulatory failure (e.g. sepsis, drug overdose). Survival has been quoted as being <50% in this age group, but with increasing experience this is probably now closer to 80%. In the United Kingdom, ECMO is now being performed on comparable numbers of older children and neonates.

Types of ECMO

Veno-arterial (V-A) ECMO

Most ECMO experience has been gained using this method, and it is still the approach of choice in neonates. Blood is removed from the right atrium via a line in the internal jugular vein and returned to the ascending aorta via a line in the common carotid artery.

The advantage is that it provides near-total cardiopulmonary support and is therefore the method of choice in myocardial insufficiency. The disadvantages are that carotid artery flow is interrupted during bypass and the artery is usually ligated after ECMO. There is also potential for systemic embolization of clot or air from the circuit.

Variations   A second internal jugular venous catheter placed toward the head may provide further cephalad venous drainage and avoid cerebral venous congestion.

In older children and adults venous drainage may be from the inferior vena cava via a femoral venous cannula.

In patients with a very poorly functioning myocardium, additional left heart decompression may be required using a left atrial or ventricular catheter.

Some centres are now attempting carotid artery repair after ECMO.

Veno-venous (V-V) ECMO

This method is increasingly used in older children with respiratory failure. Blood is removed from the right atrium as for V-A ECMO, but is returned to the systemic venous circulation, into the iliac vein via a femoral cannula in older children. In younger children both removal and return of blood can be achieved with a large double lumen, flow directed catheter in the right atrium.

The advantage is that there is no cannulation of the carotid artery. The disadvantages are that systemic delivery of oxygenated blood depends on myocardial function, and there is some recirculation of oxygenated blood through the extracorporeal circuit.

Veno-arterial ECMO should always be available in case an increase in support is suddenly necessary. At placement of the venous cannula, the carotid artery is identified and a sling passed around it to aid emergency arterial access.

Low-frequency positive pressure ventilation with extracorporeal CO_2 removal (LFPPV-ECCO2R)

This is a form of extracorporeal life support used in older children and adults with respiratory disease. Essentially, V-V ECMO is instituted, but at much lower flows, at which the circuit membrane is efficient at CO_2 removal, but not at oxygenation. Systemic oxygenation is achieved by ventilating the patient with a high F_IO_2, high positive end expiratory pressure (PEEP) and very low rate.

Cannulae

The ECMO cannulae used vary in size from 8 to 14 French gauge. The biggest catheter that is practical is used to maximize flow, particularly since venous drainage is dependent on gravity alone. The new double lumen V-V ECMO cannulae attempt to direct returning blood through the tricuspid valve to reduce recirculation.

ECMO circuit

An ECMO circuit is shown in Fig. 7.2.

Circuit components

Bladder box and venous return monitor (VRM)
The bladder is a reservoir of venous blood drained from the patient by gravity. If the rate of bladder emptying by the circuit pump exceeds the rate of filling, the fall in bladder volume is detected by the VRM which sounds an alarm and stops the pump.

Pump
A roller head pump is used to draw blood from the bladder and advance it through the circuit in a non-pulsatile fashion. The pump flow dictates how much blood passes through the oxygenator, and is the most important determinant of patient oxygenation. In the event of a power failure the pump

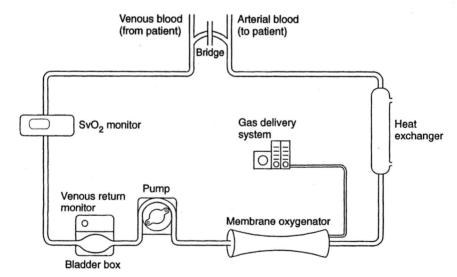

Fig. 7.2 Veno-arterial circuit.

can be hand-cranked. The tubing between the pump and the membrane oxygenator is subjected to the highest pressures in the circuit.

Membrane oxygenator

The oxygenator is a silicone membrane bilayer held apart by a plastic spacer screen. This membrane 'envelope' is then spirally wound around a polycarbonate spool and encased in a cylindrical outer cover. Gas flows between the two membrane layers of the envelope and blood flows between the turns of the spiral in a countercurrent direction.

Oxygen diffuses from the gas compartment, through the membrane into the blood, with CO_2 diffusing in the opposite direction.

Oxygen exchange is governed by:

- permeability of the membrane to O_2
- driving pressure (PO_2 in gas $-PO_2$ in venous blood)
- membrane surface area
- time of blood/gas interface.

The membrane has a high diffusion coefficient for (permeability to) CO_2—approximately six times greater than that for O_2. CO_2 exchange is therefore more efficient, despite a lower driving pressure.

Circuit pressures are constantly monitored before and after the membrane by in-line transducers.

Gas delivery system

The gas delivery system consists of an air/oxygen blender, an O_2 flowmeter and a CO_2 flowmeter. The outlets of these feed into the gas inlet port of the membrane oxygenator, with a safety blow-off valve to prevent excessive pressure in the gas phase in the event of obstruction to exhaust gas.

The F_1O_2 supplied to the membrane determines the driving pressure for O_2 diffusion into blood. This is adjusted to obtain a post-membrane oxygen saturation of approximately 95%.

The gas supplied to the membrane should contain a low concentration (usually ~5%) of CO_2. At this level, CO_2 removal is adequate, but the $PaCO_2$ of post-membrane blood is not so low as to suppress respiration in the weaning patient.

Gas flow should always be kept higher than 1 l/min to prevent condensation on the membrane ('wet membrane').

Heater

Distilled water is warmed by an electronic heater before being passed through a cylindrical countercurrent heat exchanger. Blood passes in the opposite direction through the heat exchanger and is warmed to 36.5–37 °C, before being returned to the patient.

ECMO—practicalities

Priming the ECMO circuit

The circuit is meticulously filled with normal saline, the bubbles are removed at high pump flow rate. 100 ml of 25% albumin is added to the circuit and allowed to circulate at high flow for 5 min. This prevents further adherence of circulating proteins to the prosthetic surfaces of the circuit. The circuit is then primed with 1.5–2 units of packed red cells. 5 ml of 8.4% $NaHCO_3$ and 5 ml of 10% calcium gluconate are added for each unit of red cells used (to correct acidosis and calcium depletion in stored, citrated blood).

Cannulation

The carotid artery is isolated under general anaesthesia, a loading dose of heparin (50–100 iu/kg) is given and the artery is cannulated under direct vision. The internal jugular vein is isolated, then cannulated and a chest radiograph is taken to confirm the cannula tip position. The arterial, then venous cannulae are connected to appropriate, clamped, circuit connections. The arterial clamp is opened, the bridge is clamped off and the venous clamp is opened. Hypotension is common at this point, and should be treated with volume expansion using blood and plasma protein solution. The circuit flow is slowly increased so that the desired flow is reached in about 20 min and the ventilator is turned to rest settings.

Extracorporeal membrane oxygenation flows

Extracorporeal membrane oxygenation flows are as follows:

- neonate = 140 ml/kg/min
- infant = 100–120 ml/kg/min
- child = 90 ml/kg/min
- adult = 70 ml/kg/min.

These flows are designed to match approximately the resting cardiac output (e.g. neonate 200 ml/kg/min, adult 70 ml/kg/min). Higher flows may be necessary in high output states, e.g. sepsis.

Ventilator 'rest settings'

Ventilator rest settings are as follows:

- Peak inspiratory pressure (PIP) = 15–20 cmH_2O
- PEEP = 5–10 cmH_2O
- Rate = 10 min
- F_IO_2 = 0.21.

Monitoring

Monitoring should consist of:

- patient arterial blood gas 2–4 hourly, and more frequently if making changes
- activated clotting time (ACT) at cannulation, half-hourly until stable, and hourly thereafter
- blood sugar 4 hourly
- electrolytes (including calcium) 8 hourly
- cranial ultrasound daily
- CXR daily (often complete whiteout for first few days after going onto ECMO and after changing membrane).

Sedation

The patient is not paralysed during ECMO, and will breathe and move spontaneously. Continuous, adequate sedation is vital, and is usually achieved using a morphine infusion, with additional doses of morphine or midazolam as required.

Nutrition

Total parenteral nutrition, including lipid, is required. Enteral feeding is only occasionally reinstituted whilst on ECMO.

Physiotherapy

This is very important for the recovery of lung function. Frequent chest vibration and drainage should be done, along with 'sigh bagging' every 1–2 h.

Anticoagulation

At cannulation, this consists of heparin 50–100 iu/kg loading dose. On bypass, use heparin 50 iu/kg/h by constant infusion. Aim for:

- ACT 180–200
- ACT 160–180 if at high risk for bleeding
- ACT 200–220 at low flows (<200 ml/min).

If ACT >300 during bypass, slow heparin infusion down to 5–10 iu/kg/h until ACT returns to desired level. Do not stop the infusion as this may lead to clot formation.

Diuresis or platelet transfusions will increase the heparin requirement.

In patients at very high risk of bleeding, or in whom bleeding occurs, aprotinin is used. Give a loading dose of 1 ml/kg, followed by an infusion at 1 ml/kg/h.

Heparin bonded circuits are being developed in an effort to eliminate the need for systemic anticoagulation. These are not yet in general use.

Oedema

Salt and water retention are common, as renin secretion is elevated on ECMO. Diuretics are often needed to promote urine excretion. Urine output should be kept greater than 1 ml/kg/h.

A haemofiltration unit can easily be incorporated into the circuit, if necessary.

Hypertension

This is a frequent problem and is usually treated acutely with hydralazine. Captopril is used for those patients who require ongoing treatment.

Blood products

Blood, platelets, cryoprecipitate and fresh frozen plasma (FPP) can all be transfused into the circuit. Platelets, cryoprecipitate, and FP should all be given into the circuit beyond the oxygenator because of concerns about adherence to the membrane.

Aim for:

- Hb 12–14

- prothrombin time: normal

- platelets >100 000.

Free haemoglobin

Damage to red blood cells by the pump and also by double lumen V-V ECMO cannulae can cause an elevation in plasma-free Hb. This should be estimated every 48 h, and should not rise above 50 mg/100 ml.

Access to circuit

There are multiple access ports in the circuit:

- venous samples: withdrawn from pre-bladder port

- circuit arterial blood gases: withdrawn from post-oxygenator port

- heparin, drugs, TPN: infused post-bladder, pre-pump

- blood, PPS, drugs: infused into bladder

- platelets, cryoprecipitate, FFP: infused post-oxygenator.

Weaning

Veno-arterial ECMO

Flow rates are weaned by a maximum of 20 ml/min at a time, maintaining venous saturation >75%. When flow is 10% of cardiac output ('idling'), maintain this level of support for 48 h. It is important to wean the blender setting when flows are dropping, or supersaturation of blood and bubbling will occur. Therefore when the flow is down to 100 ml/min, wean the blender to 90% and concomitantly with flow thereafter. For idling flow of 10% of cardiac output, a blender setting of 10% is appropriate. The ventilator F_IO_2 is increased when flow is at 30% of cardiac output.

Veno-venous ECMO

Flow rates are weaned as above to ~50% cardiac output. For 'trial off', disconnect the gas flow to the membrane so that bypass continues through the circuit that no longer contains an oxygenator.

For patient CO_2 retention while weaning, it is important to obtain a post-oxygenator blood gas from the circuit if the patient's gas shows an elevated $PaCO_2$. If circuit $PaCO_2$ is low, patient hypoventilation will be causing the CO_2 retention. The CO_2 flow to the membrane should be increased. If the circuit $PaCO_2$ is also high, decrease the CO_2 flow to the membrane. Consider wet membrane or membrane failure as a cause.

Decannulation

The wound is opened under general anaesthesia, the internal jugular vein and venous cannula are isolated and the venous cannula is clamped. The bridge is opened, the arterial cannula is clamped and a manual breath on the ventilator is held on inspiration. With pressure on the liver, the venous cannula is removed and the vein is ligated. The carotid artery and arterial cannula are isolated and after removal of the cannula, the artery is ligated. Protamine 1 mg intravenously is given and the wound is closed.

Emergency removal from bypass

The procedure is as follows:

- clamp venous line, open bridge, clamp arterial line

- stop pump

- increase ventilator settings

- remove gas flow to membrane

- stop infusions to circuit.

Once off bypass, the patient's ACT will fall and cannulae are at risk of clotting, so monitor ACT and administered small doses of heparin if necessary.

Venous return monitor (VRM) alarm

The following are causes for alarm:

- possible obstruction to venous drainage (malpositioning/kinking of catheter, catheter too small for flows)

- possible hypovolaemia.

Membrane failure

Signs include CO_2 retention and decreased PaO_2 in post-oxygenator blood. Causes include wet membrane (high $PaCO_2$, normal PaO_2); clot (high $PaCO_2$, low PaO_2); and defective manufacture.

Decreased patient PaO_2

Causes are hypovolaemia, pneumothorax and membrane failure.

Increased patient PaO_2

Causes:

- hypoventilation (post-oxygenator $PaCO_2$ low)

- inadequate sweep gas flow/CO_2 flow to membrane too high—post-oxygenator $PaCO_2$ high.

Pump failure

Hand crank pump until power can be reconnected.

Air in circuit

Come off bypass.
Venous air—?leak in venous tubing/catheter connection. Aspirate air from nearest port.
Arterial air—?from membrane. Remove patient from bypass immediately. Membrane may need replacing.

Intra-aortic balloon pumps

Augmentation of left ventricular output by intra-aortic balloon counter-pulsation is a common form of circulatory support in adults with cardiogenic shock. Experience with such devices in paediatrics is increasing and, despite inherent technical difficulties, this can be a useful technique, particularly in older children.[31-33]

A sausage-shaped balloon is placed in the descending aorta. This is inflated and deflated in synchrony with the patient's heartbeat. Helium is used as the inflating gas because of its low density and rapidity of response. The balloon inflates during diastole, at aortic valve closure, and deflates immediately prior to systole. The beneficial effects of this are:

- displacement of blood distally in the aorta, improving peripheral circulation

- displacement of blood proximally into the coronary circulation

- creation of negative aortic pressure on deflation, reducing left ventricular afterload.

The intra-aortic balloon pump (IABP) works in series with the left ventricle, and relies on some left ventricular output. It is not an effective3 means of support in right ventricular failure.

The following factors limit the use of IABPs in small children:

- the small size of the aorta, necessitating a small balloon

- increased aortic elasticity, decreasing the effectiveness of the counter-pulsation

- rapid heart rates

- small stroke volume.

Intra-aortic balloon pumps—practicalities

These are made of polyurethane and come in a range of volumes.

The balloon selected should have a volume of approximately 50% of estimated stroke volume. The balloon is placed via the femoral artery, either percutaneously or by cut-down in smaller children. The balloon should sit in the descending aorta, above the diaphragm. This minimizes the risk of ischaemia in the renal and splanchnic circulations. The balloon should inflate on closure of the aortic valve and deflate just prior to aortic valve opening. This is synchronized by a set of electrocardiograph electrodes attached to the pumping unit. The arterial tracing indicating optimal counterpulsation is shown in Fig. 7.3. Systemic heparinization is necessary to prevent thrombus formation.

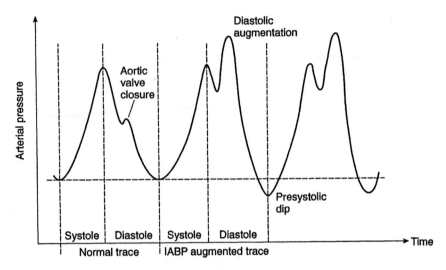

Fig. 7.3 Intra-aortic balloon pump arterial tracing.

Complications

Complications include:

- limb ischaemia

- interference with renal perfusion

- bleeding.

Left ventricular assist devices

Left ventricular assist devices work in parallel with the left ventricle by pumping a proportion (up to 100%) of left atrial blood into the aorta. In paediatrics they have mainly been used in post-cardiotomy cardiogenic shock and, less successfully, as a bridge to transplantation.

Although variations exist to provide support for the right ventricle, most devices are left-sided and will do little to help in right ventricular failure. Difficulties in miniaturization of devices have been a major obstacle to their use in small children.

The devices vary in design, but all have an inflow tract and outflow tract which must be surgically positioned. The driving mechanism is either a centrifugal extracorporeal pump providing non-pulsatile flow, or a pneumatic pump compressing a paracorporeal blood sac in a pulsatile fashion. Systemic anticoagulation is necessary.

LEARNING POINTS

1. Invasive cardiovascular monitoring should be introduced early in the management of children with an unstable circulation.

2. Pharmacological circulatory support should be delivered by central venous lines where possible and carefully titrated.

3. Mechanical circulatory support is being increasingly used with good results in children of all ages.

REFERENCES

1 Wetzell RC, Tobin JR. Shock. In *Textbook of pediatric intensive care*, 2nd edn (ed. MC Rogers), pp. 563–613. Williams & Wilkins, New York, 1992.

2 Perkin RM. Shock states. In *Pediatric critical care* (ed. BP Fuhrman, JJ Zimmerman), pp. 287–298. Mosby Year Book, St Louis, 1992.

3 Advanced Life Support Group. *Advanced paediatric life support—the practical approach*. BMJ Publishing group, London, 1993.

4 Hantsch TA, Soifer SJ. Congestive heart failure. In *Textbook of pediatric critical care* (ed. PR Holbrook), pp. 316–326. WB Saunders, Philadelphia, 1993.

5 Tynan M. The ductus arteriosus and its closure. *New England Journal of Medicine* 1993; **329**: 1570–1572.

6 Ganong WF. Synaptic and junctional transmission. In *Review of medical physiology*, 14th edn (ed. WF Ganong), pp. 67–92. Appleton and Lange, New York, 1989.

7 Foëx P, Fisher A. Catecholamines and their derivatives. In *Oxford textbook of medicine*, 2nd edn (ed. DJ Weatherall, JGG Ledingham, DA Warrel), pp. 111–114. Oxford University Press, Oxford, 1987.

8 Hoffman BB. Adrenoreceptor activating drugs. In *Basic and clinical pharmacology*, 5th edn (ed. BG Katzung), pp. 109–129. Appleton and Lange, New York, 1992.

9 Nottermann DA. Cardiovascular support—pharmacological. In *Textbook of pediatric critical care* (ed. PR Holbrook), pp. 279–283. WB Saunders, Philadelphia, 1993.

10 Seri I. Cardiovascular, renal, and endocrine actions of depamine in neonates and children. *Journal of Peditrics* 1995; **126**: 333–344.

11 Thomson BT, Cockrill BA. Renal-dose depamine: A Siren song? *Lancet* 1994; **344**: 7–8.

12 Nottermann DA, Greenwald B, Moran F *et al.* Dopamine clearance in critically ill infants and children: Effect of age and organ system dysfunction. *Clinical and Pharmacological Therapy* 1990; **48**: 13.

13 Colucci WS, Wright RF, Braunwald E. New positive inotropic agents in the treatment of congestive heart failure. *New England Journal of Medicine* 1986; **314**: 349–358.

14 Skoyles JR, Sherry KM. Pharmacology, mechanisms of action and uses of selective phosphodiesterase inhibitors. *British Journal of Anaesthesia* 1992; **68**: 293–302.

15 Stevenson DK *et al.* Refractory hypoxaemia associated with neonatal pulmonary disease: The use and limitations of tolazoline. *Journal of Pediatrics* 1979; **95**: 595–599.

16 Ward RM, Daniel CH, Kendig JW *et al.* Oliguria and tolazoline pharmacokinetics in the newborn. *Pediatrics* 1986; **77**: 307–315.

17 Rossaint R, Pison U, Gerlach H *et al.* Inhaled nitric oxide: Its effects on pulmonary circulation and airway smooth muscle cells. *European Heart Journal* 1993; **14** (Suppl. 1): 133–140.

18 Vallance P, Collier J. Biology and clinical relevance of nitric oxide. *British Medical Journal* 1994; **309**: 453–457.

19 Miller OI, Celermajer DS, Deanfield JE *et al.* Very-low dose inhaled nitric oxide: A selective pulmonary vasodilator after operations for congenital heart disease. *Journal of Thoracic and Cardiovascular Surgery* 1994; **108**: 487–494.

20 Kam PCA, Govender G. Nitric oxide: Basic science and clinical applications. *Anaesthesia* 1994; **49**: 515–521.

21 Association of the British Pharmaceutical Industry. *Data sheet compendium 94–95.* Datapharm Publications, London, 1994.

22 Shann F. *Drug doses,* 8th edn. Collective Pty, Melbourne, 1994.

23 Trissel LA, ed. *Handbook of injectable drugs,* 8th edn. American Society of Hospital Pharmacists, 1994.

24 Pennington DG, Swartz MT. Circulatory support in infants and children. *Annals of Thoracic Surgery* 1993: **55**: 233–237.

25 Bartlett RH. Extracorporeal life support for cardiopulmonary failure. *Current Problems in Surgery* 1990; **27**: ??

26 Butt W, Beca J. Extracorporeal circulatory support in children in intensive care. *Critical Care Medicine* 1993; **21** (Suppl.): S381–S382.

27 Dalton HJ, Thomson AE. Extracorporeal membrane oxygenation. In *Pediatric critical care* (eds BP Fuhrman, JJ Zimmerman), pp. 545–558. St Louis, Mosby Year Book, 1992.

28 Short BL, Brans YW. Extracorporeal membrane oxygenation: pro and con. *Current Opinion in Pediatrics* 1990; **2**: 308–314.

29 Klein MD, Whittlesey GC. Extracorporeal membrane oxygenation. *Pediatric Clinics of North America* 1994; **2**: 365–384.

30 Royal Hospital for Sick Children, Glasgow ECMO Training Manual. 1994.

31 Veasy GL, Blalock BA, Orth JL *et al.* Intra-aortic balloon pumping in infants and children. *Circulation* 1983; **68**: 1095–1100.

32 Glenville B. Mechanical support for the failing heart. *Hospital Update* 1991; Feb: 89–97.

33 Park SB, Liebler GA, Burkholder JA *et al.* Mechanical support of the failing heart. *Annals of Thoracic Surgery* 1986; **42**: 627–631.

FURTHER READING

Baskett PJF, Dow A, Nolan J, Maull K. *Practical procedures in anesthesia and critical care.* Mosby, London, 1995.

Davey A, Moyle JTB, Ward CS. *Ward's anaesthetic equipment,* 3rd edition. Saunders, London, 1992.

8

Fluid, nutritional, metabolic and haematological support in critically ill children

N.S. Morton and F. Munro

FLUID SUPPORT

Developmental factors

Developmental changes in body fluid composition and distribution

The composition of the intracellular and extracellular compartments changes significantly during fetal and neonatal life and for a considerable period thereafter (Fig. 8.1). The preterm infant has a very high proportion of its total body weight as water, with two-thirds residing in the extracellular fluid compartment.

As the cells grow and multiply and organs develop, the intracellular proportion of the total body water increases with a corresponding reduction in the extracellular water.

The proportion of fat is very low in the preterm and is relatively low at birth with much of the body lipid residing in the central nervous system. Thus term and preterm neonates have little fat insulation and few reserves of metabolically available fat stores to call upon during times of cold stress and starvation.

Development of renal function

Maturation of renal function occurs throughout fetal life and for the first 12 months of postnatal life. Glomerular filtration rate in the newborn is 1/4 that of the adult and renal tubular function is inefficient. Concentrating ability is limited so lack of fluid intake or loss of fluids leads to problems much more rapidly. Sodium balance is dependent on sodium intake in neonates and daily sodium requirements increase with degree of prematurity. Giving sodium free fluids will more readily produce hyponatraemia and sodium excretion after a sodium load is not very efficient in neonates.

Fluids and the cardiovascular system

Fluid loads are well tolerated in older healthy children but not by neonates and heart failure can be precipitated. In premature babies, excessive fluid administration delays closure of the arterial duct.

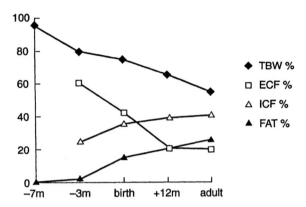

Fig. 8.1 Changes in body composition with age. TBW = total body water; ECF = extracellular fluid; ICF = intracellular fluid.

Fluid restriction is not well tolerated by younger children because their higher metabolic rate is associated with high water turnover. Dehydration can occur rapidly in small babies and intravascular volume depletion, hypoperfusion, hypotension and circulatory failure may ensue.

In children with persistence of the fetal circulation or in those with congenital abnormalities of the circulatory system, judging fluid and electrolyte balance can be very difficult and more intensive review of the volume and composition of fluid intake and output must be carried out, in some cases hourly.

Maintenance fluid requirements

Rational basis for volume of fluid

The starting point for fluid maintenance requirements is the basal metabolic rate which varies with age. Superimposed upon this are factors such as body temperature, ambient temperature, thyroid status, sedation, anaesthesia, and losses of fluids of various types and from various sites.

The neonate uses about 30 kcal/kg/d if it is in a neutral thermal environment and this increases over the first week of life and thereafter as the child grows and becomes more active. The healthy neonate may need up to 150 kcal/kg/d to cope with the additional metabolic demands imposed by trying to maintain its body temperature and to support anabolism. Beyond the neonatal period, 100 kcal/kg/d are adequate for the first 10 kg, 50 kcal/kg/d for the next 10 kg and 20 kcal/kg/d thereafter. This simplifies to 4, 2 and 1 kcal/kg/h respectively (Table 8.1).

As normal basal water losses equate to about 1 ml/kcal (Table 8.2) basal fluid maintenance can follow the same simplified 4, 2, 1 formula (Table 8.3).

Table 8.1 Daily and hourly basal caloric intake

Weight (kg)	kcal/kg/day	kcal/kg/h
<10	100	4
10–20	$((kg - 10) \times 50) + 1000$	$((kg - 10) \times 2) + 40$
>20	$((kg - 20) \times 20) + 1500$	$((kg - 20) \times 1) + 60$

Table 8.2 Normal water losses

Fluid losses	ml per 100 kcal
Urine output	+70
Skin insensible loss	+30
Respiratory insensible loss	+15
Extra intake due to metabolism of 100 kcal	−15
Total net fluid loss	100 ml/100 kcal (= 1 ml/kcal)

Table 8.3 Daily and hourly basal maintenance fluids

Weight (kg)	ml/kg/day	ml/kg/h
<10	100	4
10–20	$((kg - 10) \times 50) + 1000$	$((kg - 10) \times 2) + 40$
>20	$((kg - 20) \times 20) + 1500$	$((kg - 20) \times 1) + 60$

Factors which *reduce* the maintenance fluid requirements to about 70% of basal are high antidiuretic hormone levels (e.g. due to controlled ventilation, brain injury or morphine), high room humidity, use of humidified inspired gases and hypothyroidism. In renal failure restriction of fluid intake is more aggressive, down to 30% of basal plus the urine output. After cardiopulmonary bypass, fluid intake is often restricted to around 50% of basal and in hypothermia fluid input should be reduced by 12% per degree Celsius below 37 °C. Sedation and anaesthesia reduce basal metabolic rate and therefore fluid requirements.

Factors which *increase* the basal fluid needs by 50% are use of radiant heaters, phototherapy, surgery on a body cavity, hyperthyroidism and normal activity. Preterm neonates or children who are hyperventilating may need 20% above basal rates. Pyrexia increases the fluid requirement by 12% per degree Celsius and very hot ambient temperatures over 31 °C may mean the child needs 30% more fluid per degree Celsius above 31. Burn injuries result in an increased fluid requirement of about 4% per percent of burn on the first day reducing to 2% per percent burn area on the second day. Vomiting, diarrhoea,

bowel obstruction, and surgical manipulation of the bowel can all lead to excessive gastrointestinal fluid losses which must be made good.

Rational basis for composition of fluid

The composition of fluids given depends on the deficits of fluid and electrolytes, the nature and volume of ongoing losses and the appropriately adjusted maintenance rate. Electrolytes, water, osmolarity, and caloric content must be considered. The aim is to provide fluid and electrolytes to prevent the kidneys having to conserve or excrete large amounts of either component. To maintain electrolyte balance, for every 100 ml of water, about 2.5 mmol each of sodium and potassium and 5 mmol chloride are needed.

In the newborn, sodium is required at a rate of 2–6 mmol/kg/d because the immature kidney has limited capacity for sodium conservation and this is even more evident in the premature infant. Potassium, 2–4 mmol/kg/d, should also be given provided the urine output is 0.5 ml/kg/h or more. These rates are maintenance rates and do not take into account deficits that may have accumulated or ongoing losses.

The sugar content of fluids should be enough to spare breakdown of proteins and to prevent ketosis while avoiding hyperglycaemia. This is particularly important in children who have undergone the stress of major surgery, trauma, burns, or sepsis. The neonate's renal transport maximum for glucose is lower than the older child or adult and excess glucose tends to spill over into the urine causing an osmotic diuresis and ultimately, dehydration. However, these small babies are particularly at risk of hypoglycaemia because they have low stores of glycogen and impaired gluconeogenesis.

Administration of crystalloids or colloids may be considered for intravascular volume replacement where losses are in the form of exudate, transudate, blood, or third space losses especially where these are rapid and ongoing. For each litre of crystalloid given the intravascular volume is expanded by about 300 ml while the interstitial fluid volume increases by 700 ml. To replace blood loss, therefore, crystalloids need to be given in a volume of three times the measured blood lost. In contrast, colloids expand intravascular volume on a millilitre for millilitre basis and also have a much longer intravascular half-life.

Fluid and electrolyte balance in the PICU

To restore and maintain fluid and electrolyte balance in all PICU patients is a difficult practical problem and various strategies are used depending on the primary disease process and secondary complications. Frequent estimation of plasma electrolyte concentrations, acid–base status and osmolarity and of urinary electrolyte concentrations and osmolarity will be needed several times per day in critically ill patients. Fluid intake and output should be charted in

Table 8.4 Correction of electrolyte abnormalities

Abnormality	Calculation of deficit	Intervention	Comments
Low sodium (<130)	Na desired – Na actual × kg × 0.6	Slow correction with Na (or diuretics if low Na due to excess H_2O)	Maximum correction 2 mmol/l per hour
High sodium		Restore intravascular volume and urine output; slow correction over at least 24 h	Avoid rapid correction as cerebral oedema and seizures may occur
Low potassium	K desired – K actual × kg × 0.3	Slow correction with frequent checks; correct concurrent low chloride; beware low urine output when K being given	Maximum correction 0.4 mmol/l per hour with ECG monitoring
High potassium		Stop K,§ monitor ECG, alkalinize, calcium, dextrose + insulin, ion exchange resin	Rapid intervention necessary; may need to consider dialysis early

detail and the volume and composition of the fluid intake should be titrated against losses and laboratory results. Hourly urine output should be maintained at 0.5–1.0 ml/kg/h and daily weighing of the patient can help in judging fluid overload. Gross abnormalities of plasma electrolytes should be corrected but there are dangers in too rapid correction of conditions such as hyponatraemia or hypokalaemia. Gross hyperkalaemia however must be corrected rapidly using alkalosis, calcium, dextrose and insulin and ion exchange resin. Peritoneal or haemo-dialysis may have to be considered (Table 8.4).

NUTRITIONAL SUPPORT

There are a number of differences between children and adults which significantly affect the provision of nutritional support.

Nutritional reserve

Children are less able to withstand starvation than adults; the smaller the child, the shorter his or her energy stores will last. A healthy adult might be expected to withstand 90 d of starvation, in contrast a preterm neonate

weighing 1 kg has reserves for only 4 d, a 3.5 kg term neonate for 32 d and a 1-year-old for 44 d. Hence, particularly in the preterm infant, provision of nutritional support is a matter of great urgency.

Growth and development

In the child nutrients are not only required to meet basal needs but also for incorporation into growing tissues. Growth rates are maximal in the first year and in early adolescence. Deprivation at these times may have serious effects on growth. This may be particularly a problem in adolescence as there is limited time for 'catch-up' growth at this age. As well as requirements for energy substrates and protein the need for minerals such as phosphorus and trace elements will be higher at these times of maximal growth. This is particularly so in the first year.

Brain growth

The brain is rapidly growing and developing in the first year of life and is particularly sensitive to malnutrition. Long-term intellectual and developmental impairment may result.

Nutrient requirements

As well as quantitative differences in nutrient requirements there are qualitative differences. For example, histidine is an essential amino acid in infancy but not in adulthood. In addition, in the preterm infant, the amino acids cysteine, tyrosine, and taurine also become essential. Hence amino acid profiles in parenteral nutrition preparations have to be adapted.

NUTRITIONAL ASSESSMENT

There are four components to the nutritional assessment of a child: (1) clinical history and examination, (2) dietary history and evaluation, (3) anthropometric measurements, and (4) laboratory assays.

The medical history should include social history, growth and developmental milestones, gastrointestinal symptoms and drug history. Physical examination findings will not usually be gross and findings suggestive of nutrient deficiencies are usually non-specific and require to be backed up by confirmatory laboratory investigations.

Dietary history should allow an evaluation of past feeding and present intake.

As growth is a characteristic of children, serial anthropometric measurements are of great value in assessment of nutritional state. Weight gives an

indication of present nutrition whilst height reflects better the long-term dietary intake. Growth charts are available with population means and centiles; these are helpful in interpreting height and weight data and following trends over time. An accurate gestational age is vital to the use of such charts in the first year of life. Head circumference is another important measurement, giving an indication of brain growth, and should be recorded particularly in infants. Measurement of triceps skin fold thickness gives an assessment of subcutaneous fat stores whilst mid-arm circumference, in conjunction with triceps skinfold thickness, gives a measure of arm muscle area and hence skeletal muscle mass.

Laboratory investigations provide an objective assessment of some aspects of nutritional state. They are particularly valuable in the detection of specific deficiencies of minerals, trace elements and vitamins. Plasma albumin concentration is a useful assessment of protein energy malnutrition. It has the advantage of being a readily available assay but the disadvantage of a long plasma half-life and so it will not reflect acute changes. Other plasma proteins such as transferrin and retinol binding protein have a shorter half-life but may not be routinely available in all laboratories. Transferrin has the additional disadvantage of being raised in iron deficiency, making interpretation potentially difficult.

NUTRITIONAL REQUIREMENTS

Energy requirements

Preterm

The preterm infant has a resting energy expenditure (REE) of 50–75 kcal/kg/d. A significant proportion of this energy expenditure occurs in maintenance of body temperature and keeping such infants in a thermoneutral environment will result in an REE at the lower end of this range. For growth to occur 90–100 kcal/kg/d must be provided by the parenteral route or up to 130 kcal/kg/d by the enteral route. There are greater energy requirements for enteral nutrition because of an approximately 20% loss of delivered energy in the stools. Delivery of these energy requirements may be difficult in the preterm newborn infant. Glucose may be poorly tolerated and excessive intravenous fluid volumes may lead to problems such as reopening of the ductus arteriosus and cardiac failure.

Infants and older children

Energy requirements for paediatric patients are summarized in Table 8.5. It must be emphasized that these figures are only a guideline and do not take into account any additional needs. Each patient must be assessed individually and their response to nutritional support should be constantly reassessed.

Table 8.5 Paediatric energy requirements

Age (years)	Enteral kcal/kg/d	(kJ/kg/d)	Parenteral kcal/kg/d	(kJ/kg/d)
0<1	105–135	(440–570)	90–120	(380–500)
1<7	85–100	(360–420)	75–90	(315–380)
7<12	65–85	(275–360)	60–75	(250–315)
12<18	45–65	(190–275)	30–60	(125–250)

Table 8.6 Factors increasing energy requirements

	Per degree C above 37 °C
Fever	12%
Cardiac failure	15–25%
Major surgery	20–30%
Sepsis	40–50%
Burns	Up to 100%
Protein energy malnutrition	50–100%

Measurement of REE in paediatric intensive care patients by indirect calorimetry is feasible but this technique is not routinely available and its use remains primarily a research tool. A number of factors increase energy requirements significantly and these are listed in Table 8.6. Some of these factors can be gathered together under the umbrella of the stress response to injury or sepsis. Increases in REE and negative nitrogen balance have long been recognized following surgical trauma and burns. Much interest has focused recently on the regulation of this response and the role of cytokines, particularly tumour necrosis factor and interleukin-6, as mediators. Arachidonic acid metabolites also appear to be important mediators of the stress response and there is the potential for influencing the response by modifying dietary lipid profiles.

The neonate appears to be different from older children with regard to the stress response, which is of a much shorter duration. REE has been shown to return to normal within 12 h of surgery. It is postulated that a diversion of energy from growth to the stress response may occur with no overall increase in energy requirements and it would therefore seem there is no need to provide more than basal requirements in the immediate post-surgical period in the neonate.

Protein requirements

Protein is needed in the diet to provide amino acids for the synthesis of body proteins. Eight amino acids are 'essential', that is they cannot be produced by transanimation and must therefore come from the diet. In addition, in infancy several other amino acids are considered 'semi-essential' as amino acid metabolic pathways are immature and incapable of meeting the body's full needs. The balance of amino acids in a protein source is therefore critical in determining its usefulness in promoting positive nitrogen balance and growth. Human milk has the ideal balance for the newborn infant, and infants can sustain normal growth on a human milk protein intake of 1.8 g/kg/d. In the same age groups artificial formulas should provide around 2.2 g/kg/d or provide about 10% of the total energy content as protein.

Carbohydrate requirement

Glucose is the preferred energy source of the central nervous system, red blood cells and the haemopoietic system. Glucose may be derived from dietary carbohydrate, glycogen stores or gluconeogenesis. In order to prevent ketosis and diversion of amino acids to gluconeogenic pathways then carbohydrate is essential in the diet. Most formula milks and human breast milk will provide 35–50% of the total energy in the form of carbohydrate.

Fat requirement

Dietary fats provide energy, fat-soluble vitamins and essential fatty acids (EFA). For infants and children the two essential fatty acids are linoleic and linolenic acids. Requirements are estimated at 1.2–3% of supplied energy. EFA deficiency is rare except in the instance of small infants being parenterally fed without lipid, it is manifest by scaly dermatitis, hair loss and growth retardation. It has been suggested that massage of oil onto the skin might be an effective means of delivering EFA particularly in the preterm neonate, however there is little evidence of significant absorption by this route.

Mineral, trace element and vitamin requirements

If a vitamin supplement is required in a patient on an artificial diet then a full vitamin supplement such as Ketovite should be used as other multivitamin preparations may not supply a broad enough range.

ENTERAL FEEDING

The gut is the preferred route for nutritional support in the paediatric intensive care patient. The only reason for not using the enteral route is if the

gut is not functioning, for example following major abdominal surgery, in gastroschisis, obstruction or pseudo-obstruction and in preterm infants with necrotizing enterocolitis (NEC). The enteral route avoids the risks of sepsis associated with central venous catheters. Cholestasis frequently occurs in paediatric patients receiving parenteral nutrition but is not a problem with enteral feeds and indeed even partial gut feeds of no nutritional significance may reduce the incidence of cholestatic jaundice in total parenteral nutrition (TPN).

In recent years the gut has been recognized as a potential source of sepsis in critically ill patients. Loss of gut mucosal integrity leads to translocation of bacteria and endotoxin into the portal circulation. Interaction of endotoxin with hepatic macrophages causes release of the cytokines thought to be responsible for mediating the systemic inflammatory response syndrome and multi-organ system failure. There is evidence that gut mucosal atrophy occurs with starvation, an effect that is not prevented or reversed by TPN. Patients being supported with TPN may thus be at increased risk of translocation and its sequelae. Enteral feeding, however, maintains integrity of the gut mucosa. This seems in part due to the provision of glutamine which plays a central role in enterocyte energy metabolism and is absent from commercial parenteral amino acid preparations. There is evidence that in surgical patients the early provision of enteral feeds and the avoidance of TPN is associated with fewer septic complications and reduced mortality though in other patient groups benefits are not yet proven.

Complications of enteral feeding are in general less serious than with TPN, an exception being the increased risk of NEC seen in enterally fed preterm neonates. In addition to these advantages enteral feeding is cheaper and less labour intensive to provide for the paediatric intensive care patient.

DELIVERY SYSTEM

The commonest site of delivery of enteral feeds is to the stomach via a nasally inserted tube. These may be made of either polyvinyl choloride (PVC) or silicone, the latter being preferred as it is softer. The tube should be of the smallest diameter possible to minimize discomfort and, in small infants, to avoid nasal obstruction. For the latter reason orogastric tubes may be preferred in preterm infants. Tube position must be confirmed by aspiration of acid gastric juice or auscultation over the stomach and by X-rays in all cases before commencing feeds. Tube malposition may occur with the tip in the oesophagus or the bronchial tree. Bronchial incubation is not protected against by the presence of an endotracheal tube and may in fact be made more likely. Perforation of the oesophagus and trachea is possible following insertion of feeding tubes stiffened by a central wire stillette.

Some patients, particularly in the intensive care unit (ICU) setting, are at increased risk of enteral feed regurgitation and aspiration. In these patients, and those with impaired gastric emptying, then a nasoduodenal or nasojejunal tube might be considered. Placement of such tubes can however be problematic. Simple measures such as 'freezing' the tube to stiffen it, lying the patient on the right side and the use of prokinetic drugs such as metoclopramide may produce success in about 50% of patients. Insertion under fluoroscopic control is more reliable, achieving appropriate placement in more than 80% of cases. In adults, endoscopic assisted placement also achieves a high success rate and might be useful in older children if the expertise is available. If a decision has been made that jejunal feeding is required then positioning of a tube under fluoroscopic control, at the earliest opportunity, is recommended.

Some patients undergoing upper gastrointestinal tract surgery, for example tracheo-oesophageal fistula repair or duodenal atresia repair, may have a transanastomotic feeding tube placed at the time of surgery allowing early enteral feeding. In occasional circumstances surgical insertion of a jejunostomy tube may be indicated if jejunal feeding is desirable but attempts at passage of a nasojejunal tube fail.

In some ICU cases long-term enteral nutrition support may be required. In these circumstances the use of a percutaneous endoscopic gastrostomy (PEG) has advantages and might be considered at the same time as a tracheostomy in selected patients. It removes the need for tubes in the pharynx and traversing the gastro-oesophageal junction. This reduces the risk of infections in the upper airway, for example sinusitis, and should improve the competence of the lower oesophageal sphincter reducing reflux and retrograde pharyngeal colonization.

Apart from problems with malposition of enteral feeding tubes the commonest problems are accidental removal or blockage. A routine of at least twice daily flushing with water or saline will minimize the latter problem.

CONTINUOUS VS BOLUS ADMINISTRATION

Bolus administration of enteral feeds has been the traditional method with large volumes being given every 3 or 4 h. Evidence suggests, however, that continuous administration has a number of advantages. There is a lower incidence of diarrhoea, bloating and aspiration with continuous feeds. Less nursing time is required and errors should be less likely. Enteral feeding is associated with an increase in energy expenditure, this is lower with continuous feeds than with bolus, so more of the delivered energy is available for other energy requiring processes and growth. Both bolus and continuous administration have similar effects in promoting bile flow and preventing cholestatic jaundice and bile sludging in the gall bladder. Delivery of continuous feeds

requires some form of infusion controller, a syringe driver is suitable for neonates and there are several pumps available for use in older children.

STARTER REGIMES

In children who have previously tolerated normal feeds and who have no gut pathology there should be no need to grade the introduction of enteral feeds either by diluting the feed or reducing feed volumes. This merely delays the provision of an adequate calorie intake and does not reduce the incidence of problems such as diarrhoea. However, where there are abnormalities of either gut motility or absorptive capacity, for example following NEC or with 'short gut' then graded introduction of feeds perhaps using semi-elemental formulae may be required. In the ICU gut motility may be altered by opiate sedatives and this may necessitate a gradual introduction of enteral feeds. Muscle relaxants do not affect gut smooth muscle function and do not preclude enteral feeds.

FEED TYPES

Neonates

The preferred feed is breast milk from the infant's mother. This offers protection against the development of NEC, and has a high content of utilizable non-protein nitrogen in the form of urea. Alternatively a standard infant formula is adequate for babies with a normal gastrointestinal tract, providing 0.66 kcal/ml. For preterm infants a variety of special formulae are available with an increased calorie and protein content, a greater proportion of essential amino acids and increased concentrations of vitamin E, calcium, phosphorus and iron.

Older children

A variety of commercially available nutritionally complete feeds are available usually providing 1–1.5 kcal/ml.

Special feeds

Semi-elemental formulae (e.g. Pregestamil, Pepti-Junior) contain protein hydrolysate, dipeptides, and medium chain triglycerides (MCT) reducing the requirement for intraluminal digestion. Pregestamil is also lactose free. These feeds are useful in patients with short gut, mucosal damage; for example,

post-NEC, and with lactose intolerance. The osmolality of these feeds is low allowing concentration to achieve 1 kcal/ml if required. Feeds high in MCTs are also useful in reducing chyle flow in the management of chylothorax post cardiac surgery. Full elemental feeds (e.g. Neocate) are also available but have the disadvantage of high osmolality. Persistent severe malabsorption may necessitate the use of modular feeds. Glucose, amino acid and MCT components are provided separately starting with amino acids and adding glucose and then fats as tolerated. These feeds also have a very high osmolality and very gradual introduction is necessary to avoid diarrhoea. Parenteral nutrition support will be required during the introduction of such feeds.

MONITORING

Accurate recording of fluid balance is essential as is regular weighing of the patient. In neonates and infants the head circumference should also be recorded as an index of brain growth. Both weight and head circumference should be plotted on growth charts to compare achieved with expected growth. Haematological and biochemical parameters should be monitored daily initially, but in the stable patient weekly measurements should suffice. Particular attention must be paid to glucose, potassium and phosphate, especially in the early stages with severely malnourished patients. In the longer term monitoring of trace elements and vitamins may be required if clinical indications arise. Serial albumin levels give a useful indication of protein status.

COMPLICATIONS

Complications relating to tube placement have already been mentioned. Displacement of gastric tubes may lead to oesophageal infusion and an increased risk of aspiration. Inadvertent passage of the tube through the pylorus may lead to onset of diarrhoea. Perforation of the gut can occur when PVC tubes are left in place for more than 8 days. The presence of a nasoenteric tube may predispose to the development of ear, nose and pharyngeal infection. Reflux with or without aspiration may occur. Prokinetic drugs such as cisapride have been suggested as a means of reducing this problem but as yet these are unproven. Hypertrophic pyloric stenosis has been reported as a complication of the use of transpyloric feeding tubes in neonates.

Although infection is a lesser risk with enteral than parenteral feeds, none the less contamination of feeds can and does occur, leading to clinically significant infections. Continuous feeding using closed systems, strict asepsis, and a 'hang time' for feeds of less than 24 h should minimize this problem.

The commonest problem is of diarrhoea particularly in those with an abnormal gut or in those in whom the osmolality of the feeds is increased by

additives such as potassium supplements. This is best managed by a reduction in the concentration or volume of the feed followed by gradual building back up. MCT feeds may also be associated with troublesome diarrhoea because of rapid hydrolysis of MCT by pancreatic liase and subsequent osmotic overload.

Metabolic complications are rare but close monitoring is nevertheless essential.

PARENTERAL NUTRITION

Indications

The only absolute indication for parenteral nutrition is an inability to provide feeding by the enteral route. It must be remembered, however, that even if only partial enteral feeding is possible this is beneficial in maintaining the gut mucosa and reducing the incidence of parenteral nutrition associated cholestasis and it should therefore be continued alongside parenteral feeding. Other indications for parenteral feeding such as in preterm infants with respiratory distress syndrome or children with severe burns are recognized but parenteral feeding in these circumstances has not been the subject of controlled trials and superiority over enteral feeds is open to doubt.

Access

Peripheral

It is possible to provide intravenous feeds via peripheral veins. The major drawback is rapid production of thrombophlebitis by hypertonic solutions and because of this the maximum glucose concentration that can reasonably be used is 10%. This means that unless large amounts of lipid are used it is not possible to provide sufficient energy to support normal growth. The life of peripheral infusions can be maximized by using the smallest possible cannula and siting it in the largest available vein. This maintains bloodflow and delays the onset of thrombophlebitis. Other techniques such as the use of transdermal nitrates and non-steroidal anti-inflammatory drugs have been studied in adults but there is no experience in children. The use of filters in the infusion line to remove microparticles may also prolong infusion life. Because of the requirement for frequent re-siting of infusions venous access may soon become difficult and there is the risk of significant skin necrosis if extravasation of hypertonic solutions occurs.

The value of the peripheral route is therefore limited but it does have a place when only short-term nutritional support is required and long-term promotion of growth is not of concern.

Central

Siting a cannula in a large central vein allows the rapid dilution of infused fluids. This means hypertonic solutions can be used without the same risk of thrombophlebitis. It should however be realized that in small babies a central venous cannula may be so large in relation to the size of the veins that blood-flow may be severely reduced and dilution may not occur. With this caveat, central delivery of TPN in children will be able to provide suffficient energy and nutrients for normal growth and development to occur. There are a number of methods of siting central venous catheters in infants and children which may be appropriate in the ICU. In general the catheter used to deliver TPN should be dedicated to that purpose and not used for intermittent injections, other infusions or blood sampling. If multi-lumen catheters are used then the same principles should apply to the lumen used for TPN.

Many patients in a paediatric ICU will already have had a percutaneous central line inserted for monitoring purposes. These may subsequently be used for the delivery of TPN but because they are frequently accessed and may have been inserted with less than scrupulous asepsis there is a high rate of infection. This means that the initial central line is rarely able to remain *in situ* for more than a week or so and if parenteral nutritional support is required beyond that time then a dedicated TPN line should be strongly considered. There are essentially two options.

The first option is central placement of a fine silicone catheter (Epi-cath) through a peripheral vein. These lines are widely used in preterm and term neonates and can provide satisfactory long-term access. Preferred placement sites are the antecubital fossa, temporal veins and the long saphenous vein at the ankle or knee. Catheter position must be confirmed radiologically as complications from malposition do occur, albeit rarely. These catheters have also been used in adults to provide full parenteral nutrition. The catheter tip in these circumstances is not truly central but in the large veins in the arm or axilla. Nevertheless catheter lifespan equivalent to a central line is reported. This may be an option therefore in provision of TPN in larger children as well as neonates.

The second option is surgical central venous catheter (CVC) insertion. A tunnelled silicone rubber catheter may be used. These catheters have a Dacron cuff which is positioned in the subcutaneous tunnel and once tissue ingrowth occurs (usually 2–3 weeks) this fixes the catheter preventing accidental removal. This type of CVC is usually inserted by a surgical cut-down onto the external or internal jugular vein but percutaneous placement via the subclavian vein using the Seldinger technique and a peel-away sheath is possible even in neonates. Skin tunnelling was not thought to reduce the incidence of catheter sepsis but more recently catheters have been produced with a silver impregnated cuff which does seem to reduce the incidence of infection via the skin tunnel. Tunnelling does help to secure the catheter and allows it to exit at a convenient point on the chest wall or axilla. It must be remembered that

some form of fixation to avoid early accidental removal is needed, such as a suture or adhesive dressing until fibrosis fixes the cuff.

A number of totally implantable venous access devices are available (e.g. Portacath) but there would seem to be few indications for their use in ICU patients.

Infusion pumps

A volumetric infusion pump should be used to deliver parenteral nutrition in children. A peristaltic type of pump is sufficiently accurate for delivery of fluid volumes in excess of 5 ml/h but below this flow rate, for example lipid infusion in neonates, a syringe pump is preferable. Most modern infusion pumps incorporate comprehensive monitoring, protection against air embolism and occlusion alarms.

Solutions

Carbohydrate

Glucose is the carbohydrate in current TPN solutions, providing 3.4 kcal/g of dextrose. Unfortunately, the ability of neonates to metabolize intravenous glucose is limited and in preterm infants even more so. This leads to some difficulties with its use in these groups.

In term neonates glucose infusion should be begun at 7–8 mg/kg/min and increased slowly to 12–14 mg/kg/min. This should avoid problems with hyperglycaemia. In one study of low birthweight infants 8.1 mg/kg/min was tolerated but 11.2 mg/kg/min produced hyperglycaemia in 50% and 14 mg/kg/min in 100%. In this context 10% dextrose at 150 ml/kg/d is equivalent to 10.4 mg/kg/min. Hence one would expect in many low-birthweight babies that 10% dextrose may not be tolerated, at least initially. Administration of exogenous insulin in these circumstances is not helpful as there appears to be a degree of insulin resistance and blood glucose may become very unstable and difficult to control. The preferred approach is a gradual increase in glucose concentration allowing a response of endogenous insulin. Close monitoring of blood and urine glucose is obviously vital during the initiation of TPN in neonates.

Glucose as a sole energy source is associated with two problems. First, excessive hepatic lipogenesis may be stimulated. Fat is produced faster than it can be exported from the liver leading to fatty infiltration. Second, metabolism of glucose produces more CO_2 than metabolism of fat. This may lead to respiratory acidosis and is thus of significance in patients with respiratory failure.

In newborn and preterm infants hepatic gluconeogenesis has a reduced capacity and abrupt cessation of TPN infusions in this group causes rebound hypoglycaemia. If TPN has to be withdrawn because of problems with

Table 8.7 Daily protein requirements for parenteral nutrition

	g/kg/d
Preterm and term infants	2.0–2.5
Older infants	2.5–3.0
Older children	1.5–2.5
Adults	1.0–1.5

central lines then a peripheral infusion of 10% dextrose must be started immediately.

Protein

Protein is provided by solutions of crystalline L-amino acids. Protein is usable as an energy source and provides 4 kcal/g. It is not however usually provided as an energy source but rather for incorporation into body proteins, to reverse negative nitrogen balance and to promote growth. Daily protein requirements for different ages are listed in Table 8.7.

For efficient utilization of administered protein adequate non-protein calories must be provided. Current recommendations suggest 150–200 non-protein kcal/g nitrogen (1 g N_2 = 6.25 g protein). These calories should be a combination of carbohydrate and fat with fat providing approximately 40% of the energy.

'Adult' amino acid solutions may not be appropriate in preterm and term infants. In these groups histidine is an essential amino acid and cysteine, tyrosine and taurine are 'semi-essential'. A specifically formulated amino-acid solution such as Vaminolact (Pharmacia) is therefore preferable.

If excessive amounts of amino acid solutions are administered then hyper-aminoacidaemia, hyperammonaemia, uraemia and cholestatic jaundice will develop.

Fat

Fat is provided by preparations of soya bean oil emulsified with purified egg phospholipids and glycerol (e.g. Intralipid). These contain large amounts of the essential fatty acids linoleic and linolenic acid. Infused fat is cleared from the circulation in a fashion similar to natural chylomicrons, a process dependent on lipoprotein lipase. It has been suggested that heparin might improve uptake of fat by stimulating lipoprotein lipase but in practice this has not proven to be of use.

Tat emulsions are isotonic and hence can be infused peripherally. Fat is a rich energy source providing 9 kcal/g when metabolized by beta-oxidation. Unfortunately the capacity to metabolize intravenous lipid is limited; the maximum tolerances at various ages are summarized in Table 8.8.

Table 8.8 Maximum tolerances of intravenous fat

	g/kg/day
Preterm/low birthweight	3.0
Term neonate	4.0
Children	2.0

Like glucose fat infusions should be started in small amounts. 0.5 g/kg/d for preterm infants and 1 g/kg/d for term infants and older children, and thereafter increased in increments of 0.5 g/kg/d up to the maximum levels. If visible lipaemia occurs in the serum then the rate of fat infusion should be reduced.

Glucose is also required for the efficient utilization of fat as an energy source and overall fat should not provide more than 50–60% of the total energy intake. As mentioned previously, a combination of fat and carbohydrate is optimum in promoting a positive nitrogen balance. Carnitine is essential for the transport of free fatty acids (FFAs) into mitochondria for oxidative metabolism. It is not provided in fat emulsions and measurable falls in carnitine levels occur during TPN. Newborn infants in particular seem to have limited carnitine reserves and it has been suggested that supplementation should be used. As yet however there is insufficient evidence to recommend this as routine practice.

Administration of fat emulsions may be continuous over 24 h or over 18 h with a 6-h break in the infusion. The latter has the advantage of allowing lipid to clear from the blood before samples for electrolytes are drawn, as lipid may interfere in some assays. It has also been suggested that a period free from lipid might allow regeneration of enzymes in metabolic pathways but this is unproven.

With currently available solutions, incompatibilities prevent formulation of all in one bags. Lipid must therefore be infused separately although mixing close to the point of infusion is not a problem. Furthermore, filters are commonly used in the amino acid/dextrose line and these may destabilize the lipid emulsion. Lipid must therefore be infused into the line beyond these filters.

A number of problems are recognized with lipid infusions in the paediatric age groups, as follows.

Unconjugated hyperbilirubinaemia
The FFA released during parenteral feeding with lipid may displace bilirubin from binding sites on albumin with the theoretical risk of precipitating kernicterus in newborn infants. Lipid should probably therefore be avoided if there is unconjugated hyperbilirubinaemia in a neonate which is more than half the exchange transfusion level.

Hypoxaemia

Lipid infusion has been associated with hypoxia and rises in pulmonary artery pressure. It was initially thought this was due to lipid deposition in the pulmonary vasculature but more recently it has been postulated that changes in prostaglandin production in the pulmonary blood vessels occur in response to lipid infusion and that these account for the changes in vascular tone. Problems only seem to arise with rapid infusion of lipid and as long as the daily requirement is given over 18–24 h there should be no deleterious effects.

Lipid overload

If lipid is given in excess of metabolic capacity a syndrome of hyperlipidaemia, fever, lethargy, liver injury and coagulopathy has been reported both in adults and children.

Other problems

Hypersensitivity reactions are reported but are very rare. Falls in platelet numbers and abnormal platelet function can also occur. Preexisting severe thrombocytopenia may therefore mitigate against the use of lipid emulsions.

Trace elements and vitamins

Requirements for trace elements and vitamins during parenteral nutrition in children are not well defined. Supplements have been formulated (e.g. Ped-el, Solivito and Vitlipid—Kabi Pharmacia) in accordance with the best information available.

Solivito and Vitlipid contain water- and fat-soluble vitamins respectively. They are both usually administered dissolved in the lipid emulsion part of the feed. Additional vitamin supplements are not generally required.

Ped-el contains calcium, magnesium, iron, zinc, manganese, and copper. Additional iron is frequently given in the form of blood transfusions as anaemia not uncommonly develops during TPN, particularly in the ICU patient with significant iatrogenic blood loss from blood sampling. Selenium supplementation may be considered in addition if long-term TPN is required. Recently there has been some concern that recommended quantities of manganese may be excessive. Manganese levels should therefore be periodically monitored and if problems arise a trace element supplement with lower concentrations (Peditrace) substituted.

Complications of parenteral nutrition

Complications of CVC placement

Complications of percutaneous central line placement are well known and are described in detail elsewhere (see Chapter 9).

Catheter-related sepsis

The commonest and most serious complication of parenteral nutrition is catheter-related sepsis which can occur in up to one-third of patients. Common infecting organisms are coagulase negative staphylococci (*S. epidermidis*) and enterococci. Other possibilities include *S. aureus*, gram negative bacilli and *Candida albicans*. Catheter-related sepsis can present in many ways, including fever, metabolic acidosis, thrombocytopenia, and glucose or lipid intolerance at previously tolerated concentrations. Some patients may present with overt septic shock. It is important to remember that most episodes of fever in patients on TPN are not due to catheter sepsis and other sites of infection should also be actively sought. Definitive diagnosis hinges on quantitative peripheral and through line blood cultures, a five- to tenfold higher colony count in the central line culture indicating a high likelihood of catheter infection.

Colonization of the catheter exit site will inevitably occur with all catheters. As long as there is no evidence of invasive infection this is probably of little importance. Organisms at the exit site are more likely to be involved in catheter sepsis with percutaneous rather than tunnelled lines. Certain organisms particularly *S. aureus* and *C. albicans* are more worrying at the exit site and may be an indication for removal of a percutaneous line. The best dressing for the exit site is a matter of controversy. Clear semipermeable dressings have the advantage of allowing visualization of the site but are associated with increased growth of skin organisms under the dressing when compared with dry gauze dressings.

In most cases catheter infection seems to emanate from colonization of the catheter hub or line connections. Occasionally infection may arise from contaminated feeds but with preparation under sterile pharmacy conditions this is now very rare.

Ideally the management of suspected or confirmed catheter sepsis would be immediate removal of the catheter and reestablishment of central venous access via an alternative site. This in practice may however be extremely difficult and has led to attempts at catheter salvage, particularly of surgically inserted cuffed catheters. In patients with septic shock, evidence of septic emboli or infection with either *S. aureus* or *C. albicans* this would be inappropriate and the catheter should be removed as soon as possible. In other cases if vascular access is difficult and there is a continued need for TPN then an attempt at sterilizing the catheter seems reasonable. Vancomycin is the mainstay of treatment as this antibiotic is active against the commonest infecting organisms. Gentamicin or netilmicin may be added to give additional cover against gram negative bacilli. Vancomycin is stable in heparinized saline and in TPN solutions. It can therefore simply be added to the TPN although a 'lock' in the catheter appears more effective at least under experimental conditions. The addition of urokinase has been suggested to remove infected fibrin and clot

from the catheter lumen. Studies have shown that catheter salvage rates of 70–90% are achievable by these means.

Prevention of sepsis is clearly better than cure. Measures that reduce the risk of catheter sepsis include, wrapping the catheter hub with an iodine impregnated sponge, minimizing line connections and taps, training of specialist nurses and the establishment of nutrition teams and catheter care protocols.

Catheter occlusion

A sheath of fibrin is deposited on the outside of the intravascular portion of most CVCs. If this extends over the catheter tip it may act as a valve allowing injection but preventing aspiration. It may also cause infused fluids to track back between the fibrin sheath and catheter to leak from the exit site or into the subcutaneous tissues. Such obstructing fibrin sheaths may be lysed by continuous infusion of urokinase (200 U/kg/h). Complete obstruction of the catheter lumen may be caused by blood clot, deposits of lipid or calcium salts. Blood clot can be lysed with urokinase. Occlusion by lipid deposits can be removed by locking or flushing with 70% alcohol and deposits of calcium with 0.01 M hydrochloric acid. If blockage has occurred close to the catheter hub this may, as a last resort, be cut off and replaced using a catheter repair kit.

Central vein thrombosis

Clots commonly occur either on catheters themselves or on the walls of the cannulated veins. Usually they are asymptomatic but on occasion thrombotic occlusion of the central veins may occur. Thrombosis of the SVC may propagate up the innominate vein to obstruct flow of chyle in the thoracic duct leading to generalized oedema and chylothoraces. Suspected central vein thrombosis can be confirmed by ultrasound, echocardiography, or venography. Such thromboses may be successfully lysed with urokinase or tissue plasminogen activator if recognized early.

Cholestasis

Cholestasis is associated with the prolonged use of TPN in children to a greater extent than adults. In most cases it is reversible on stopping TPN but in some it may progress to cirrhosis or even in rare instances to hepatocellular carcinoma. Up to 17% of newborn infants given TPN for more than 14 days develop cholestasis (defined as bilirubin > 40 μmol/l).

Risk factors for the development of cholestasis include preterm birth, failure to tolerate enteral feeds and sepsis. The absence of taurine from amino acid preparations has also been implicated. In animal models taurine supplements reversed cholestasis, but the advent of amino acid preparations containing taurine (e.g. Vaminolact) whilst raising taurine levels in the blood has yet to show a fall in the prevalence of TPN associated cholestasis in patients.

Unfortunately it is rarely feasible to stop TPN if cholestatis develops and a number of strategies, including reducing the parenteral load, cycling TPN over only part of the day, the use of antibiotics and phenobarbitone and the introduction of even minimal enteral feeds, have been suggested. Probably the only approach that can be commended both to try to prevent and to treat cholestasis is the introduction of at least partial enteral feeding either bolus or continuous.

A problem related to cholestasis is the development of gallbladder sludge and occasionally stones. This is attributed to bile stasis as a consequence of low cholecystokinin levels whilst on TPN. Once again enteral feeding should help to reduce this problem.

Metabolic complications

Metabolic complications relating to the glucose, protein and fat content of TPN have been covered already as have abnormalities of water and electrolyte balance. In the absence of large abnormal losses of fluid, for example from small bowel fistulae or stomas, then serious or unexpected metabolic abnormalities are unusual. One exception is hypophosphataemia which is seen not infrequently when feeding begins with severely malnourished children. With longer-term TPN then either deficiencies or more rarely accumulation of trace elements or vitamins may arise.

Monitoring

Monitoring of infants and children receiving TPN should consist both of frequent assessments of nutritional state and growth and biochemical screening for metabolic abnormalities.

Weight should be recorded daily if possible or at least twice weekly in more stable patients. Head circumference should be measured weekly in infants. A suggested laboratory monitoring protocol is set out in Table 8.9. It should be borne in mind that the volumes of blood required for these tests may become significant, particularly in the small infant. A record should be kept of cumulative blood sample volume.

METABOLIC SUPPORT

Renal support

Renal failure is quite commonly seen to varying degrees on initial presentation of children to intensive care. Good basic resuscitation and optimal post-resuscitation management can correct renal dysfunction or ameliorate damage to the kidneys but some children present in established renal failure. It is important to check at an early stage whether the child has normal urinary

Table 8.9 Suggested biochemical monitoring protocol for parenteral nutrition

	Pre-TPN	Daily (unstable)	Twice weekly (stable)	Weekly	3 weekly
Glucose	X	X	X		
Electrolytes	X	X	X		
Ca/PO$_4$				X	
Liver function tests	X			X	
Blood count				X	
Trace elements (Fe, Cu, Zn, Se, Mn)					X

Table 8.10 Common causes of paediatric renal failure

Cardiac surgery	Sickle cell disease
Cardiac arrest	Glomerulonephritis
Sepsis	Drug toxicity
Haemolytic uraemic syndrome	Congenital abnormalities
Oncology	High intra-abdominal pressure

anatomy as congenital abnormalities may predispose to renal failure. Other diseases such as coarctation of the aorta may also predispose to renal failure. The prognosis of renal failure is probably better in children than in adults and non-oliguric renal failure probably has a better outlook.

Early management priorities are to ensure correction of intravascular volume depletion, fluid overload, and hyperkalaemia. Diuretics, inotropes, vasodilators, and vasopressors should be given as appropriate depending on the results of the clinical examination, invasive intravascular monitoring, urine output and serial biochemistry. Meticulous attention to fluid and electrolyte balance, treatment of high blood pressure, infection control, antacid prophylaxis, and restriction of protein intake are vital supportive measures in the child with established renal failure.

Dialysis is required in severe volume overload, cardiac failure, severe metabolic derangement (hyperkalaemia, severe acidosis, rapidly rising urea and creatinine, severe hypocalcaemia, neurological impairment) or in the hypercatabolic patient. Peritoneal dialysis is relatively efficient in children and can achieve up to 50% of the nitrogenous clearance of haemodialysis. Modern PD access kits are very easy to use and can be inserted at the bedside in the PICU under local anaesthesia using a Seldinger technique. Cycle volumes of

20 ml/kg are used initially and increased to 40 ml/kg if tolerated. The dextrose, electrolyte, and bicarbonate content of the dialysate must be individualized and titrated against serial biochemistry results. Intraperitoneal infection, catheter blockage, bowel perforation, diaphragmatic splinting, and pleural effusion may be seen when this technique is used in critically ill children. Haemodialysis for small children is quite possible with the advent of better kits for vascular access and specifically designed paediatric dialysis membranes. Double lumen catheters can be placed in femoral, subclavian or jugular veins and pumped veno-venous haemofilitration and/or dialysis can be performed. Continuous arteriovenous haemofiltration and/or dialysis is favoured by some and in small babies a pumped arteriovenous system is preferred by some centres. Haemofiltration is being used in some complex cases of sepsis syndrome as kinins and cytokines may be removed and body temperature can be controlled using this system. Filtration is used for fluid clearance and to make space for nutritional fluids and/or coagulation factors and blood products. Dialysis is used to achieve biochemical correction and clearance.

Liver support

The commonest reasons for liver failure in children are drugs, infections, or Reye syndrome. Paracetamol, iron, isoniazid, non-steroidal anti-inflammatory drugs, antibiotics and anticonvulsants are most often associated with acute hepatic necrosis. Primary hepatic infections such as hepatitis A, B and non-A–non-B, or secondary toxic or ischaemic damage as part of the sepsis syndrome can all cause liver failure in children. Accurate diagnosis, meticulous fluid and electrolyte management to avoid hypovolaemia, hypoglycaemia, hyponatraemia, and hypokalaemia, prevention and treatment of stress bleeding, encephalopathy, cerebral oedema, infection, respiratory failure, coagulation failure, and hepatorenal syndrome are all vitally important. If the child deteriorates rapidly, referral for transplantation should be considered at an early stage.

Inborn errors of metabolism and endocrine disorders

Inborn errors of metabolism

Neonatal presentation of inborn errors of metabolism often corresponds with the start of protein containing feeds. Presentation later in infancy is more insidious and non-specific with signs which are often interpreted as indicating sepsis. Failure to thrive, vomiting, lethargy, coma, hyperventilation, hypotonia, seizures, and apnoea may be seen. Jaundice, liver enlargement, and dysmorphism are also clues. The disorders can be of two main types: (1) those due to metabolic toxicity from high levels of ammonia, organic acids, amino acids, galactose or fructose; (2) those due to energy failure in the brain, heart, liver

or muscle may be due to defects in gluconeogenesis, fatty acid oxidation, microsome function or utilization of lactate.

On admission, at the time when the child is very sick, samples of blood, urine and CSF (if no cerebral oedema) should be taken to assist in the detective work. Ammonia, pH, blood gases, calcium, sodium, potassium, choloride, bicarbonate, base deficit, glucose, lactate, urea, and creatinine results can be obtained relatively quickly. Liver enzymes, bilirubin, full blood count and coagulation studies should be measured. Plasma should be saved for amino acids, carnitine, and organic acids. Urinalysis for pH, electrolytes, ketone bodies, microscopy, culture and sensitivities should be carried out acutely with further samples saved for analysis of amino acids, carnitine, organic acids and orotic acid. From these initial screening tests the presence of a metabolic acidosis, very high plasma ammonia, hypoglycaemia and renal failure are important to identify and treat. Good basic paediatric intensive care management with careful correction and maintenance of fluid, electrolyte, nutritional and acid–base balance are vitally important. Peritoneal dialysis or haemodialysis may be used to assist this process and are useful in correcting high ammonia levels, acidosis, and other electrolyte anomalies particularly if renal dysfunction is present. Sometimes specific defects can be treated or bypassed by giving compounds such as arginine or biotin. Sodium benzoate and sodium phenylacetate can be used to divert ammonia from the urea cycle to be excreted in the urine.

Some common inborn errors of metabolism

Defect	Typical effects
urea cycle defects	high ammonia
organic acidaemias	high ammonia, metabolic acidosis, neutropenia, thrombocytopenia
amino acid disorders	ketosis, ketonuria
carbohydrate defects	hypoglycaemia, lactic acidosis, ketonuria
defective steroidogenesis	hyponatraemia, hyperkalaemia

Disorders of glucose metabolism

Diabetic ketoacidosis

The child with an acute presentation in diabetic ketoacidotic coma may be severely dehydrated, shocked and deeply unconscious with loss of airway control due to cerebral oedema. It is important to stress that the principles of basic and advanced life support are followed in such cases and the metabolic and biochemical disorders are corrected gradually. The airway must be maintained and secured if necessary, ventilation and oxygenation should be optimized and shock corrected by intravascular volume expansion. Fluid and electrolyte deficits are calculated and replaced over about 36–48 h and an

intravenous insulin infusion is started and carefully titrated against serial blood sugar estimations. An example protocol is shown below.

Protocol for management of severe diabetic ketoacidosis

Fluids
> Treat shock 10 ml/kg colloid or 0.9% saline over 30–60 min; may need one repeat.
> Calculate fluid deficit from normal weight and % dehydration and give over 36 h (48 h if plasma osmolality 380 mosm/l or more).

Calculate hourly maintenance fluid requirement using 4, 2, 1 formula.
Measure continuing hourly losses, e.g. due to vomiting.

Electrolytes

Sodium
> If <150 mmol/l use 0.9% saline.
> If >150 mmol/l use 0.45% saline (0.45% saline in 5% dextrose once glucose <14 mmol/l).

Potassium
> If <5 mmol/l give 20–30 mmol KCl per litre of fluid.

Bicarbonate
> Only give if pH <7.00 and shocked.
> Give (kg × base deficit × 0.3)/2 mmol over 60 min.

Recheck electrolytes and osmolality 2 hourly initially.

Insulin
> Make up a solution of 1 unit insulin per millilitre 0.9% saline.
> Check Glucostix hourly.
> If glucose >30 mmol/l infuse at 0.1 units/kg/h.
> If glucose ≤30 mmol/l infuse at 0.05 units/kg/h.
> If glucose falls at >5 mmol/l/h then reduce rate of insulin infusion.
> Once glucose is in the range 4–14 mmol/l keep insulin infusion at the rate current at that time; if the glucose then falls to <4 mmol/l halve the insulin infusion rate; if glucose rises to >14 mmol/l double the insulin infusion rate.

Keep insulin and fluids going intravenously until child is drinking well and able to tolerate food.

Cerebral care
> If the child is old enough to talk but has difficulty in conversing, then they should be considered as having severe cerebral impairment. Headache, confusion, irritability, deterioration in conscious level, respiratory impairment, and seizures are indicators of cerebral oedema.
> Exclude hypoglycaemia.

Give mannitol 0.25–0.5 g/kg over 15 min.
Restrict maintenance fluids to 2/3 and replace calculated deficit over 72 h instead of 36 h.
Control ventilation and oxygenation.
Avoid hypovolaemia.
Consider CT scan and ICP monitoring.

Gastric aspiration
Ensure stomach is emptied hourly and chart and replace losses.
Keep child nil by mouth for 12 h then if conscious level normal allow gradual introduction of oral fluid intake.

Hypoglycaemia

Neonates are prone to hypoglycaemia though this is usually transient but persistence of low blood sugars suggests disorders of carbohydrate or amino acid metabolism, insulin excess or deficiency of growth hormone, cortisol, or ACTH. Hypoglycaemia in older infants and children has a huge multiplicity of causes including lack of available glucose, increased glucose utilization, defects in hepatic glucose formation, and release and toxicity from drugs such as aspirin or paracetamol.

If blood glucose is <2.5 mmol/l, give bolus of dextrose 1 g/kg (2 m/kg 50% dextrose), start 10% dextrose infusion at 6 ml/kg/h. If no IV access give IM glucagon 1 mg (0.5 mg if <6 years). If blood glucose is 2.5–4 mmol/l, give oral glucose; if vomiting give 10% dextrose at 6 ml/kg/h.

BLOOD TRANSFUSION, BLOOD PRODUCTS AND COAGULATION SUPPORT

Bleeding

Children who are bleeding can rapidly be assessed by history, clinical examination and measurement of haematocrit, platelet count, prothrombin time, activated partial thromboplastin time, and fibrinogen or fibrin degradation products. Surgical bleeding, trauma and some blood vessel disorders are usually obvious causes of bleeding. Low platelet numbers or functionally abnormal platelets can cause bleeding while coagulation factors may be deficient due to impaired liver production, due to consumptive coagulopathy or because of a congenital defect.

In the PICU bleeding is most commonly seen in children after cardiac surgery, after trauma, in those with sepsis and in oncology patients. After cardiac surgery, surgical sources should be dealt with and residual heparinization from cardiopulmonary bypass checked for and reversed with additional protamine. Platelets, 1 unit per 5 kg should be given and fresh frozen

plasma 10 ml/kg. Cryoprecipitate 1 unit per 3 kg can be helpful and repeated doses of all these products should be used by titration against serial coagulation test results. The same approach can be used in sepsis and early involvement of senior haematology staff is extremely helpful in complex cases.

SAFE OPERATION OF INFUSION DEVICES

All paediatric infusions should be considered as 'high risk' because even simple solutions given wrongly can have serious adverse effects. Thus syringe drivers and volumetric pumps must comply with modern safety regulations in terms of their safety features, alarm functions, accuracy, and electronic quality. It is vitally important that staff who are using these devices are trained on each individual device so that they know how to set the device up correctly, what settings are appropriate for that particularl patient and how to troubleshoot the device. All paediatric infusion devices must be monitored along with observations of the patient to check for overinfusion, under-infusion, malfunction of the pump or occlusion, or misplacement of the delivery system. Pumps should be set up so as to avoid the possibility of retrograde flow up concurrent infusion lines and free flow into the patient. Free flow or siphonage can occur if the infusion syringe is more than 1 m above the patient, if the syringe is not located properly in the syringe driver or if the syringe barrel or plunger has a leak. All these problems can be identified by careful checking and rechecking of the pump set up, pum settings, syringe, residual volume, delivery system, infusion site, and response of the patient.

LEARNING POINTS

1. Fluid balance must be meticulously adjusted in critically ill children.

2. Nutritional management should have a high priority in critically ill children, with the enteral route being used whenever possible.

3. Metabolic monitoring must be undertaken with an intensity according to the severity and complexity of the illness.

9

Monitoring techniques in paediatric intensive care

M. Robson

Monitoring the paediatric patient relies on the same basic equipment and underlying physical principles as in adult practice. However, differences are present particularly in relation to their size, physiology and underlying medical conditions (persistent fetal circulation, congenital heart defects) which are important in interpreting values and positioning of monitoring lines.

The doctor in the PICU must be aware of the specific requirements of each patient and limit the use of invasive techniques with their inherent risks during insertion and increased risk of infection. The cost of monitoring is very important especially with more sophisticated equipment being introduced and uncertainty as to whether this increased cost reduces patient morbidity and mortality.

Increasing the amount of monitoring does not reduce the need for close observation and clinical examination of the patient by the ICU nurse and medical staff.

MONITORING THE RESPIRATORY SYSTEM

Clinical signs

The presence of central cyanosis is often difficult to detect and requires at least 5% reduced haemoglobin. Ambient light, drape, and bed cover colour can all interfere with its detection. When present it indicates dysfunction of blood oxygenation which may be respiratory or cardiovascular in origin. Respiratory rate is a very good indicator of respiratory insufficiency. Increasing respiratory rate in any pathology indicates increased work and when accompanied with the use of accessory muscles may indicate the need for assisted ventilation. Tracheal tug, flaring of the nares, intercostal and sternal recession and paradoxical movement of the abdomen indicate airway obstruction. The presence and severity of inspiratory stridor reflect the degree of upper airway obstruction. Biphasic or expiratory stridor is suggestive of intrathoracic obstruction. Signs of hypercarbia may include an increasing pulse rate and blood pressure, associated with a bounding pulse. If respiratory acidosis develops

cardiac output can be reduced and often the child will appear mottled, cold and peripherally shut down. This may be seen during overenthusiastic weaning of the ventilated child with cardiac problems.

Severe respiratory insufficiency is suggested by a passive and silent infant who is fatigued, hypoxic and/or hypercarbic and requires immediate assisted ventilation. Auscultation of the chest can be difficult and may not detect problems within the chest. However, reduced breath sounds, decreased chest wall movement, hyperresonance and tracheal shift are suggestive of pneumothorax. Changes in the size of the electrocardiogram (ECG) complexes has also been reported as an early sign of pneumothorax. Wheeze is associated with small airways disease, cardiac failure and foreign body aspiration. The history will suggest the likely cause.

The above clinical observations are often all that is required when deciding to secure the patient's airway and institute assisted ventilation.

PULSE OXIMETRY

Pulse oximetry is a non-invasive method of measuring the arterial oxygen saturation. The underlying principles are the Beer–Lambert Law and the different absorption spectra of oxygenated and deoxygenated blood. Light of two wavelengths, red (660 nm) and infra-red (940 nm) is emitted from two light-emitting diodes (LEDs). The intensity of light after passing through the tissues is measured by a photodiode. The absorption by the tissues and non-pulsatile elements is assumed to be constant, the pulsatile arterial flow gives a variable absorption. The oxygen saturation is estimated from the ratio of the difference in these measurements at the two wavelengths of light. The photodiode is unable to detect which wavelength of light the signal is generated from. To overcome this the LEDs are turned on in sequence with a period when neither is on to obtain an absorbency due to external light sources. This sequence is repeated many times a second and the absorbency due to external light is subtracted from the values due to the LEDs. In this way the oximeter tries to reduce the effect of external light sources. The above wavelengths of light are chosen as they optimally calculate the proportion of deoxyhaemoglobin and oxyhaemoglobin which are used to calculate the functional saturation. If other haemoglobin species are present an error is introduced. This is especially true with carboxyhaemoglobin which can result in a normal recorded saturation in the presence of severe carbon monoxide poisoning. In patients with high HbF, carboxyhaemoglobin values are inappropriately elevated, leading to a decreased measured saturation.

The monitors are calibrated in the factory using human volunteers who are desaturated to known levels (in the range of 80–100%). This limits the accuracy of the monitors at levels of oxygen saturation below 75%. Some monitors will also measure a saturation even when not attached to the patient

and one is always reminded to check the source of the information before acting on it. The other problem in this respect is the monitoring probe used on the paediatric population. Size of probe, method of attachment, and position can all influence the accuracy and consistency of readings, and it is important to ensure that the photodiode is directly opposite the LEDs.

Technical and clinical factors affecting pulse oximetry

Common causes of error include:

- connection
- arrhythmias
- dyes
- dyshaemoglobins
- anaemia

- peripheral vasoconstriction
- motion artifact
- neon or infra-red light
- oxygen dissociation curve
- nail polish.

Connection

False readings can occur from oximeter probes which are poorly attached to the patient because of added light and motion artifact. Good connection is often accompanied by close correlation between the oximeter pulse rate and that recorded by the electrocardiograph (ECG). Delay in response time of the oximeter also results from poor connection as the signal is averaged out over a longer period of time.

Arrhythmias

The variation in beat-to-beat arterial pulse wave due to atrial fibrillation, atrial flutter and ventricular ectopics can result in a variable oxygen saturation being recorded.

Dyes

Methylene blue and indocyanine green both cause a fall in the recorded saturation.

Peripheral vasoconstriction/low perfusion states

This results in a very low pulsatile signal which the oximeter has to amplify in order to obtain a reading. In doing this the noise signal is also equally amplified for both red and infra-red light which results in an absorbance ratio near to one and a pulse oximeter reading near 85%. Oximeters may incorporate an automatic cut-off when the ratio of pulsatile signal-to-noise signal reaches a certain level and will not display a value. Other oximeter devices display a waveform which the user can interpret as to the quality of the signal. However,

this waveform does not represent flow and indeed a saturation can be calculated when peripheral bloodflow has fallen to 10% of normal.

Anaemia

At haemoglobin levels below 5 g/dl the pulse oximeter may not be able to detect the pulsatile changes.

Clinical uses

Pulse oximetry is a useful method of non-invasive oxygen monitoring in children with cardiorespiratory disease, those who are ventilated and during the transfer of patients between hospitals and within the same hospital. The limitations which arise are often due to the clinical condition of the patient in terms of poor peripheral circulation and placement of the oximeter probe.

The oxygen saturation has limitations as a physiological value due to the shape of the oxygen dissociation curve. Arterial oxygenation has to fall below 80 mmHg (10.5 kPa) before the saturation drops below 97%. The oxygen dissociation curve is influenced by physiological conditions and this should be remembered when interpreting the SaO_2. For example, acidosis shifts the curve to the right while alkalosis shifts the curve to the left. In the acutely ill infant the proportion of HbF may also influence the ability of the SaO_2 to predict the arterial PO_2 because of the different shape of its oxygen dissociation curve.

Arterial oxygen saturations can be determined accurately by pulse oximetry in infants and children with cyanotic congenital heart disease. In infants with acute cardiorespiratory problems, pulse oximetry is unreliable in reflecting PaO_2, but may be useful in detecting clinical deterioration.

Transcutaneous oxygen monitoring

This device is used less often now that pulse oximetry is more widely available. However, it still has a place in the close control of oxygen therapy in neonates and young infants. The monitoring device is basically a Clark electrode with a heating coil. The skin is heated to 43 °C which arterializes the capillary blood. Heating the skin has two effects: (1) the heated blood in the capillaries has a reduced oxygen solubility, and (2) the oxygen dissociation curve is shifted to the right with a reduction in oxygen affinity. The oxygen tension is therefore increased which counteracts the increase in oxygen metabolism (due to heating the skin) and the diffusion gradient through the skin. Transcutaneous PO_2 is a close approximation of arterial PO_2. Transcutaneous PO_2 is affected by skin bloodflow which is influenced by both physiological factors and pharmacological agents.

Transcutaneous carbon dioxide monitoring

The Severinghaus sensor is used to measure transcutaneous PCO_2. It comprises pH sensitive glass and a silver/silver chloride reference electrode. Heating the skin is not essential but this decreases the response time. Skin surface CO_2 measurements reflect peripheral gas tensions and not arterial tensions. The value is influenced by both ventilatory and haemodynamic changes and in combination with transcutaneous PO_2 can be a useful monitor of circulatory function and oxygen delivery.

Apnoea monitors

A simple pneumograph picks up chest wall movement and allows a graphic and rate display. This may be of use in conjunction with pulse oximetry when monitoring young children on opioid infusions and alert staff to the presence of respiratory irregularity which may herald respiratory insufficiency.

Capnography (end-tidal carbon dioxide monitoring)

Capnography has been used extensively in adult ICU and theatre practice and has been particularly welcome in detecting oesophageal intubation where the tracing falls to zero. Its use in PICU is less widespread and the values obtained are more difficult to interpret. This is a particular problem in small infants with corresponding rapid respiratory rates and small tidal volumes. Infra-red analysis of flow through gas is one method of capnography and is accurate in ventilated neonates and infants when large tidal volumes and an endotracheal tube with no air leak is used. When used in children who are self ventilating or who have a leak around the tube the values of end-tidal CO_2 may not be accurate or correlate with arterial PCO_2. Other concerns include the high sampling gas flows necessary for side arm analysis and the increase in dead space associated with the connections for the apparatus. This can now be minimized using endotracheal tube connectors with a built in gas sampling port. Their place in the ICU may be in the child requiring prolonged ventilation to reduce the need for invasive arterial sampling.

Principles of CO_2 measurement

There are four physical methods of measuring CO_2 concentration in respiratory gases. Mass spectrography, Raman spectrography, infra-red spectrography and photoaccoustic spectrography. A brief description of infra-red spectrography and photoacoustic spectrography will be given as these are the main methods used in clinical monitoring.

Infra-red spectrography

The infra-red gas analyser works on the principle that molecules with two or more dissimilar atoms absorb infra-red radiation between one and 15 micrometres. In this respect oxygen (O_2) does not absorb radiation but CO_2 does.

The different atomic masses and molecular bonds create dipole moments which oscillate at a natural frequency and absorb infra-red radiation creating an absorption spectrum characteristic of the molecule. Carbon dioxide selectively absorbs infra-red light with a wavelength of 43 micrometres. The amount of light absorbed is proportional to the concentration of CO_2 present and can be compared to a standard. Two sources of error in the infra-red analyser come from (1) the slight overlap of the absorption spectrum of nitrous oxide and CO_2, and (2) collision broadening when the presence of other gases in the analysed sample alters the absorption spectrum of the analysed gas. This can be overcome by calibration of the analyser with a sample of the background gas which is assumed to be constant or by introducing a constant correction for an assumed concentration of background gas such as nitrous oxide.

Photoacoustic spectrography (PAS)

Acoustic techniques for gas measurement are based on the fact that gas will expand when energy is applied to it. If infra-red light is applied to a gas in a pulsatile manner the resulting pressure change will fluctuate. If the pressure changes lie in the audible range these can be detected by a microphone as a sound wave. The amplitude of the signal caused by the pressure changes is directly proportional to the concentration of gas present.

The main difference between the two techniques is that in the standard infra-red analyser, the energy absorbed by the gas sample is measured indirectly by comparing it to a standard absorption. With PAS the amount of infra-red light absorbed is measured directly. Calibration is not required as there is no acoustic signal when no gas is present.

The location of the CO_2 sensors can differ. These can be sidestream capnometers or mainstream sensor capnometers.

Sidestream analysers

These involve the aspiration of gas from the breathing circuit via a length of narrow tubing. The gas is aspirated at a rate between 50 and 250 ml/min. High rates are required to achieve accurate measurements of peak expired end-tidal CO_2 as the sample of gas is subjected to dispersal caused by convection and diffusion during transit down the tube. This results in the loss of the peak and trough gas concentrations and results in an underestimate of peak expired end-tidal $P_{ET}CO_2$ especially in children. This accounts for the

shape of the capnograph trace often seen in children which is different from the classical trace seen in adults. A water trap is required to collect the condensation before the sample is analysed. This condensation can also cause blockage of the sample tube and an increase in the transit time. Other sources of error with side sampling are:

- increase in the length and width of the sample tubing

- reduced sample flow rate

- higher breathing frequency of patient.

Mainstream sensor capnometer

The sensor is placed between the endotracheal tube and the breathing circuit. These have to be heated to prevent accumulation of condensation. They are heavy, difficult to support, and can pull on the endotracheal tube.

The response time of the analyser is made up by the transit time and the rise time. The rise time is the time taken by the output from the capnometer to change from 10% of the final value to 90% of the final value in response to a step change in PCO_2. The rise time is dependent on the size of the sample chamber and the gas flow. When the response time of the analyser is greater than the respiratory cycle time of the patient PET CO_2 may be under-estimated.

The characteristic capnograph tracing is made up of four phases:

- exhaled dead space gas

- mixture of dead space and alveolar gas

- mixed alveolar gas

- inhalation, rapid descent of graph to zero CO_2.

The capnograph gives information on the following aspects of the patient:

- airway

- mechanical ventilatory function

- lung function

- cardiovascular function

- metabolic function.

The arterial PCO_2 is normally 2–5 mmHg (0.3–0.7 kPa) higher than the capnograph reading.

The use of the capnograph in the ICU helps in the control of ventilation, weaning from the ventilator and as a general indicator of cardiorespiratory

function. It is not accurate if there is severe lung or heart disease or if there is a large leak around the child's endotracheal tube.

Inspired oxygen tension

Modern ventilators have oxygen monitors incorporated in the machine with automatic alarm systems if the preset level drops by 5%. These monitors need to be calibrated and serviced regularly and modern machines often have an automatic calibration function.

Airway pressure

The use of pressure limited ventilation in infants has been the norm because of the difficulty in accurately measuring small tidal volumes. However, the peak pressure measured on the inspiratory limb is not the pressure delivered to the alveoli and can not be used to work out the tidal volume directly. The endotracheal tube introduces a significant resistance which is directly proportional to its length and inversely proportional to the fourth power of its radius. Significant changes can occur in this resistance due to kinking of the tube or partial obstruction due to secretions. As a result the tidal volume delivered is reduced. Adequacy of ventilation has to be gauged from observation of the chest wall, breath sounds, capnography, and arterial gas analysis.

Airway pressures have to be monitored to avoid barotrauma to the lungs and gauge the progression of diseases where high airway pressures are encountered, namely asthma, acute respiratory distress syndrome, and thermal lung injury.

Ventilator volumes

The volume of each breath delivered can be measured by some machines. Some can separately measure the volume during inspiration and the volume during expiration. The difference between these values is then calculated as the leak round the endotracheal tube. From the ventilator rate and the inspired and expired volume of each breath the machine can calculate the minute volume of ventilation. All these recordings can have alarm limits set around them automatically to detect changes quickly.

Arterial blood gases and acid–base status

The presence of small blood gas analysers in the ICU allows quick and reliable estimation of arterial blood gases and the main electrolytes, sodium, potassium and calcium. This is of particular use in the shocked patient, after cardiopulmonary bypass, and in those with metabolic upset.

The blood gas machine has three main components: the Clark PO_2 electrode, the Severinghaus PCO_2 electrode, and the Sanz pH electrode.

Clark PO_2 electrode

This electrode measures the voltage which results from the electrochemical reduction of oxygen at a platinum cathode, with a silver/silver chloride anode providing the electrons.

Severinghaus PCO_2 electrode

This electrode comprises two silver/silver chloride electrodes, bicarbonate solution and pH sensitive glass. The change in pH caused by the diffusion of CO_2 across the permeable membrane is proportional to the partial pressure of the CO_2 in the sample.

Sanz pH electrode

This electrode works on the principle that pH sensitive glass will generate an electrical potential if placed between a solution of known pH and the sample solution. The potential difference is measured by a silver/silver chloride electrode and compared using a reference electrode composed of mercury and mercurous chloride or calomel.

Handling of the sample

Small volumes of blood, approximately 240 micrometre, are required for analysis. However, a larger sample is required to be taken to dilute the heparin which is present in the sample syringes. An excess of heparin tends to reduce the PCO_2 and pH measured. Air bubbles should be removed as they will cause diffusion of the gases from high to low partial pressure areas. A well oxygenated sample will give a lower PO_2 than expected if full of air bubbles. Delay in analysing the sample can result in a lower PO_2 and increased PCO_2 due to ongoing metabolism by the red cells and leukocytes. The sample should be placed in ice if there is to be a delay in analysis.

Interpretation of results

Blood gas analysis gives information on the adequacy of oxygenation, ventilation and acid–base balance. It is important to remember that the pH is dependent on the ratio of HCO_3 to CO_2 and not the actual value of either.

Hypoxaemia can be the result of the following:

- hypoxic mixture
- hypoventilation

- mismatch of ventilation and perfusion

- shunt.

Hypoxaemia as a result of hypoventilation is due to an increase in alveolar PCO_2 and the alveolar to arterial oxygen gradient is normal. In all cases other than shunt increasing the inspired oxygen content will improve the arterial PO_2. The arterial blood gases should be interpreted in association with the cardiovascular status of the patient as cardiac output and blood pressure influence lung perfusion and oxygen delivery.

The adequacy of alveolar ventilation is based on the $PaCO_2$ and there is a direct relationship between the alveolar minute ventilation (VA) and the $PaCO_2$ assuming constant CO_2 production. Using the equation $V_1 * PaCO_2 = V_2 * PaCO_2$, fairly accurate adjustment of minute ventilation can be made to obtain the desired $PaCO_2$.

The pH should be considered next:

- Normal pH = 7.36–7.44

- Acidosis = pH <7.36

- Alkalosis 5 pH >7.44

Base excess/deficit is the number of milliequivalents of fixed acid or base needed to restore the pH of 1 litre of blood to a pH of 7.4 when the PCO_2 is held constant at 40 mmHg. It gives a quantitative index of the non-respiratory metabolic component of acid–base upset. Acid–base calculations assume that changes only take place in the extracellular space.

Consider the PCO_2 in connection with the pH to determine the respiratory component of any acidosis or alkalosis. Then consider the base deficit and bicarbonate to establish any metabolic component. Then decide if the ventilatory and metabolic events are primary or secondary. Compensatory mechanisms never completely correct the underlying upset but mixed pictures of acidosis and alkalosis often coexist in the ICU patient.

Capillary blood gases can be used if arterial samples are not available. These are taken after a heel stab and a glass capillary tube is filled. Their accuracy is influenced by the ease of obtaining the sample but they do give useful information on acid–base status rather than absolute values of PO_2 and PCO_2.

Monitoring the cardiovascular system

Clinical signs

The principle of cardiovascular monitoring is to assess the adequacy of organ perfusion and oxygen delivery. The cardiovascular system should always be assessed in combination with the respiratory system and not in isolation. Remember, hypoxia is the main cause of cardiac arrest in children.

When assessing a child's cardiovascular status colour, temperature and capillary return are important. Cyanosis is clinically detectable when there is greater than 5 g/dl of deoxyhaemoglobin, and can be central or peripheral. Peripheral cyanosis results from poor peripheral perfusion caused by vaso-constriction or low cardiac output resulting in increased oxygen removal from the blood available. Peripheries may be cool as well as cyanosed. Central cyanosis is due to a failure of blood oxygenation and can be respiratory or cardiac in origin. Cardiac causes may be due to poor cardiac output, or a right to left shunt. Respiratory causes may be due to hypoventilation, and venti-lation–perfusion mismatch and should respond to supplementary oxygen therapy (unlike right to left shunt). Skin temperature and in particular core/peripheral temperature difference is a useful indicator of peripheral perfusion. In general the core peripheral gradient should not be greater than 2 °C. However, this may not be the case in patients with septic shock or those who have received peripheral vasodilators (phenoxybenzamine, sodium nitraprusside) where perfusion may not be adequate despite a small core/peripheral gradient and other parameters need to be assessed such as acid–base status and urine output.

Capillary return is often assessed by squeezing the pulp of a finger or toe and looking at the rate of return of colour. Greater than 3 s is abnormal.

The presence of oedema in children in the ICU is often multifactorial and not necessarily because of right heart failure. Fluid overload, leaky capillary in association with septic syndrome, prolonged cardiopulmonary bypass and hypoalbuminaemia can all contribute. The loss of spontaneous movement due to sedation and paralysis contributes significantly to fluid retention.

Assessment of peripheral pulses for both timing and volume can aid in diagnosis, particularly of coarctation. Displaced apex beat is suggestive of left ventricular hypertrophy and parasternal heave suggestive of right ventricular enlargement. Presence of a triple rhythm and enlarged liver is indicative of congestive failure.

ECG monitoring

Standard three lead monitoring is the most useful in the paediatric popula-tion. Heart rate is the main contributor to cardiac output in the compliant infant heart and should be closely monitored. The occurrence of arrhythmias particularly in the postcardiac surgical patient is common. Interference with the conduction pathway can result in varying degrees of heart block. Over-filling and handling of the atria may contribute to the development of atrial fibrillation. Ischaemic changes on the electrocardiograph are less common in comparison to adult practice but can occur after arterial switch or other operations involving the aortic root.

Blood pressure monitoring

The mean blood pressure is the product of cardiac output and systemic vascular resistance. Its value is important in that it determines the perfusion of the vital organs (brain, heart, liver, kidneys). Although these vascular beds autoregulate, their ability to do this in conditions of physiological disturbance is greatly reduced and bloodflow through the organs is directly related to mean blood pressure.

Blood pressure can be measured by invasive and non-invasive techniques.

Non-invasive methods

Non-invasive methods of blood pressure measurement involve occlusion of an artery (most often brachial) and a method of detecting pulsation distal to the occlusion. Detection devices include palpation by the fingers, Doppler probe and pulse oximetry. These measurements give an indication of systolic blood pressure in relation to the detection of bloodflow. The mercury sphygmomanometer in combination with auscultation uses the Karotkoff sounds to determine the systolic and diastolic pressures. In all these methods it is important to use the correct cuff size. Bladder width should be approximately 40% of the circumference of the extremity, as too small a cuff results in a high reading and too large a cuff results in a low pressure reading.

Automatic measurement using oscillometry (Dinamap) is frequently used when direct arterial pressure measurement is not required. A single bladder cuff with two tube connections is used. One tube is used to inflate the cuff, the other detects the pressure changes as the cuff is automatically deflated. In this way systolic, diastolic and mean pressures are measured. This technique tends to over-read at low pressures and under-read at high pressures. It is troubled by motion artefact, irregular rhythms (atrial fibrillation) and rapidly changing blood pressures.

Finapres is a non-invasive device which has been developed to give continuous blood pressure measurements. The device uses a photoplethysmograph (similar to a pulse oximeter) and a pneumatic finger cuff to maintain the finger volume constant by a cuff pressure equal to intra-arterial pressure. In this way a waveform of cuff pressure can be analysed to determine systolic and diastolic pressure. The area under the curve will be equal to diastolic pressure. It has been found that in critically ill adults it could not be used as an alternative to intra-arterial monitoring.

INDICATIONS FOR INVASIVE ARTERIAL PRESSURE MONITORING

Invasive arterial pressure monitoring should be undertaken in cardiac surgery, surgery where rapid blood loss is anticipated, in the shocked, unstable patient,

in inotropic, vasodilator manipulation of the cardiovascular system, and where there is a requirement for frequent blood sampling.

The technique is not without risk and distal ischaemia, tissue necrosis and infection have all been described. The incidence of complications is related to the length of cannulation, age of the patient (less than 1 year) and weight. Clear labelling of the line and cannula should prevent inadvertent injection of drugs.

The system requires a cannula, plumbing system and a transducer which converts the pressure waveform into an electronic signal. The cannula should be made of a non-irritant, flexible material which does not kink. Tubing should be rigid, wide and as short as possible to avoid distortion of the waveform in travelling to the transducer. Disposable transducer systems are routinely used now as they reduce infection and avoid the requirement for sterilization. A continuous heparinized flush system prolongs the life of the cannula. In small infants, this should be via a syringe driver at a controlled low rate of 0.5–1.0 ml/h.

CENTRAL VENOUS PRESSURE MONITORING

Monitoring the central venous pressure (CVP) can give useful information regarding the intravascular volume and right sided filling pressures. There are conditions where the absolute value obtained may be inaccurate (tricupsid regurgitation, elevated sympathetic tone, increased intrathoracic pressure due to positive pressure ventilation), but it is the change in pressure accompanying volume administration which is of greater clinical use. Catheter placement is achieved most commonly by the internal jugular or subclavian route using a 4 or 5 French catheter of appropriate length, usually 5 or 8 cm. The ease of placement is influenced by the weight and age of the patient. Correct placement should be confirmed by free back flow of blood and a plain chest radiograph.

Insertion technique and approaches

The Seldinger technique (needle, guidewire, catheter) is the most common method for insertion of multi-channelled lines. Some practitioner prefer the catheter over the needle when placing single lumen catheters which will not be in place for a long period.

Internal jugular cannulation has been described using many different approaches. The favoured approach which is suitable for all paediatric age groups is a mid-level approach. The child is positioned suprine with 10° head down tilt, a roll or small sandbag under the shoulders and the head turned 45° to the opposite side. The most reliable landmark for the internal jugular vein is the apex of the triangle formed by the sternal and clavicular heads of the

sternomastoid muscle. The vein can often be ballotted here and sometimes the venous pulsation can be visualized. A useful cross-check is to make sure that this landmark falls along the expected line of the vein running from the mastoid process to the sternoclavicular joint. A higher approach has a lower incidence of pneumothorax but a higher incidence of carotid puncture in infants. If the carotid is palpated and the medial border of sternocleidomastoid identified the insertion site is between the two. Aiming away from the carotid accidental puncture should not happen. The operator should always be cautious of moving medially when locating the internal jugular. It must be appreciated that the pressure of the fingers on the carotid should be minimal as it is enough to completely compress the internal jugular vein and enables the needle to pass through the vein without any flashback. In patients with low CVP the pressure exerted by the needle as it passes through the skin is enough to compress the vein and this is especially the case with some of the short-bevelled needles provided by manufacturers. A brief pause once through the skin will allow the vein to fill again. Once located with the needle the syringe should be removed and the flow of blood observed. A steady flow indicates that the needle is within the lumen of the vein and not partially in. Pulsatile flow strongly suggests arterial puncture and the needle should be removed. However, colour and pressure are not always helpful in the severely shocked patient or in the child with cyanotic congenital heart disease. The guide wire should pass easily and not be advanced too far. The assistant should observe for arrhythmias induced by the wire hitting the atrial wall. The dilator should pass easily, and should not be passed more than 1 cm, a slight give indicating that the dilator has passed into the vein. Once the catheter has been passed check for easy aspiration of blood, or free back flow when attached to a line held below heart level. A portable chest X-ray should be taken to ensure correct placement.

Subclavian approach

The subclavian route is more common for long-term cannulation but has a higher incidence of catheter malposition than the internal jugular approach. It becomes particularly difficult in the oedematous patient when land marks are poorly identified. Attempted cannulation in patients with a coagulopathy is not recommended due to the difficulty in applying pressure to the subclavian artery if accidental puncture occurs. Placing a roll longways down the back allows the shoulders to fall back and helps in needle placement between the first rib and clavicle. The patient should be placed head down, with the head turned away from the site of entry. The sternal notch, angle of the clavicle, subclavian artery and the deltopectoral groove are identified before needle insertion. Entry 0.5 cm lateral and below the mid-third of the clavicle makes it easier to pass between the clavicle and first rib. Once through the skin it is important to keep the needle parallel to the skin to avoid lung puncture. The

needle should be advanced with negative pressure on the syringe aiming for the triangle formed by the clavicular and sternal heads of sternocleidomastoid muscle. The same measures as outlined above should be taken to ensure venous puncture.

Femoral vein

The femoral vein is easily located and is most often used in the emergency situation. There have been questions raised about the incidence of infection and the occurrence of femoral thrombus when used for a prolonged period. It can not be relied upon for accurate measurement of CVP although it is an alternative route for passing a pulmonary artery catheter (see below). It is the route of choice for catheterization studies in children with congenital heart disease.

A useful method of cannulating the vein is to use the Seldinger technique having located the vein with a 21 gauge butterfly winged needle. Once free flow of blood is observed, the small extension tubing is cut off and the guide wire is passed via the butterfly needle.

Points to pick out on the AP chest X-ray after line placement

After line placement, the X-ray should be studied to ensure that:

- the catheter tip is in the superior vena cava and not the atrium, inferior vena cava or subclavian vein—on the AP film the tip should not be below a line drawn between the lower border of the medial ends of the clavicles.

- the catheter is not in the pleural cavity

- there is no pneumothorax or haemothorax.

The soft tissues in the neck should also be checked if carotid puncture occurs.

Complications of internal jugular cannulation

Complications include:

- carotid artery puncture

- pneumothorax

- air embolism

- sepsis

- incorrect placement (extra vascular/intra-thoracic/thoracic duct mediastinal vessels)

- nerve damage.

Table 9.1 Values which can be obtained or calculated from the PA catheter

Stroke volume	SV = CO/HR	50–80 ml
Cardiac index	CI = CO/BSA	3.5–5.5 l/min/m^2
Systemic resistance	SVRI = 80(MAP–CVP)/CI	800–1600 dyn s/cm^5/m^2
Pulmonary resistance	PVRI = 80(MPAP–PCWP)/CI	80–240 dyn s/cm^5/m^2

Pulmonary artery catheters

The use of pulmonary artery catheters other than those placed under direct vision during cardiac surgery is rare in paediatric practice. The reason for this reluctance is related to technical difficulty in floating the catheter into the pulmonary artery, potential complications such as pulmonary artery rupture and until recently the availability of small enough catheters. Routing the catheter from the left subclavian or femoral veins helps. Preforming the catheter tip into a gentle curve by wrapping it round the finger prior to insertion is useful in steering the catheter around the acute angles within a small heart.

The following points are important when inserting these catheters:

1. Before passing the catheter check the integrity of the lumens and ensure that the balloon inflates beyond the end of the catheter. Check the volume required to inflate the balloon (0.5 ml for 5Fr catheter).

2. Check that the PA transducer is attached and working before passing the catheter.

3. Inflate the balloon once you have advanced the catheter into the superior vena cava. Only advance the catheter with the balloon inflated. Only pull the catheter back with the balloon deflated.

4. Make a note of the distances at which the various pressures are found.

5. Once the catheter wedges, deflate the balloon to ensure that a normal PA pressure tracing is obtained.

6. To ensure accuracy of the pulmonary artery wedge pressure check the position of the catheter on chest X-ray. It should lie in the lower lung zone where mean LA pressure is greater than alveolar pressure. Make the wedge reading at end expiration.

7. Ensure that the catheter does not become wedged accidentally. Always inflate the balloon slowly and stop inflating once it has wedged. The catheter can lengthen as it heats up and the position of wedging should be rechecked.

The indications for pulmonary artery catheter placement are not dissimilar to those guiding adult practice:

- global cardiac dysfunction as found in severe septic shock
- disparity between left and right ventricular function
- pulmonary hypertension
- serial cardiac output determination
- changes in pre-/afterload resulting in left ventricular dysfunction.

Directly placed PA catheters after complex cardiac surgery (e.g. Fontan, Glenn) in combination with a left atrial line give valuable information in relation to fluid management and ventricular function. Rising pressures may be due to fluid overload, ventricular failure or mechanical obstruction of bloodflow. Obstruction may be surgical in origin or due to pulmonary vasoconstriction or pulmonary artery stenoses.

Pulmonary capillary wedge pressure and left atrial pressure will correlate with left ventricular end diastolic pressure in cases with no mitral valve disease and normal ventricular compliance. This enables therapy to be directed towards preload enhancement or after load reduction. The calculation of cardiac output by thermodilution is useful in the tailoring of inotropic therapy and is discussed below. The latest catheters have oximetric capability which allows the measurement of mixed venous saturation. The trend of this measurement rather than the actual figure may help in assessing global cardiovascular function.

Complications associated with the PA catheter

The complications include:

- dysrhythmias
- air embolus
- coiling/knotting in the left ventricle
- thrombus at the catheter tip
- balloon rupture
- pulmonary infarction
- perforation of heart or great vessel.

Cardiac output measurement

There are three techniques of measuring cardiac output directly:

- Fick

- dye dilution

- thermal dilution.

Thermal dilution is the most practical technique for clinical practice. The Fick method requires measurement of oxygen consumption and arterial and mixed venous O_2. Dye dilution has the problem of distal blood sampling, and recirculation which reduces the frequency of repeating the method. Thermodilution is accurate and reproducible enough for clinical use but the accuracy of the technique falls off as smaller volumes of injectate are used. One millilitre is the minimum injectate volume for most paediatric systems. Volume overload and cooling are theoretical problems most likely to occur in the small infant due to repeated injection for cardiac output measurement. The time of injecting the cold injectate can influence the results obtained and it is best to time the injections with end expiration.

Another development in adult practice is a continuous CO catheter which uses thermodilution principles but operates by heating the blood passing a miniature element. This minibolus of blood is then detected by a sensor. The heat/cold cycle is very rapid and controlled by a microprocessor to give a continuous readout.

The wish to measure cardiac output by a non-invasive technique has led to the development of Doppler techniques. The principle used is that sound waves are reflected from a moving object at a different frequency. The sound-waves are directed towards the aorta from one of the following positions: (1) suprasternal notch, (2) trachea, (3) oesophagus, and (4) probe applied directly to the aorta during surgery. The sound waves are reflected by the moving blood cells and their mean elocity can be calculated. The flow can be determined by measuring the cross-sectional area of the aorta. The problem with the external probe placements is that the exact cross-sectional area of the aorta can not be determined. Since it is elastic in nature the aorta changes in area between systole and diastole. Using pulsed Doppler the beam can be focused and therefore the depth at which the measurement is being made is known and a more accurate cross-section determined. In situations where the aortic diameter can be measured directly the accuracy is increased. The accuracy of a trans tracheal probe in post cardiac adults has been investigated and it was found that the technique was not accurate or reliable enough to compare it to thermodilution cardiac output. The *trend* of the value obtained by Doppler techniques or acute changes in the value are probably more useful than the actual reading and in this way may be of value in altering treatment.

Monitoring the central nervous system in the ICU

Monitoring the central nervous system is particularly important in the treatment of patients with the following disorders:

- head injury as a result of trauma

- hypoxic, ischaemic cerebral insult
- encephalopathy/Reye syndrome
- meningitis
- status epilepticus
- metabolic upset.

Glasgow Coma Scale

The Glasgow Coma Scale (GCS) was devised to enable standardized assessment of the head trauma patient for referral to neurosurgical units. The GCS can be used in children over 4 years of age but for younger children a modified scale has to be used (see Table 9.2). Initial GCS should not be assessed until hypotension or hypoxia have been stabilized thus ensuring that the score is due to the brain trauma. In the ICU where patients are often intubated, paralysed and sedated the GCS is not easily scored. A GCS score should be obtained on as many ICU admissions as possible but if the patient is paralysed or sedated and there is an accurate GCS score obtained before such treatment (and no reason to suspect that the patient's neurological status has changed) the previous GCS score can be carried forward to the current day. If there is the suspicion that the patient's neurological status has changed substantially from a previous determination, and the sedation or the paralysis can be safely reduced for a short time, a repeat neurological evaluation without sedation should be done. If there is neither an earlier GCS determination, and the sedation or paralysis cannot be reduced, the GCS score should be recorded as normal. Intubated patients should be given a verbal pseudoscore of one and the fact that they are intubated noted. Patients with severe periorbital swelling should be given an eye-opening pseudoscore of one and the swelling documented. It is important to have a consistent method of scoring patients who have been paralysed, intubated and sedated before admission to hospital and using the above guidelines moves some way towards that.

The GCS is used as a guide to the requirement of ventilatory support in traumatic head injury. Patients with a score less than or equal to 8 should be intubated and ventilated. Patients with a deteriorating GCS score who require transfer to another centre should have their airway secured and ventilation controlled. Coma in children who have suffered traumatic head injury increases the risk of clot 200-fold, compared with a fully conscious patient. The GCS score may be limited in predicting outcome in children with traumatic brain injury in the absence of hypoxic–ischaemic injury. With aggressive neuroresuscitative measures a significant number of children with GCS scores of 3–5 can be expected to function independently if they survive.

Table 9.2 Glasgow Coma Scale

Activity	Best response	Score
Glasgow Coma Score		
Eye opening	Spontaneous	4
	To verbal stimuli	3
	To pain	2
	None	1
Verbal	Oriented	5
	Confused	4
	Inappropriate words	3
	Non-specific sounds	2
	None	1
Motor	Follows commands	6
	Localizes pain	5
	Withdraws to pain	4
	Flexes to pain	3
	Extends to pain	2
	None	1
Modified Coma Score for Infants		
Eye opening	Spontaneous	4
	To speech	3
	To pain	2
	None	1
Verbal	Coos and babbles	5
	Irritable cries	4
	Cries to pain	3
	Moans to pain	2
	None	1
Motor	Normal spontaneous movements	6
	Withdraws to touch	5
	Withdraws to pain	4
	Abnormal flexion	3
	Abnormal extension	2
	None	1

EEG

The electroencephalogram (EEG) is a recording of the summation of excitatory and inhibitory postsynaptic action potentials in the underlying neurons. The frequency and amplitude of the waveforms seen on the EEG are outlined in Table 9.3. The arrangement of the electrodes on the scalp is known as the montage. The full montage of the International Ten Twenty System uses 21

Table 9.3 EEG wave forms

Waveform	Frequency	Amplitude
Beta	14–30 Hz	$<20\ \mu V$
Alpha	8–13 Hz	$20–50\ \mu V$
Theta	4–7 Hz	$20–50\ \mu V$
Delta	1–4 Hz	$>50\ \mu V$

Beta: awake, alert, eyes open, produced by barbiturates, benzodiazepines, phenytoin, alcohol.
Alpha: awake relaxed, eyes closed.
Theta: normal in children and the elderly. Produced by hypothermia, may indicate neuronal dysfunction by disease or drugs.
Delta: normal during sleep and deep anaesthesia, indication of neuronal dysfunction.

accurately placed electrodes and generates a large volume of information which is difficult to interpret. In an attempt to simplify the information displayed the cerebal function monitor (CFM) and later the cerebral function analysing monitor (CFAM) were developed.

The CFAM uses three monitoring electrodes. It displays the frequency and amplitude of the waves. The amplitude analysis is charted on a logarithm scale showing the mean, 10th centile, 90th centile and the absolute maximum and minimum amplitudes. The frequency analysis shows the proportion of each frequency band present (alpha, beta, theta, delta) and the relative amount of scalp muscle activity. An indication of burst suppression may also be shown. The monitor will also display the raw EEG which is being analysed.

Application of the EEG in the ITU

The EEG is used mainly to monitor coma and the treatment of status epilepticus when the clinical appearances of the fit are hidden by sedation and paralysis. Characteristic temporal discharges can be seen in herpes encephalitis, although a non-specific flattening of the EEG is often seen in severe bacterial meningitis. Cerebral contusion and ischaemic areas after traumatic head injury can result in EEG changes and epileptiform discharges. Post-traumatic epilepsy can occur within 24 h of head injury in children. Acute cerebral ischaemia shows up initially with high amplitude beta waves which will progress to predominantly low amplitude theta and delta activity and eventual electrical silence if this is not corrected.

Intravenous anaesthetics can be used to give cerebral metabolic protection and can be titrated until the patient shows burst suppression on the CFAM. Monitors are currently being developed to measure depth of sleep, sedation and anaesthesia and these will need careful evaluation in different age and diagnostic groups.

Intracranial pressure monitoring

There are four methods of measuring intracranial pressure (ICP): (1) intra-ventricular catheter, (2) subarachnoid screw, (3) extradural catheter, and (4) intracerebral catheter tip transducer.

The intraventricular catheter is the gold standard and has the advantage of being able to remove cerebrospinal fluid (CSF) for acute decompression. The indications for measuring ICP are not universally agreed and monitoring is often not undertaken because of the lack of on site expertise. There is a relatively high infection rate (15–20%) and reliable measurements can not always be obtained for more than a few days. A recent study of 19 paediatric ICUs indicated that 2% of children admitted to these units received ICP monitoring.

Monitoring systems which show a wave trace as well as an actual mean pressure are more useful than an isolated number. The normal ICP is less than 15 mmHg and should show arterial pulsation on top of cyclical respiratory changes. The ICP should not be looked at in isolation in patients who have lost the ability to autoregulate cerebral bloodflow. This happens after trauma, cerebral infection, and hypoxic injury. The cerebral perfusion pressure in such cases is the driving pressure and is equal to the mean arterial pressure minus the ICP. When the cerebral perfusion pressure is less than 40 mmHg cerebral perfusion can be expected to be compromised and cerebral ischaemia likely. Cerebral bloodflow is either normal or slightly below normal shortly after head injury and in such circumstances the use of hyperventilation may induce cerebral ischaemia as a result of cerebral vasoconstriction. It would appear that measurement of cerebral bloodflow or flow velocity in conjunction with jugular venous saturation values should show true hyperaemia before profound hyperventilation in head-injured children is started.

The outcome over a 2-year period of patients who underwent ICP monitoring has been studied in two broad groups: (1) hypoxia or ischaemic injuries (HII), and (2) non-hypoxic or non-ischaemic injuries (NHII). Patients with NHII faired better and may benefit from ICP monitoring and treatments aimed at reducing ICP. The benefit of ICP monitoring in Reye syndrome where brain swelling is thought to be cytotoxic in origin is more widely agreed on. It was also felt that ICP monitoring may be of benefit in children with bacterial meningitis who are in coma or have evidence of brain swelling on computed tomography. The poor outcome in children with HII probably reflects the severity of the hypoxic or ischaemic insult at the time of injury.

Peripheral nerve stimulator

The peripheral nerve stimulator is a useful monitor for assessing the extent of neuromuscular block in patients receiving paralysing agents on the ICU. In

particular children who are receiving infusions of muscle relaxants should have their train of four response monitored to avoid profound prolonged paralysis. This can be a problem in patients with renal dysfunction where excretion of relaxant is impaired. Intermittent boluses of a relaxant titrated to the train of four response avoids such a problem. When paralysis and sedation are weaned it is important not to under sedate a partially sedated patient and the train of four response and post-tetanic count should be normal before sedation is reduced. It is also worth excluding residual neuromuscular block in a previously paralysed patient before ventilation is weaned.

Monitoring renal function

In the acutely ill child and post-surgical patient renal monitoring is directed towards maintaining an adequate volume and composition of extracellular fluid and the prevention of acute parenchymal renal failure. Analysis of the urine can help in the detection of systemic disease namely haemolysis, rhabdomyolysis, and ketoacidosis. The presence of haemoglobin in the urine in the absence of red blood cells suggests the presence of haemolysis or rhabdomyolysis. Bedside tests for the presence of haemoglobin do not distinguish between red blood cells and free haemoglobin or myoglobin. Myoglobin is the haem pigment present in muscle cells which can be released into the circulation after muscle injury. Haemoglobinuria and myoglobinuria are both associated with a high risk of acute renal failure.

Glycosuria occurs when the renal absorption threshold is passed and should lead the clinician to check plasma glucose. If the plasma level is normal then proximal tubular epithelium function needs to be assessed. Ketoacids are rapidly transported from the plasma into the tubular fluid by the proximal tubule and ketonuria precedes significant elevation of plasma ketone bodies.

Serum creatinine in itself is not a particularly accurate indicator of renal function. Changes in its level are influenced by its rate of production and the extracellular fluid volume. The rate of creatinine production is directly proportional to muscle mass which declines rapidly in critically ill patients. Creatinine is largely eliminated by glomerular filtration although tubular secretion of creatinine increases as serum creatinine increases. Thus creatinine clearance represents the maximum likely glomerular filtration rate (GFR). Changes in plasma creatinine reflect changes in renal function which are hours to days old.

Hourly urine output is easily measured if a catheter is *in situ*. This is always another source of possible infection and the risk benefit should always be assessed. The presence of a urine output at the rate of 1–1.5 ml/kg/h does not always guarantee good renal function especially if diuretics and dopamine are in use. The development of complete anuria should always make the clinician suspicious of catheter blockage, which should be excluded before other measures are taken.

Ultrasound evaluation can be helpful in detecting renal tract obstruction, renal vascular supply and drainage problems and in looking for fungal deposits in the renal pelvis.

Temperature

The monitoring of body temperature is very important in the paediatric patient as they are prone to hypothermia because of their large body surface area to weight ratio (0.075 m²/kg in the neonate, 0.025 m²/kg in the adult). Maintaining normothermia can put increased demands on the respiratory and cardiovascular systems and infants should be nursed under overhead heaters. Care must also be taken not to overheat them and the heater should be placed at an appropriate level above the infant. Premature neonates need specialist incubators to minimize heat loss.

The most common sites of measuring core temperature are the rectum, lower third of the oesophagus (which reflects cardiac temperature), and the nasopharynx (reflecting cerebral temperature, important for cerebral protection). During cardiopulmonary bypass and topical cooling of the myocardium a temperature probe inserted in the ventricle allows more accurate application of topical cooling and better myocardial protection. A mercury bulb thermometer placed over the axillary artery will generally be approximately 1 °C below core temperature.

IMAGING IN THE PICU

Chest radiograph

The chest radiograph is the most frequent image obtained in the PICU often as a routine investigation and part of the initial work-up of any acutely ill child. The maximum information obtained from the investigation is when the ICU clinician and the radiologist work closely together and communicate well. The position of tubes and lines, changes in lung parenchyma, pleural fluid or air, heart size and shape and unexpected cardiopulmonary changes are revealed. It is important to check specifically for pneumothorax which in the supine patient may be difficult to see. Remember anterior pneumothorax may require a shoot through lateral film to see clearly because on the AP film it may only be evident as a difference in opacity between the two hemithoraces. A subpulmonary pneumothorax can also be difficult to visualize.

COMMON TUBES WHICH ARE IDENTIFIED
ON THE CHEST X-RAY.

Airway tubes

OTT/ETT

The most important point in tube position (other than correct placement in the trachea) is its length. If too long, endobronchial intubation can result in contralateral lung collapse and obvious deterioration in respiratory function. Too short a tube means that the patient is at risk of accidental extubation. The tip of the ETT should sit in the midthoracic portion of the trachea approximately 1–1.5 cm above the carina. It is important that the head is in the neutral position and not artificially over extended or flexed when the X-ray is taken. Tracheostomy tubes should be assessed for length and position within the tracheal lumen. Pneumomediastinum and pneumothorax should be looked out for and bronchial obstruction should be excluded after initial placement.

Thoracostomy tubes

The position of mediastinal and pleural chest drains should be noted. The side holes of the chest tubes should be identified by interruption of the radio-opaque line and confirmed to be intrapleural. Subcutaneous placement of the chest tube is identified because the non-radiopaque edge of the tube is not silhouetted by the subcutaneous tissue.

CVP lines

Chest radiographs are requested after insertion of central monitoring lines to check the position of the line and look for immediate complications of insertion, namely pneumothorax, haemothorax and haematoma (mediastinal or neck). The operator should have a high index of suspicion if there was any difficulty in inserting the line. In order to monitor the CVP accurately the line tip should be beyond the venous valves and in an intrathoracic location. The last venous valves are located distal to the anterior first rib on the chest radiograph and a good guide is a line drawn through the lower border of the medial end of the clavicles. Subclavian lines are often seen to pass into the ipsilateral internal jugular vein or the contralateral brachiochephalic vein. It is important that the tip of these lines is not within the heart cavities, as perforation could lead to cardiac tamponade.

PA catheters

PA catheters are inserted via the internal jugular or the femoral vein and used as described earlier for pulmonary pressure monitoring, PAWP and cardiac

output. The position of the PA catheter should be within zone II of the lung field and not positioned too peripherally.

Coiling and knotting within the right ventricle should be excluded.

Complications of PA catheters, mainly pulmonary artery haemorrhage or pulmonary infarction, can be picked up on plain film.

Nasogastric tube

The tip of the nasogastric tube should be beyond the gastro-oesophageal junction and below the diaphragm (diaphragmatic hernia in trauma patients). The path of the tube should be traced to exclude placement in the bronchial tree because the presence of an endotracheal tube does not prevent passage of the tube into the trachea.

Atelectasis

This commonly occurs in patients who are sedated and ventilated. It has been noted in chest radiographs in 85% of patients after thoracic surgery and approximately 20% of patients after extrathoracic surgery.

Most atelectasis is caused by reabsorption of gas from the alveoli as occurs after acute bronchial obstruction. This is often seen in bronchiolitis where areas of atelectasis are seen in association with hyperinflation of other areas. With increasing F_IO_2 collapse occurs more rapidly as nitrogen diffuses out very quickly and may be apparent radiographically within minutes. This may account for the appearance of areas of collapse after electively intubating and ventilating children with primary respiratory pathology. The right upper lobe often collapses in ventilated children because the right upper lobe bronchial origin is dependent and acts like a sump for secretions.

The common occurrence of left lower lobe atelectasis after cardiac surgery may be related to the use of topical cooling of the heart. The left phrenic nerve is positioned between the pericardium and the mediastinal pleura and cooling can result in temporary paralysis of the left leaf of the diaphragm with subsequent left lower lobe infiltrate or atelectasis. Extensive mediastinal dissection always carries the risk of phrenic nerve damage and elevated hemidiaphragm should always be looked out for. This may also account for difficulty in weaning from the ventilator.

Signs of lobar collapse include displacement of interlobar fissures and increased radio-opacity. Various indirect signs include:

• deviation of the trachea

• narrowing of the rib-cage

• elevation of ipsilateral hemidiaphragm

- compensatory over aeration of uninvolved lung

- hilar displacement.

The left hilum is higher than the right in 97% of the normal population. The right hilum is never normally higher than the left.

Pulmonary oedema

Pulmonary fluid balance depends on the equilibrium between hydrostatic and plasma oncotic pressures, and normal capillary wall permeability. Disturbance of this balance results in pulmonary oedema which may be cardiogenic or due to increased permeability in ARDS.

Appearances on an erect chest film in cardiogenic pulmonary oedema include:

- cephalad redistribution of pulmonary venous flow

- interstitial oedema, peribronchial fluid accumulation

- septal lines

- pulmonary alveolar oedema.

In infants with obstruction of their pulmonary venous drainage varying degrees of pulmonary congestion occur appearing as bilateral interstitial oedema. Unilateral oedema can occur in children who have excessive flow through a systemic to pulmonary shunt. In ARDS (increased permeability pulmonary oedema), there is usually bilateral interstitial and alveolar consolidation. Oedema tends to be in a more peripheral distribution than cardiogenic alveolar oedema. As the condition progresses the patchy consolidation can coalesce with widespread air-space consolidation. Features of pleural effusion in the supine position include:

- increased homogenous density across the lung field

- loss of the normal silhouette of the hemidiaphragm

- blunting of the costophrenic angles

- apical capping

- elevation of the hemidiaphragm.

Abdominal radiograph

A checklist for evaluation of plain abdominal films would include the following questions:

- are the catheters in a satisfactory position?

- what is the bowel gas pattern?
- is all the air in the bowel lumen?
- is there abnormal calcification?

Ultrasound scanning

Cranial ultrasound can be carried out on infants under 18 months of age before closure of the anterior fontanelle, scanning through the posterior fontanelle can give good definition of the posterior fossa. Ultrasound is valuable in the diagnosis of hydrocephalus and intraventricular and periventricular haemorrhage and is used to screen infants on extracorporeal life support who are at increased risk of cerebral bleeds. Ultrasound gives clear images of the ventricular system and allows recognition of a wide range of congenital malformations. It will be of use in assessing infants who have suffered head trauma.

Free fluid in the thorax can be accurately located and guided aspiration reduces morbidity in small infants. The renal tract can be clearly visualized looking for polycystic disease, urinary tract obstruction, and pyelonephritis. Doppler ultrasound can be used to assess renal arterial and venous flow and is valuable in assessing the kidney after transplant.

Abdominal ultrasound is useful in locating free fluid and organ rupture after trauma but should not delay laparotomy in children with cardiovascular instability despite ongoing resuscitation.

Ultrasound of muscle groups may be used before biopsy in cases of possible myopathy.

CT scan

CT scan is the investigation of choice in children with altered consciousness following trauma, encephalitis or Reye syndrome.

Intracerebral or extracerebral haemorrhage will be identified and an assessment of brain swelling can be made. This may influence the decision to monitor ICP or the safety of carrying out a lumbar puncture. In intractable status epilepticus sequential computed tomography scans may show progressive brain atrophy and help in management decisions in such cases.

Magnetic resonance imaging (MRI)

Magnetic resonance imaging (MRI) is becoming more readily available and may be the investigation of choice in many neurological conditions.

LEARNING POINTS

1. The principles of monitoring critically ill children are the same as for adults but the size and different disease processes impose limitations on the use of some techniques.

2. Invasive monitoring should be used whenever the benefits outweigh the risks.

3. Full haemodynamic monitoring should be employed more often in critically ill children to guide therapy.

4. Intracranial pressure and neurological monitoring techniques need to be further studied in critically ill children.

5. Modern imaging techniques can greatly assist management of critically ill children.

FURTHER READING

Baskett PJF, Dow A, Nolan J, Maull K. *Practical procedures in anesthesia and critical care*. Mosby, London, 1995.

10

Sedation and analgesia for critically ill children

T.G. Hansen and N.S. Morton

Critically ill children undergoing mechanical ventilation frequently require sedation and/or analgesia.[1-4] The main purpose of this treatment is to improve the efficacy of mechanical ventilation but sedation and analgesia are also required to alleviate unpleasant experiences faced by children in the paediatric intensive care unit (PICU) (Table 10.1). Sedation and analgesia can also be used as therapy in patients with increased intracranial pressure, status asthmaticus, status epilepticus and to attenuate pulmonary hypertension.[1,2,5-8] Sedation should always be performed without compromising the child's haemodynamic stability.

Both non-pharmacologic and pharmacologic means can be used to improve mechanical ventilation in children, and in recent years ventilator technology has improved with new modes of ventilation which substantially decrease the need for pharmacologic intervention.

MONITORING OF SEDATION AND ANALGESIA

Children's need for sedation and analgesia varies widely. Some do not need sedation or analgesia, some need one but not the other while others need both sedatives and analgesics. Some children have a modest requirement while others require large doses to achieve satisfactory sedation and pain control.[1,2,9,10] The duration of treatment varies too. Occasionally only short-term sedation is necessary, but often sedation is required for many hours or days

Table 10.1 Goals of sedation and analgesia in PICU

Reduce fear, pain and stress responses
Prevent removal of drains, catheters, tubes etc.
Facilitate ventilation (synchronization, barotrauma, oxygen consumption and CO_2 production)
Control the pulmonary and cerebral circulation
Secure day/night cycle with appropriate sleep

Table 10.2 Different sedation scales

Alder-Hey Sedation Scale

1. No response to suction
2. Cough and slight limb movements in response to suction
3. Agitation with significant limb movements or crying in response to suction
4. Awake and moving but not agitated when not disturbed
5. Awake or restless or distressed when not disturbed

Addenbrooke's Sedation Scale

0. Agitated
1. Awake
2. Arousable
3. Awake by suction
4. Non-arousable
5. Paralysed
6. Asleep

and, more rarely, for weeks or months. In addition, the need for sedation and analgesia changes with time as the child recovers, deteriorates or becomes tolerant to the effects of the drugs used. It is clear that proper sedative and analgesic treatment requires that the level of sedation and analgesia is assessed regularly in a manner appropriate to the child's age. Appropriate doses of sedatives and analgesics are titrated against these assessments.

Numerous subjective scales have been described for use in the PICU for scoring sedation and/or analgesia (e.g. Ramsay's, Addenbrooke's, Cook's, Alder-Hey, Comfort, Bion, CRIES)[1,2,9,10] (Table 10.2). Many of these are too complicated for clinical use, some are useless in intubated children and none can reliably be used in paralysed children. They are behavioural observational scales, correlating different levels of sedation with the responses to verbal or physical stimulation, including medical or nursing procedures such as suctioning. Objective methods to evaluate levels of sedation are similar to those which attempt to measure levels of anaesthesia. These are based upon the processed electroencephalograph (EEG), for example the cerebral function monitor (CFM), cerebral function analysing monitor (CFAM), power spectral analysis of EEG (PSA), or upon measurement of lower oesophageal contractility or the frontalis electromyogram. None of these methods are used routinely in the PICU, as they are difficult to interpret and influenced by other factors than merely the level of sedation.[9,10]

In most ventilated, non-paralysed children, a simple behavioural observer scale will do (e.g. Comfort, Alder-Hey, Ramsay's) supplemented by the well

known physiological signs of the stress response such as changes in heart rate, blood pressure, oxygen saturation, pupils and sweating.

NON-PHARMACOLOGIC INTERVENTION

The fear, stress and discomfort experienced by children in the PICU are caused by many factors (Table 10.3). However, simple practical interventions can reduce the child's need for sedation. It is essential to comfort the child by involving parents in their care, avoiding hunger or thirst, providing warmth and human contact, ensuring a child-friendly environment with the child's own toys, music, videos, etc. Nasotracheal tubes are more comfortable and easy to manage and fix than orotracheal tubes. Ensuring that the endotracheal tube is not near the carina is also an important contributor to comfort and safety. Use of patient-triggered ventilator modes and avoiding hypercapnia and hypoxia all reduce the sedative requirements. Intravascular catheters used for haemodynamic monitoring can of course be used for blood sampling to minimize needling procedures (Tables 10.4 and 10.5).

Table 10.3 Causes of children's fear and discomfort in the PICU

Mechanical ventilation
Endotracheal tube
The causative disease
Different invasive procedures
Physiotherapy
Change of dressings
Disrupted sleep
Unfamiliar people and equipment
Separation from parents

Table 10.4 Reasons for excessive sedation requirement

Inadequate ventilation
Endotracheal tube near carina
Pain
Full bladder
Abnormal movements
Stimulant drugs (beta-2 agonist, theophylline, steroids, morphine-3-glucuronide)

Table 10.5 Non-pharmacological means which can reduce children's need for sedation

Presence of familiar people and objects (toys, clothes, etc.)
Normal day/night rhythm
Ensure the child's comfort (temperature, clothes, bed)
Regular verbal contact and human touch
Music, videos
Patient-triggered ventilation modes

PHARMACOLOGICAL INTERVENTION

Frequently some form of pharmacological intervention is required for ensuring sedation and pain relief. Many different drugs have been used (Table 10.6). However none of these fulfil the criteria for the ideal sedative (Table 10.7).[1,2] No drug alone can be expected to be efficient in all children. The combination of two or more drugs is usually necessary and hence detailed knowledge of several sedative drugs is important. Thus if a drug turns out to be inefficient or its use is associated with too many side-effects, try some of the alternatives rather than using ever increasing doses of a single agent.

Table 10.6 Guidance on intravenous dosing schemes for the most popular sedatives, analgesics and neuromuscular blocking agents in the PICU

Drugs	Bolus dose (mg/kg)	Infusion rate (mg/kg/h)
Midazolam	0.05–0.10	0.03–0.20
Morphine	0.05–0.10	0.01–0.03
Fentanyl		
Low dose	0.002–0.004	0.001–0.005
High dose	0.050–0.100	0.010–0.015
Ketamine	1.0–2.0	0.5–2.5
Pentobarbitone	1.0–3.0	1.0–5.0
Thiopenthone	2.0–5.0	2.0–4.0
Neuromuscular blocking agents		
Atracurium	0.30–0.60	0.30–0.60
Vecuronium	0.05–0.10	0.06–0.60

Table 10.7 Features of the ideal sedative agent

Quick onset/offset

Predictable duration of activity

No active metabolites

Effects dissipate when agent discontinued

Multiple options for route of delivery

Easy to titrate by continuous infusion

Limited effects on cardiorespiratory function

Effects and duration not altered by renal or hepatic disease—no interference with effect or metabolism by other drugs

Wide therapeutic index

No interference with the adrenal–pituitary axis

Basic pharmacology

Children differ from adults in the way they respond to drugs and exhibit a striking variability in pharmacokinetic and pharmacodynamic responses, especially when newborn or preterm.

Pharmacokinetics

In the PICU most drugs are administered intravenously, hence the absorption of drugs is always rapid and complete. The child's relative body composition varies with age. Neonates and especially preterm infants have a larger total body water compared to older children and adults. The preterm infant's total lipid content is lower than that of the neonate.

In the neonate the cardiac output is twice that of an adolescent (200 ml/kg/min vs 100 ml/kg/min). Thus, most drugs are distributed to and from their sites of action more rapidly in the neonate. The relative size of the brain in newborns and infants is larger and it receives a greater percentage of the cardiac output than in adults. Indeed the neonatal brain constitutes a significant target organ for lipid-soluble drugs but the neonate's ability to redistribute these drugs to muscle or fat tissue is limited. In normal children and adults the brain capillaries are relative impermeable to most ionized and hydrophilic molecules due to a lack of fenestrations between the endothelial lining of brain capillaries. In the neonate this barrier is poorly developed resulting in an increased penetration of partly ionized and/or hydrophilic drugs such as morphine and neuromuscular blocking agents (NMBs).

The protein binding capacity in neonates is reduced due to both a reduced concentration of plasma proteins (albumin, alpha-1-acid glycoprotein, gamma-globulins) and a reduced affinity for drugs. Furthermore, increased concentrations of free fatty acids and unconjugated bilirubin compete with acidic

drugs for binding sites. Most opioids and local anaesthetics are bound by alpha-1-acid glycoprotein.

The neonatal liver and kidneys are immature in function, thus influencing the rate of elimination and excretion of most drugs.[11] However, children from the age of 1–5 years eliminate lipid-soluble drugs much more quickly than older children and adults, presumably because these children have a larger liver-to-bodyweight ratio and/or increased liver bloodflow.[12]

Pharmacodynamics

In terms of drug/receptor relationships, the action of a particular drug can be influenced by developmental changes within the number, type, affinity, and availability of the different receptors. This seems particular important in the neonatal period. Evidence is emerging that in the neonatal brain the presence of most subtypes of opioid receptors is different compared to older children and adults. In addition the selectivity of mu-receptors for mu-specific ligands changes with age. These differences in number and affinity of the different opioid receptors may, at least in part, explain the increased susceptibility of neonates to opioid-induced respiratory depression.

The GABA receptor is presumed to be responsible for mediating the action of the benzodiazepines, the barbiturates and most anaesthetics. In the neonatal brain the numbers of GABA receptors are much lower than in adults. Furthermore, the GABA receptors present have lower affinity for benzodiazepines. This may also influence the potency of those drugs expressing their effect via the GABA receptor.

At the neonatal nicotinic acetylcholine receptor located at the neuromuscular endplate there is a highly significant reduction in the release of acetylcholine from nerves. This may explain the increased sensitivity to the effect of non-depolarizing neuromuscular blocking agents in the neonate.

Routes and techniques of administration

In most cases, the main route of administration is intravenous but if prolonged sedation is required alternative routes may be considered in certain circumstances (such as per oral, per rectal, nasal, transcutaneous, and inhalational).[1,2,13]

Since neonates and preterm infants show a wide pharmacokinetic and pharmacodynamic diversity it is logical to use a bolus infusion technique in these children, particularly when an infusion is to be commenced. The amount of drug which one wants to give as a bolus is infused for 30–60 min while monitoring the child's level of sedation, analgesia and vital functions. If the desired level of sedation is obtained before the total amount of sedative is infused, or undesired side-effects occur, the bolus infusion is stopped and the child is observed until sedation again is needed. This technique is useful in

evaluating each child's individual requirements. The time interval between two consecutive bolus infusions will often vary considerably.

Children suffering solely from respiratory insufficiency usually do not have the same need for analgesia compared to children following surgery. In the acute phase of these children's illness when endotracheal intubation, resuscitation, and insertion of intravascular catheters are performed, the combined use of sedatives, analgesics and NMB is often required. When the child is stable, it is essential to titrate the infusion rate of the chosen sedative towards the child's individual needs, monitored by means of a simple behavioural observer scale.[13]

Usage of opiods strictly for sedation is currently being widely debated. It is the authors' opinion that opioids should be used as *analgesics* or as a *supplement* to sedatives otherwise tolerance may develop.[2,13,14]

SPECIFIC PHARMACOLOGY

Benzodiazepines

The benzodiazepines are the most widely used sedatives in the PICU.[15-18] These drugs exert their effects via GABA-receptors within the limbic system in the brain and produce sedation, anxiolysis, amnesia, and peripheral muscle relaxation. The different benzodiazepines differ in terms of potency, efficacy, and selectivity of their effects. In some children, the sedative effect of benzodiazepines is unpredictable and they can produce disinhibition and restlessness. They have no analgesic effect at all and should not be used alone in the child in pain. Coadministration of an opioid or local anaesthesia is essential.

For many years diazepam was the most widely used benzodiazepine in the PICU. The terminal elimination half-life of diazepam is prolonged following repetitive dosages or infusion and it is metabolized into the pharmacologically active n-desmethyl-diazepam, whose elimination half-life can be up to 100 h in some individuals.[1,2]

Midazolam is a water-soluble imidazo-benzodiazepine. Following intravenous administration midazolam has a quick onset and a relatively short half-life of 2–4 h, but reaching 12 h in neonates and preterm infants.[18,19] For intensive care sedation, a continuous infusion is often required. The potency of midazolam is 2–4 times that of diazepam. Midazolam undergoes hepatic metabolism. Heparin competes with midazolam for protein-binding sites and hence increases the free plasma fraction of midazolam. Cimetidine inhibits the metabolism of midazolam. Patients with renal failure also have decreased protein binding and hence an increased free fraction. Prolonged sedation is often seen in children following termination of a long-term midazolam infusion even in patients without liver or kidney failure. This phenomenon is due to active metabolities: 1-hydroxy-midazolam, 4-hydroxy-midazolam and

1,4-hydroxy-midazoplam. These metabolites accumulate even more during renal and hepatic failure. A variety of routes of administration can be used for midazolam, e.g. oral, rectal, nasal, sublingual and intravenous. Use of midazolam is normally associated with cardiovascular stability as long as rapid or large bolus doses are avoided and caution is exercised in the hypovolaemic patient.[19,20] Midazolam does not affect the adrenal–pituitary axis. The literature concerning sedation with midazolam in the PICU mainly relates to older children in whom an infusion rate of 0.05–0.2 mg/kg/h is usually adequate. In preterm ventilated infants with respiratory distress syndrome (RDS), Jacqz-Aigrain *et al.*[18] showed in a randomized double-blind placebo-controlled design involving 46 preterm infants, that the use of a low-dose midazolam infusion technique satisfied the demands for sedation in these infants. Children with a gestational age older than 33 weeks received 60 micrograms/kg/h during the entire study period (5 d), whereas children younger than 33 weeks received 60 micrograms/kg/h for the first 24 h and thereafter only 30 micrograms/kg/h for the remaining periods of time. This regimen produced acceptable levels of sedation without compromising the baby's cardiovascular status. The course of the RDS was not influenced by the midazolam sedation, although a trend was seen towards a reduction in the incidence of persistent pulmonary hypertension of the newborn infant. In neonates who in addition to midazolam receive fentanyl as part of a sedative regimen a long-lasting hypotension requiring inotropic support has been reported.[20]

Tolerance during midazolam infusion as well as withdrawal symptoms following discontinuation of the infusion is common, especially in the smallest infants. Following long-term infusion, a slow reduction in infusion rate is advisable, rather than an abrupt discontinuation. A specific midazolam withdrawal syndrome comprising impaired social contact, poor feeding, confusion, hallucinations, choreoathetoid movements, dystonia and convulsions has been described in small infants sedated with midazolam. This syndrome is seen within a few hours following cessation of an infusion and disappears within 48–72 h.[21]

Opioids

Opioids have been used for sedation and analgesia in the PICU for many years. Morphine and fentanyl are the most investigated drugs.[1,2,22–25] In recent years it has been argued that opioids should not be used as sedatives in the ICU unless there is a specific need for analgesia or in cases where sufficient sedation cannot be obtained using midazolam or other sedatives. The half-life of morphine is dependent on the child's age: 14 h in the preterm infant, 9 h in the neonate, 2–4 h in the older child.[26,27] Morphine has considerably less analgesic effect than its metabolite morphine-6-glucuronide. Indeed morphine can be regarded as a prodrug of morphine-6-glucuronide which has a

much longer half-life than that of morphine in all age groups. In neonates, the half-lives of both morphine and morphine-6-glucuronide are prolonged due to immaturity of hepatic enzyme systems. In the immediate neonatal period a large proportion (10–30%) of neonates are unable to metabolize morphine to the more potent 6-glucuronide and so they do not obtain the same analgesic effect from a given dose of morphine.[26] Convulsions have been described in some neonates during morphine infusions which may be related to accumulation of morphone-3-glucuronide which is a central nervous system stimulant.

Morphine is being widely used for provision of safe postoperative analgesia in children. For instance following cardiac surgery a morphine infusion of 10–30 micrograms/kg/h is effective and does not significantly delay extubation.[22,28] The histamine release reported with the use of morphine can limit its use in some critically ill children, e.g. those with severe asthma or atopy. Morphine can cause immunosuppression when high doses are used for prolonged periods.[29–31] Titration of the dose against a regular reassessment of the levels of sedation and analgesia is important in order to allow the use of the minimum effective dose of opioids.

Fentanyl, a synthetic opioid, has been used increasingly for sedation in the PICU, especially in the United States.[23,24] Fentanyl is approximately 100 times as potent as morphine. It is metabolized in the liver and has no active metabolites.[32] The pK_a-value of fentanyl is less than that of morphine and the drug has a high lipid solubility. Following administration of a bolus dose, fentanyl has a quick onset and a short duration of action due to rapid redistribution. So fentanyl is generally considered to be a short-acting opioid. This is correct when fentanyl is administered infrequently and in small doses. High doses (>10–20 micrograms/kg) or prolonged administration of fentanyl reveals that in these circumstances it behaves like a long-acting drug with a terminal elimination half life of 2–5 h in older children, 8–12 h in neonates and 18 h in preterm infants.[32,33] The clearance of fentanyl is partly dependent on hepatic bloodflow. The hepatic enzyme system gradually matures within the first weeks of life. The increased clearance described in infants is a result of a larger liver to body weight ratio (extraction) and/or an increased liver bloodflow. The volume of distribution (Vd) of fentanyl is increased in infants due to a larger percentage of lipid tissue and/or an age-related increase in plasma protein binding capacity. Fentanyl is associated with cardiovascular stability even in high doses in critically ill neonates and preterm infants as long as rapid bolus doses are avoided and caution is exercised in the hypovolaemic patient. Furthermore fentanyl has a favourable effect on the pulmonary circulation in children with pulmonary hypertension where it blunts the rise in pulmonary pressures due to stimuli such as suctioning, e.g. in children with congenital diphragmatic hernia, or in those with congenital heart disease with a preoperative left to right shunt.[7,8] Low-dose fentanyl (1–5 micrograms/kg/h) is a highly effective regimen for sedation in neonates. In the older child fentanyl

has a limited sedative effect and coadministration of a sedative such as midazolam is often required. High-dose fentanyl (10–15 micrograms/kg/h), originally introduced as a postoperative continuation of intraoperative high-dose fentanyl anaesthesia has been shown to be beneficial in critically ill neonates and infants with pulmonary hypertension supplemented with 25 micrograms/kg prior to suctioning. However, with such high doses of fentanyl tolerance develops quickly resulting in the need to increase the infusion rate by 10–20% per 24 h. Discontinuation of an infusion is followed by severe withdrawal symptoms after this type of accelerating dosage schedule. Therefore following long-term sedation with high doses of fentanyl, a slow reduction in the infusion rate is required. Either a reduction in infusion rate of 10–20% per day, or starting oral methadone (0.05–0.1 mg/kg every 3–6 h) until the symptoms of withdrawal are controlled, followed by a slow reduction of methadone dosage each day is helpful.[23,24,34]

Opioids and benzodiazepines

When given in combination opioids and benzodiazepines show a pronounced synergism in terms of sedation, analgesia and cardiovascular depression.[20]

INTRAVENOUS AGENTS

Barbiturates

The barbiturates have been widely used in the PICU.[1,2] The rapid onset and recovery are because they are lipophilic and rapidly redistributed from the central nervous system to more peripheral tissues. Methohexitone, pentobarbitone, thiopentone and phenobarbitone are all metabolized in the liver.

The clearance of thiopentone in children is twice that of adults (6.6 vs 3.1 ml/kg/min) due to a significantly reduced terminal elimination half-life (6 vs 12 h). Except in neonates and preterm infants, there are no differences in volume of distribution and levels of protein binding between children and adults.

The role of barbiturates as sedatives in the PICU is limited because of their long half-life and the risks of cumulation. However, thiopentone and pento-barbitone are often used in the treatment of children with raised intracranial pressure (ICP) where they act by reducing brain cell metabolism and oxygen consumption. However, barbiturate sedation in patients with increased ICP has never been proven to influence the outcome in controlled trials. Blind treatment of an increased ICP is not an endpoint in itself. The purpose of sedation with barbiturates in children with increased ICP is to preserve cerebral perfusion and avoid tentorial herniation. Barbiturates not only influence the ICP but tend to reduce the mean arterial blood pressure. The net

effect is a reduction in cerebral perfusion. Barbiturates should therefore never be used in the haemodynamically compromised child. It has also been shown that patients with head trauma and increased ICP treated with barbiturates have an increased incidence of sepsis and acute ARDS.[35]

Sedation with barbiturates may be indicated in status epilepticus.

Recently it has been shown that the addition of pentobarbitone to long-term sedation with high dosages of midazolam and fentanyl in critically ill children on extracorporeal life support can reduce the need for other sedatives and analgesics, and in paralysed children the other drugs can be stopped. A loading dose of 2–4 mg/kg followed by a continuous infusion of 1–4 mg/kg/h is usually employed.[36]

Ketamine

Ketamine is a dissociative anaesthetic which resembles phencyclidine. The drug possesses both sedative, amnesic and analgesic properties. Ketamine is presumed to exert its effects via both central opioid and NMDA receptors. There is renewed interest in the use of low-dose ketamine as an analgesic (0.1–0.2 mg/kg; 0.1–1.0 mg/kg/h). It exists in two forms, with different effects and potency. The racemic mixture contains equal amounts of positive and negative enantiomers. Ketamine is a very lipophilic drug, which mainly undergoes hepatic elimination, primarily by *N*-methylation into nor-ketamine (which possesses one-third of ketamine's effect). Nor-ketamine subsequently undergoes hydroxylation and conjugation into a hydrophilic product which is eliminated via the kidneys. Distribution half-life is 5 min and elimination half-life is 130 min. Ketamine has not been properly studied in neonates and preterm infants.[2,6] The major advantage of ketamine is its association with cardiovascular stability primarily due to direct sympathetic stimulation. Indeed use of the drug in the PICU has been described in cases where sedation with midazolam and fentanyl was associated with severe cardiovascular depression. The pulmonary vascular resistance (PVR) and the pulmonary arterial blood pressure seem to be unaffected by ketamine in infants with or without severe pulmonary hypertension.[2] Ketamine has also been used in children with status asthmaticus who are not responding to conventional broncholytic treatment. This is due to sympathetic stimulation and bronchodilator effects.[2,6] As ketamine can produce stimulation of the central nervous system (CNS), coadministration of a benzodiazepine is recommended. Ketamine increases the secretion from salivary and bronchial mucous glands via a direct stimulation of central cholinergic receptors. This side-effect can be blocked using an antisialogogue such as atropine. Ketamine results in a significant increase in the ICP due to cerebral vasodilation and the drug should be avoided in children with increased ICP. This effect is mediated via activation of central cholinergic receptors and not as a result of increased cerebral metabolism.[2]

Propofol

Propofol is a phenol formulated in a lipid emulsion and is chemically unlike any other known anaesthetic or sedative. Propofol has primarily been investigated for short-term use as an anaesthetic, but became quickly introduced as a sedative in PICU due to its favourable pharmacokinetic profile with a short half-life. In theory it is easier to titrate, with a faster recovery time and a shorter period of weaning from the ventilator. The use of propofol has many side-effects.[2] In 1991 a series of case reports appeared to implicate propofol sedation with the deaths of children who were being mechanically ventilated for upper and lower respiratory tract infections. All children were sedated with large doses of propofol as the sole agent for several days. It is possible that the cardiac failure induced by sedation with propofol in children is due to the lipid emulsion rather than the propofol itself. The majority of these children received propofol at an infusion rate covering more than 50% of their daily fluid requirements.[37] For reasons which are still largely inexplicable, all children developed an increasing metabolic acidosis, cardiac failure with bradycardia and lipaemia and all the children subsequently died. Therefore, propofol is not recommended as a sedative drug in the PICU.

Inhalational anaesthetics

Several centres have described the use of inhalational anaesthetics such as isoflurane in the PICU. Isoflurane is extremely efficient, though the risk of patient and environmental pollution limits its more widespread use.[38] Use of these agents can be life saving in children with severe status asthmaticus, which is not responding to conventional treatment. However, these agents can cause hepatic toxicity, cardiovascular depression, arrhythmias, inhibition of hypoxic pulmonary vasoconstriction, and fluoride toxicity.[5]

Antihistamines

Promethazine (0.25–0.50 mg/kg, 8 hourly) or trimeprazine (1–2 mg/kg, 6–8 hourly) or chloral hydrate can be used to supplement opioids and midazolam. However, the use of these drugs has yet to be described in controlled studies. The use of chloral hydrate can be associated with hypotension, arrhythmias, respiratory depression, gastrointestinal bleeding, carcinogenicity, and genotoxicity. In addition the drug has a very narrow therapeutic index.

Non-steroidal anti-inflammatory drugs (NSAIDs) and paracetamol

NSAIDs can be used in postoperative patients in the PICU but care must be exercised in those at risk of bleeding, bronchospasm, renal dysfunction and gastrointestinal ulceration or bleeding. Paracetamol is frequently used to treat

pyrexia and can be used as an adjunct to opioid analgesia but accumulation of paracetamol following repeated doses can occur and care is required in children with hepatic dysfunction.

Local analgesia

Most local anaesthetic techniques can be used in children in the PICU, especially in the non-intubated/non-ventilated child. EMLA cream should be used prior to injections in the conscious child.[11]

Entonox

Inhalation of Entonox (a mixture consisting of 50% nitrous oxide and 50% oxygen) seems to be useful in the older cooperative child for analgesia for brief painful procedures such as removal of chest drains, change of dressings etc.

USE OF NEUROMUSCULAR BLOCKING AGENTS
(TABLE 10.6)

Neuromuscular blocking agents have been used extensively in the PICU, especially in mechanically ventilated neonates with RDS. The use of NMBs was instituted in an attempt to improve the oxygenation and reduce the fluctuations in haemodynamics and ICP to try to minimize the incidence of barotrauma and intraventricular haemorrhage.[39] However, the uncritical use of NMBs can increase morbidity in the critically ill, e.g. oedema, bed sores, venous thrombosis, prolonged paralysis and muscle atrophy.[28,40] NMBs are able to penetrate the blood–brain barrier and enter the CNS in patients with a non-intact blood–brain barrier (e.g. neonates, sepsis, diabetes mellitus and renal insufficiency) and very high concentrations of most NMBs have been found in the cerebrospinal fluid (CSF) of such patients. Most NMBs are convulsive. Within the CNS, the NMB can cause autonomic instability and neuronal damage. In recent years an NMB-associated polyneuromyopathy has been described, especially in patients receiving steroids and/or aminoglycosides or those having low plasma concentrations of calcium or magnesium. In several of these cases this condition was characterized by an acute quadriplegia and lack of motor-evoked potentials as well as loss of myosin.[28,40]

Tolerance is frequently associated with NMB use.

Both vecuronium and pancuronium are metabolized to 3-desacetyl metabolites which possess NMB properties and these accumulate in the presence of hepatic or renal dysfunction.

Atracurium is a mixture with a pH of 5.0. At a pH of 7.4 atracurium is subjected to Hofmann elimination to laudanosine and monacrylate as well as ester-hydrolysis. All these processes are independent of hepatic and renal

function. Laudanosine seems to be a convulsive agent, its half-life is pro-longed in the presence of renal failure and there is evidence that laudanosine may accumulate in patients with hepatic dysfunction.

Monitoring of the neuromuscular function is important whenever NMBs are used. A peripheral nerve stimulator and a train of four stimuli at 1 s intervals (TOF) is the most practical and effective means of avoiding NMB overdosing in critically ill patients, especially in those with multisystem organ failure. The aim is to see or feel at least one of four responses. If no responses are elicited, the infusion should be stopped and no bolus doses should be given until one out of four responses is seen again. Use of TOF does not pro-vide a 100% guarantee against prolonged paralysis (the neuromuscular function is being monitored not the muscle membrane function).[40]

NMB should be reserved for those patients in whom adequate ventilation can not be achieved by means of sedatives and analgesics and should never be used without adequate sedation and/or analgesia.

CONCLUSION

The wide variety of patients in the PICU (preterm infants to teenagers) and the broad spectrum of medical and surgical disorders encountered means that no cookbook of sedation and pain relief recipes can be provided. The impor-tant issue is to provide each child with a measured amount of sedation and analgesia based on the individual child's needs and a specific age-related pharmacologic knowledge. The chosen drugs should not be administered on the basis of mg/kg or mg/kg/h, rather the dose should be titrated against the desired effects (level of sedation and/or analgesia). In each case the necessary level of sedation should be decided on and regular reassessment of the level of sedation and/or analgesia should be recorded. The drug regimens should then be titrated to maintain the desired level of sedation and pain relief. In neo-nates and preterm infants bolus infusions of sedatives should be considered guided by scoring the level of sedation regularly using a simple behavioural observer scale. Children without any obvious need for analgesics should not routinely be given opioids. The use of NMBs should be reserved for those patients in whom adequate ventilation can not be obtained with sedatives and analgesics. The effect of the NMBs should be monitored by means of a nerve stimulator. Particular care is needed in patients with sepsis, diabetes mellitus, renal failure and in those patients with a compromised blood–brain barrier. If possible NMBs should not be used for more than 24 h without careful re-evaluation. There is still a need for studies regarding long-term use of seda-tives, analgesics and NMBs in the PICU in order to gain more information about their efficacy and potential long-term side-effects. Although many drugs are commonly used for sedation and analgesia in the PICU, the way in which they are used is often illogical. Careful reassessment and titration of

each drug against the desired effect for each individual child should be more widely practised.

LEARNING POINTS

1. Levels of sedation and pain should be routinely assessed in the PICU.

2. Sedative and analgesic doses should be titrated against the results of sedation and pain scores.

3. Muscle relaxants should only be used when adequate doses of sedation and analgesia are also being given.

4. The special sedation and analgesia needs of neonates, children with organ failure and those receiving extracorporeal life support need further investigation.

REFERENCES

1 Aitkenhead AR. Analgesia and sedation in intensive care. *British Journal of Anaesthesia* 1989; **63**: 196–206.
2 Arnold JH, Truog RD. Sedation in neonatal and pediatric intensive care. *Journal of Intensive Care Medicine* 1992; 7: 244–260.
3 Matthews AJ. An audit of sedation, analgesia and muscle relaxation in paediatric intensive care in the United Kingdom. *Paediatric Anaesthesia* 1993; 3: 107–115.
4 Marx CM, Rosenberg DI, Ambuel B *et al*. Pediatric intensive care sedation: Survey of fellowship/training programs. *Pediatrics* 1993; **91**: 369–378.
5 Hansen TG, Pedersen CM, Lybecker H. Severe bronchospasm in a one year old child treated with halothane. *Ugeskrift for Læger* 1994; 156: 58–59.
6 Tobias JD, Martin LD, Wetzel RC. Ketamine by continuous infusion for sedation in the pediatric intensive care unit. *Critical Care Medicine* 1990; **18**: 819–821.
7 Vacanti JP, Crone RK, Murphy JD *et al*. The pulmonary hemodynamic response to perioperative anesthesia in the treatment of high-risk infants with congenital diaphragmatic hernia. *Journal of Pediatric Surgery* 1984; **19**: 672–678.
8 Hickey PR, Hansen DD, Wessel DL *et al* Blunting of stress responses in the pulmonary circulation of infants by fentanyl. *Anesthesia and Analgesia* 1985; **64**: 1137–1142.
9 Marx CM, Smith PG, Lowrie LH. Optimal sedation of mechanically ventilated pediatric critical care patients. *Critical Care Medicine* 1994; **22**: 163–170.
10 Wang DY. Assessment of sedation in the ICU. *Intensive Care World* 1993; **10**: 193–196.
11 Hansen TG, Henneberg SW, Hole P. Postoperative pain management in children. *Ugeskrift for Læger* 1996 (in press).
12 Hansen TG, Henneberg SW, Hole P. Age-related postoperative morphine requirements in children following major surgery—an assessment using PCA. *European Journal of Pediatric Surgery* 1996 (in press).

13 Wolf AR. Neonatal sedation: More art than science. *Lancet* 1944; **344**: 628–629.
14 Wolf AR. Treat the babies, not their stress responses. *Lancet* 1993; **342**: 319–320.
15 Hartwig S, Roth B, Theisohn M. Clinical experience with continuous intravenous sedation using midazolam and fentanyl in the paediatric intensive care unit. *European Journal of Pediatrics* 1991; **150**: 784–788.
16 Rosen DA, Rosen KR. Midazolam for sedation in the pediatric intensive care unit. *Intensive Care Medicine* 1991; **17**: S15–S19.
17 Silvasi DL, Rosen DA, Rosen KR. Continuous intravenous midazolam infusion for sedation in the pediatric intensive care unit. *Anesthesia and Analgesia* 1988; **67**: 268–288.
18 Jacqz-Aigrain E, Daoud P, Burtin P *et al.* Placebo-controlled trial of midazolam sedation in mechanically ventilated newborn babies. *Lancet* 1994; **344**: 646–650.
19 Jacqz-Aigrain E, Daoud P, Burtin P *et al.* Pharmocokinetics of midazolam during continuous infusion in critically ill neonates. *European Journal of Clinical Pharmacology* 1992; **42**: 329–332.
20 Burtin P, Daoud P, Jacqz-Aigrain E *et al.* Hypotension with midazolam and fentanyl in the newborn. *Lancet* 1991; **337**: 1545–1546.
21 Bergman I, Steeves M, Burckart G *et al.* Reversible neurologic abnomalities associated with prolonged intravenous midazolam and fentanyl administration. *Journal of Pediatrics* 1991; **119**: 644–649.
22 Lynn AM, Opheim KE, Tyler DC. Morphine infusion after pediatric cardiac surgery. *Critical Care Medicine* 1984; **12**: 863–866.
23 Carr DB, Todres ID. Fentanyl infusion and weaning in the pediatric intensive care unit: Towards science-based practise. *Critical Care Medicine* 1994; **23**: 725–727.
24 Katz R, Kelly HW, Hsi A. Prospective study on the occurrence of withdrawal in critically ill children who receive fentanyl by continuous infusion. *Critical Care Medicine* 1994; **22**: 763–767.
25 Koren G, Butt W, Chinyanga H *et al.* Postoperative morphine infusion in newborn infants: assessment of disposition characteristics and safety. *Journal of Pediatrics* 1985; **107**: 963–967.
26 Chay PCW, Duffy BJ, Walker JS. Pharmocokinetic–dynamic relationships of morphine in neonates. *Clinical and Pharmacological Therapy* 1992; **51**: 334–342.
27 Choonara I, Lawrence A, Michalkiewicz A *et al.* Morphine metabolism in neonates and infants. *British Journal of Clinical Pharmacology* 1992; **34**: 434–437.
28 Elliot JM, Bion JF. The use of neuromuscular blocking drugs in intensive care practice. *Acta Anaesthesioligica Scandinavica* 1995; **39** (Suppl. 106): 70–82.
29 Tubaro E, Borelli G, Croce C *et al.* Effect of morphine on resistance to infection. *Journal of Infectious Diseases* 1983; **148**: 656–666.
30 Yeager MP, Yu CT, Campbell AS *et al.* Effect of morphine and beta-endorphin on human Fc receptor-dependent and natural killer cell function. *Clinical Immunology and Immunopathology* 1992; **62**: 336–343.
31 Krumholz W, Endrass J, Knecht J *et al.* The effects of midazolam, droperidol, fentanyl and alfentanil on phagocytosis and killing of bacteria by polymorphonuclear leucocytes in vitro. *Acta Anaesthesiologica Scandinavica* 1995; **39**: 624–627.
32 Koehntop DE, Rodman JH, Brundage DM *et al.* Pharmacokinetics of fentanyl in neonates. *Anesthesia and Analgesia* 1986; **65**: 227–232.
33 Collins C, Koren G, Crean P *et al.* Fentanyl pharmacokinetics and hemodynamic effects in preterm infants during ligation of patent ductus arteriosus. *Anesthesia and Analgesia* 1985; **64**: 1078–1080.

34 Anand KJS, Arnold JH. Opioid tolerance and dependence in infants and children. *Critical Care Medicine* 1994; **22**: 334–342.

35 Ward JD, Becket DP, Miller JD. Failure of prophylactic barbiturate coma in the treatment of severe head injury. *Journal of Neurosurgery* 1985; **62**: 383–388.

36 Tobias JD, Deshpande JK, Pietsch JB *et al.* Pentobarbital sedation in the pediatric intensive care unit patients. *Southern Medical Journal* 1995; **88**: 290–294.

37 Parke TJ, Stevens JE, Rice ASC, Grenaway CL, Brau RJ, Smith PJ *et al.* Metabolic acidosis and fatal myocardial failure after propofol infusion in children: Five case reports. *British Medical Journal* 1991; **305**: 613–616.

38 Arnold JH, Truog RD, Rice SA. Prolonged administration of isoflurane to pediatric patients during mechanical ventilation. *Anesthesia and Analgesia* 1993; **76**: 520–526.

39 Greenough A, Morley CJ, Wood S *et al.* Pancuronium prevents pneumothoraces in ventilated premature babies who actively expire against positive pressure inflation. *Lancet* 1984; **324**: 1–3.

40 Sladen RN. Neuromuscular blocking agents in the intensive care unit: A two edged sword. *Critical Care Medicine* 1995; **23**: 423–428.

11

Stabilization and transport of the critically ill child

N.S. Morton

Centralization of paediatric intensive care facilities means that more children will need to be moved to specialist units. It has been clearly shown that this results in improved morbidity and mortality rates for the sickest children[1] and that properly conducted transportation does not cause a deterioration in the patient's condition and outcome.[2] By recognizing critically ill children early, by thoroughly assessing and stabilizing their condition prior to transfer and by ensuring that appropriately experienced personnel accompany the child using appropriate equipment, secondary insults during transport can be avoided.[3]

The rank order of frequency of primary diagnoses in patients requiring transport to intensive care is different in adults and children (Table 11.1). The main reason is the higher incidence of infective causes of respiratory failure in children. This includes croup, tracheitis, epiglottitis, bronchiolitis, asthma, and pneumonia. Neurological dysfunction is a commoner reason for transport and may be due to primary central nervous system infection or secondary to sepsis, poisoning, hypoxia, ischaemia, trauma, epilepsy, or metabolic disorders.

EARLY RECOGNITION OF THE CRITICALLY ILL CHILD

As emphasized in Chapter 2, it is vital to recognize the early signs of respiratory, circulatory and neurological failure. Respiratory, circulatory and neurological status are all interlinked and failure of one affects the status of the others. A rapid clinical assessment of the work of breathing, respiratory rate and pattern, presence of stridor or wheeze, the breath sounds and the colour of the skin and mucosae will pick up the most important signs of impending respiratory failure. Pulse oximetry, capnography, capillary or arterial blood gases and pH are helpful, quick and easy to perform in all age groups. The heart rate, pulse volume, capillary refill time, skin colour, temperature and urine output are quick guides to circulatory status. Blood pressure, central venous pressure and electrocardiography provide additional information. Neurological status is determined by conscious level, posture and pupillary signs. The AVPU scale is a useful quick tool while the paediatric adaptation

Table 11.1 Range of diseases requiring critical care transport

Rank	Adult	Paediatric
1st	Trauma	Respiratory failure
2nd	Respiratory failure	Neurological dysfunction
3rd	Gastrointestinal disease or surgery	Major sepsis
4th	Major sepsis	Drug overdose or poisoning
5th	Neurological dysfunction	Burns or smoke inhalation
6th	Cardiovascular disease	Cardiovascular disease
7th	Drug overdose or poisoning	Trauma

Data from the Clinical Shock Study Group, Western Infirmary, Glasgow, and the Paediatric Intensive Care Unit, Royal Hospital for Sick Children, Glasgow.

of the Glasgow Coma Scale is an alternative.[4] More detailed assessments of severity of illness such as the paediatric risk of mortality (PRISM)[5] score or its modifications[6] or the Glasgow Meningococcal Scale[7] may be useful in decision making.

PRIORITIES BEFORE TRANSPORT

The priorities are the ABCDE of resuscitation with some important additions. The airway must be secure for transport and endotracheal intubation and stabilization of the cervical spine should be performed if appropriate. Ventilation must be controlled for transport if the patient is intubated. Bleeding must be controlled and the circulation must be optimized using fluids, inotropes, vasodilators and prostaglandins as appropriate delivered via appropriate intravascular lines and with intra-arterial blood pressure monitoring. In critically ill infants, hypoglycaemia is a possibility and should be sought and corrected. Intracranial hypertension should be treated in those at risk by controlling ventilation and by judicious use of diuretics, but urgent neurosurgical intervention may be required (see below). Prior to transfer, open wounds should be dressed and sutured if appropriate and fractures should be stabilized in suitable splints or plaster casts. For children with infectious diseases, cultures should be taken and antibiotic and antiviral chemotherapy should be started. This is especially important in meningococcal disease, meningitis and encephalitis. In small infants temperature maintenance is a major problem during transport and active warming measures, adequate covering with insulating layers and a heated incubator for neonates are important measures. Communication must be very good between the referring and receiving hospitals and adequate records of the patient and the management to date must be exchanged. The charts, clinical notes, results of investigations and copies of X-rays and scans must be passed on to the receiving hospital. A

detailed history from the parents/guardians must be obtained and parental transport and advice about the location of the receiving hospital intensive care unit should be given. Parents are usually not advised to travel along with their child but in certain circumstances this is the best option.

MONITORING DURING TRANSPORT

The most important safety feature during transportation of critically ill children is the presence of trained, experienced personnel monitoring the child and the equipment! Pulse oximetry is perhaps the single most useful monitor during transport but reliable information depends on the oximeter possessing the ability to reject artefacts due to movement. A portable electronic monitor incorporating pulse oximetry, electrocardiography, dual pressure monitoring, temperature measurement and capnography is very helpful. Non-invasive blood pressure recording is unreliable during transport as it is subject to movement artefact. Ventilation can be controlled by hand using an anaes-thetic T-piece circuit as long as a doctor who is familiar with this technique is present. A mechanical ventilator can be used but only a few transport ventila-tors are suitable for small infants (e.g. Baby Pac). Special neonatal transport incubators have built in simple ventilators which usually incorporate pressure and disconnection alarm functions.

ORGANIZATION OF PAEDIATRIC CRITICAL CARE TRANSPORT AND REFERRAL PROTOCOLS[8]

Paediatric intensive care units (PICUs) should provide a retrieval team for secondary transport of critically ill children from referring hospitals. However, at present many units are not resourced to guarantee a service and can only undertake to provide a team when staff can be released from duties at the receiving hospital. It is helpful to have a paediatric anaesthetist or intensivist and a paediatrician on the team and an experienced PICU nurse if possible. Even with dedicated transport teams, the response time is not immediate and so it is the responsibility of the referring hospital to perform the resuscitation of the child. This often involves securing the airway and vascular access and early involvement of senior anaesthetic or intensive care personnel at the refer-ring hospital is to be encouraged. The consultation and referral of critically ill children for transport to the regional PICU must be at consultant-to-consultant level and there should be an efficient telephone contact system to the duty PICU consultant involving one or at most two calls. Advice can be given by phone to assist the referring staff pending arrival of the transfer team

and portable phone contact is useful to keep the transfer team members updated on progress or deterioration and to give an estimated time of arrival. The child is the responsibility of the referring consultant until care is formally handed over to the transfer team at the bedside. Depending on the child's condition, the transfer team may have to spend some time on stabilization prior to departure. The PICU should be contacted, the most appropriate transport mode discussed and an estimated time of return given. It may not be possible to stabilize sufficiently some children for transport and this must be explained to relatives. Sometimes a transport team may already be on a call or may not be available and the referring staff may need to undertake the transfer but this should not be delegated to junior staff and an experienced anaesthetist should be involved in the transport in these circumstances. Head-injured children need special measures and every effort must be made to minimize delay in reaching neurosurgical care.

SPECIAL PROBLEMS OF CHILDREN WITH HEAD INJURIES[4]

Head-injured children present particular problems with some requiring immediate referral and transport for specialist neurosurgical care. In such cases it may not be appropriate to await the availability and arrival of a retrieval team and a team from the referring hospital may have to undertake the transport. An anaesthetist of suitable training and experience should be part of this team because these children often require intubation, controlled ventilation and careful monitoring. Those who need immediate intubation and controlled ventilation include those with a Glasgow Coma Score of 8 or less, those who have lost protective laryngeal reflexes, those who are hypoxaemic or hypercarbic or in whom spontaneous overventilation, periodic breathing or apnoea is noted. Some children are intubated and ventilated for the transfer and include those with deteriorating consciousness, facial or mandibular fractures, bleeding into the mouth or seizures.

Those head-injured children who require immediate referral and transport to a neurosurgeon include those with a skull fracture plus a Glasgow Coma Score <15, focal neurological signs, fits or other neurological signs; those with persisting coma; those whose conscious level is deteriorating; or those with focal pupillary or limb signs. Those head-injured children who should be referred urgently to a neurosurgeon include those in whom confusion persists for more than 6 h, those with compound depressed skull fractures, those with penetrating injuries, those with cerebrospinal fluid leaks from the ear or the nose and those with persisting or worsening headache or vomiting. Particular care is required when transporting children with head injuries to minimize changes in intracranial pressure and cerebral bloodflow due to acceleration, deceleration, hypoxaemia, and air expansion at altitude.

SPECIAL PROBLEMS OF MODE OF TRANSPORT

Road transport by ambulance carries with it the problems of acceleration and deceleration forces, movement artefact on monitors and motion sickness for staff and conscious patients. These are also problematic at sea and in air transport by fixed wing or helicopter. Temperature maintenance is a problem in small infants with all transport modes but particularly in military helicopters and at sea. Altitude is associated with a fall in ambient temperature but, more importantly with falls in both the ambient oxygen tension and the ambient pressure. This latter effect means that gas in closed spaces expands with increasing altitude and thus a given volume of air or gas in the thoracic cavity, cranium, mediastinum, pericardium, peritoneum, or obstructed viscus will try to increase in size but if contained the pressure in the cavity will rise. Unpressurized aircraft will be especially risky but even pressurized aircraft fly with cabin pressures equivalent to an altitude of around 2500 m. By special request some air ambulances can be pressurized to the equivalent of sea level but this reduces the airframe life. Helicopters produce a lot of vibration artefact on monitors and are very noisy giving communication problems. Space and visibility to work is often very limited in helicopters and fixed wing aircraft. Another important problem in all aircraft is electrical interference from medical equipment with the aircraft's electronic systems and vice versa.

ALPHABETICAL EQUIPMENT CHECKLIST FOR TRANSPORT OF THE CRITICALLY ILL CHILD

Airway

- face masks (neonatal to adult size)
- oropharyngeal airways (neonatal to adult size)
- endotracheal tubes (uncuffed sizes 2.0–6.5 mm internal diameter; cuffed sizes 6.0–8.5 mm internal diameter)
- laryngoscopes (neonatal to adult sizes and designs)
- intubation aids: Magill forceps (neonatal to adult size), bougies, introducers
- endotracheal tube fixation systems: tapes, adhesive foam, bandages, frames
- scissors
- minitracheostomy kit
- cricothyroidotomy kit
- nasogastric tubes.

Breathing equipment

- T-piece circuit
- self-inflating bags (neonatal to adult size)
- oxygen masks
- nasal oxygen speculae
- oxygen supplies (gas cylinders or portable liquid oxygen flasks)
- chest drains, valves, underwater seal drains
- suction equipment, catheters (neonatal to adult size), Yankauer suckers.

Circulatory access

- peripheral venous cannulae (14–24 gauge)
- central venous cannulae (single/double/triple lumen; 16–20 gauge)
- arterial cannulae (20–24 gauge)
- intraosseous needles
- butterfly needles
- syringes
- extension sets
- three-way taps.

Drugs

- sedatives
- analgesics
- muscle relaxants
- inotropes
- vasodilators
- diuretics
- anticonvulsants
- antihypertensives
- antiarrhythmics
- antibiotics
- antivirals
- prostaglandins
- broncholidators
- steroids
- resuscitation drugs pack.

Electrical equipment (check battery charged)

- pulse oximeter
- electrocardiograph
- invasive arterial pressure monitor
- central venous pressure monitor
- capnography
- temperature
- syringe drivers
- ventilator
- heating mattress
- insulating wrapping materials (bubble wrap, gamgee, foil wrap, foil swaddlers, baby hats)
- transport incubator for neonates.

Fluids

- saline (0.18%, 0.225%, 0.45%, 0.9%)
- dextrose (5%, 10%, 20%, 50%)
- mannitol (10%, 20%)
- colloids
- plasma.

Miscellaneous

- urinary catheters
- tape
- batteries
- bulbs
- artery forceps
- torch.

DRUGS CHECKLIST FOR TRANSPORT OF THE CRITICALLY ILL CHILD

- sedatives: midazolam, thiopentone, ketamine, etomidate, diazepam
- analgesics: morphine, fentanyl, lignocaine, bupivacaine
- muscle relaxants: vecuronium, pancuronium, suxamethonium
- inotropes: dopamine, dobutamine, enoximone, digoxin

- vasodilators: SNP, GTN, prostacyclin, phentolamine
- diuretics: frusemide, mannitol
- anticonvulsants: phenytoin, phenobarbitone, diazepam, chlormethiazole, paraldehyde
- antihypertensives: hydrallazine, labetolol
- antiarrhythmics: digoxin, propranolol, lignocaine, bretylium, adenosine
- antibiotics: benzylpenicillin, ampicillin, cephalosporins, aminoglycosides, metronidazole
- antivirals: acyclovir
- prostaglandins: PGE1, PGE2, PGI2
- bronchodilators: salbutamol, ipratropium, aminophylline, adrenaline
- steroids: hydrocortisone, methylprednisolone, dexamethasone, budesonide
- resuscitation drugs pack: adrenaline, atropine, bicarbonate, calcium, dopamine, dextrose, frusemide, lignocaine.

LEARNING POINTS

1. Paediatric critical care transport teams should be organized at a regional level and should be based at PICUs.

2. Referral of patients should be on a consultant-to-consultant basis.

3. Initial resuscitation is the responsibility of the referring hospital and should involve airway management if necessary.

4. Responsibility for the child is devolved to the transport team at a formal handover on arrival of the team.

5. Transfer teams should comprise trained and experienced personnel with equipment appropriate for paediatric patients.

REFERENCES

1 Pollack MM, Alexander SR, Clark N *et al.* Improved outcomes from tertiary center pediatric intensive care: a statewide comparison of tertiary and nontertiary care facilities. *Critical Care Medicine* 1991; **19**: 150–159.
2 Doyle E, Freeman J, Hallworth D *et al.* Transport of the critically ill child. *British Journal of Hospital Medicine* 1992; **48**: 314–319.
3 Barry PW, Ralston C. Adverse events occurring during interhospital transfer of the critically ill. *Archives of Disease in Childhood* 1994; **71**: 8–11.
4 Gentleman D, Dearden M, Midgley S *et al.* Guidelines for resuscitation and transfer of patients with serious head injury. *British Medical Journal* 1993; **307**: 547–552.

5 Pollack MM, Ruttiman PR, Getson PR. The pediatric risk of mortality (PRISM) score. *Critical Care Medicine* 1988; **16**: 1110–1115.
6 Balakrishnan G, Aitchison T, Hallworth D *et al.* Prospective evaluation of the Paediatric Risk of Mortality (PRISM) Score. *Archives of Disease in Childhood* 1991; **67**: 196–200.
7 Sinclair JF, Skeoch CR, Hallworth D. Prognosis of meningococcal septicaemia. *Lancet* 1987; **ii**: 38.
8 Paediatric Intensive Care Society. *Standards for transport of critically ill children.* PICS, London, 1995.

FURTHER READING

Oakley PA. The need for standards for inter-hospital transfer. *Anaesthesia* 1994; **49**: 565–566.
Advanced Life Support Group. *Adanced paediatric life support.* British Medical Journal Publishing Group, London, 1993.
British Paediatric Association. *The care of critically ill children.* British Paediatric Association, London, 1993.
Britto J, Nadel S, Maconochie I *et al.* Morbidity and severity of illness during interhospital transfer: impact of a specialised paediatric retrieval team. *British Medical Journal* 1995; **311**: 836–839.

12

Nursing aspects of paediatric intensive care

R. Macnab

In this chapter, general principles of paediatric intensive care nursing are outlined, and a detailed discussion of the particularly important nursing issues is presented.

Nursing assessment of critically ill infants and children, the nursing care of children in pain, the organization of nursing care, intensive support for parents and other family members and the provision for the dying child in the paediatric intensive care unit (PICU) are covered.

In addition, the peculiar stresses associated with professional life in the PICU and some management and staffing problems are examined.

PHILOSOPHY OF PICU NURSING

As a PICU nurse, you have to be a committed team worker who tries to see the impact of any advance on all members of the PICU team, children and their families.

The scientific aspects of high-tech PICU nursing will be dealt with in other chapters, but this chapter gives an opportunity to explore aspects of the art and skills of nursing in the PICU.

Strategies for coping with the many challenges faced by children and parents during a time of life crisis can be drawn from these deliberations.

A good starting point might be to identify exactly what a PICU nurse is— what she does and what makes her different from other types of nurse. She must possess some of the skills of a physiotherapist, a psychologist, a social worker, a dietitian, an anaesthetist ... The list is endless. The nature of what she does means that on behalf of the children in her care, she uses skills in the scope of practice of those professional disciplines described above to augment the care offered to those in her charge. She is, above all, an involved party in the delivery of primary care, in that she personally delivers care to children in the PICU or teaches that care or facilitates that care. She is a carer. The care that she delivers is highly specific and individually oriented towards the patient's actual and potential, physiological, psychological, spiritual and

cultural problems. This care process may begin before the child becomes her patient, for example where the child is being prepared for major surgery, or arise without time for preparation when the child is admitted to the PICU as an emergency.

The process of care will certainly involve in depth interaction between nurse, child, and family: the nurse taking steps to try to anticipate which particular care aspects will be applicable for that child and family. For families whose child is going to have major surgery on a planned basis, the phase after admission to hospital but before surgery, is a good time for the family and child to visit the PICU to see the equipment that will be used and to meet staff members. This is a point in their child's illness which parents frequently find particularly difficult as it seems to symbolize the inevitability of operation. Parents are often overwhelmed at the sight of the machines and the sounds of intensive care, but, often report that they are glad that they did take the time to come and see the unit beforehand. Parents may well require intensive support and encouragement from both PICU and ward staff to help them through this difficult time illustrating the need for the development and maintenance of strong links between nurses in PICU and other departments within the hospital.

SCOPE OF PRACTICE WITHIN THE MULTIDISCIPLINARY TEAM

The varied nature of paediatric intensive care demands cooperation and synergy among the members of the team. There is considerable variation in which clinical interventions are the domain of which staff members, for example—can the PICU nurse perform blood sampling, complete order forms for investigations or adjust ventilator settings?

The nurse's skill in direct provision of care must be dynamic and evolutionary. Nurses in intensive care units worldwide are involved in such intricacies as supervising and delivering extracorporeal membrane oxygenation (ECMO), in interpreting electrocardiographic traces and in adjusting ventilator settings within predefined limits based on blood gas results.

Nurses must examine what they do in the intensive care setting and why they do it.

The United Kingdom Central Council for Nursing, Midwifery and Health Visiting[1] urges nurses to 'maintain and improve your professional knowledge and competence', and in addition to 'acknowledge any limitations in your knowledge and competence and decline any duties or responsibilities unless able to perform them in a safe and skilled manner'. In short, be open when you do not know how to do something but take steps to learn how to do it if patients in the future will benefit as a result.

The policy document The Scope of Professional Practice[2] suggests that nurses should not simply call such tasks 'extensions of role' as, in fact, this may inadvertently be placing limitations on the role where none existed before.

Nurses in paediatric intensive care should not work in sterile isolation, but as a team with our medical and paramedical colleagues to provide optimum paediatric critical care. Territoriality and trends towards self-protection should be set aside to ensure that activities are in the best interest of our child patients and not merely a means of shifting workload.

THE PICU NURSE'S ROLE IN RESUSCITATION

Children who suffer cardiorespiratory arrest have a poorer outcome than their adult counterparts. There is a much better outcome in those children who suffer respiratory arrest compared with those who are victims of primary cardiac arrest.[5,13] This, to some extent reflects the causes of cardiorespiratory arrest in children.

Nurses working in PICUs need to be trained in basic life support and also in some aspects of advanced life support. Thus, all PICU nurses must know how to open the paediatric airway by head tilt/chin lift or jaw thrust, be able to deliver the correct rate of rescue breaths per minute either by efficient mouth to mask or bag-valve-mask ventilation, be able to position hands correctly to deliver the correct rate and depth of external chest compressions, and be aware of drugs used in resuscitation and their dosages and protocols for defibrillation.

Traditionally, in the United Kingdom responsibility for learning about and maintaining the skills associated with basic and advanced life support lies with the individual nurse in the belief that each nurse will take responsibility for her skill level and endeavour to maintain her skills in resuscitation at optimum. In many countries, employing organizations share this responsibility and consider that the provision of quality resuscitation is an organizational responsibility and to that end, actively insist that nurses within paediatric institutions regularly and systematically update their skills before they are allowed to re-register as clinical practitioners thus ensuring mandatory recertification of skills.

OBSERVATION AND ASSESSMENT

It is estimated that between 30 and 60% of children admitted to PICUs require only monitoring and observation.[3] Thus, the value of analytical observation by paediatric intensive care nurses cannot be overemphasized. This involves the physiological measurements recorded by the nurse and a general perception of the child where all the senses are used. It is not unusual for experienced

nurses in the PICU to halt in their tracks while doing something in the unit because they hear that something is unusual, for example a slowing pulse signal, a falling saturation signal or a leaking ventilator circuit.

Observation, then, takes on more than simply counting numbers of events in a minute and recording this on a piece of paper or a computer keyboard. It is an experientially developed skill, the vagueness of which makes it open to scorn, but the value of which must not be underestimated. The level of observation in many cases may be only as good as the experience and skill of the observer. Hence, awareness of behavioural and developmental norms in children should be increased by means of formal and informal teaching sessions as well as the more widely accepted educational needs of the new staff nurse, e.g. ventilation, resuscitation and unit policies and procedures. This holistic approach to the child in the PICU is the most vital patient monitor.

INITIAL IMPRESSION

The child's colour, skin perfusion, level of activity, level of responsiveness, and preferred position of comfort are indicators of general well-being.[4] These factors must be quickly but systematically assessed by the nurse on first meeting the child. Rapid evaluation of these factors leads to a 'looks good' or 'looks bad' feel for the PICU nurse.

Sample scenario

A 3-year-old boy is admitted to the PICU at 18.30 h with a brief history of shortness of breath and pallor. The PICU is in the throes of a respiratory syncytial virus bronchiolitis epidemic. The child is lying quietly on a trolley which is wheeled through the doors of the PICU. The little boy's mother is walking along beside the trolley talking quietly to her son and holding his hand. The child looks frightened. Nurses are instinctively behaving in ways to calm and reassure mother and child.

The child and his mother are separated so that the child can be intubated. The mother, sobbing, is led away by a nurse.

The child does not resist separation from his mother. This 'looks bad' to an experienced PICU nurse.

The child demonstrated no stranger anxiety and did not react to separation from his mother which suggests he is quite unwell and unable to object.

Intuitive assessment by the PICU nurse indicates that there is more to a situation than is immediately apparent. A better approach may have been to allow the mother to be with her child until he was anaesthetized whilst recognizing that the child is critically ill.

VITAL SIGN MONITORING

The monitoring and evaluation of vital signs in children in the PICU is an important nursing skill. Yet, knowledge of norms is crucial if PICU nurses are going to be involved in assessing physiological compromise in their paediatric patients.

It is more useful to record vital signs when the child is at rest, so that any changes in vital sign parameters in response to stress or exercise, including oral feeding, may be identified. Heart rate, blood pressure, body temperature and respiratory rate may deviate from normal in the PICU as a result of pain, illness, surgery or other precipitators of physiological stress.

Cardiovascular assessment

As cardiovascular performance affects all body systems, it follows that the effects of cardiovascular compromise must be observed for using a variety of approaches. It is important that PICU nurses are cognisant not only with normal cardiovascular parameters for age, but also with the normal development and behavioural milestones for all age groups of children.

Heart rate

It is routine practice to monitor continuously cardiac rate and rhythm in critically ill children so that changes can be detected and analysed as soon as they occur, and so that the child is not interrupted frequently and is allowed to rest.

Blood pressure

Blood pressure is usually measured in the PICU either by the placement of an intra-arterial catheter or by the use of a non-invasive blood pressure (NIBP) cuff system. If an intra-arterial catheter is *in situ* for pressure measurement and sampling purposes, it is important that the limb supplied by the artery in which the cannula is sited is observed closely for signs of reduced perfusion and that the line itself is labelled in some way, so as to prevent inadvertent infusion of substances intended for intravenous use. Also, the site itself should not be covered by clothing or bed clothes as significant blood loss can occur from a displaced arterial line in a very short time. Following some cardiovascular surgical procedures involving rerouting arterial supply from limbs, the pressure measurement recorded on that limb may be inaccurate (e.g. Blalock-Taussig shunt).

If NIBP devices are used, care must be taken of the skin beneath the cuff and regular change of cuff position is desirable.

The nurse must appreciate that a fall in blood pressure must be reported promptly and treated vigorously.

The paediatric intensive care nurse, as well as monitoring vital signs such as these, must continuously observe the children for other signs of cardiovascular compromise.

The American Heart Association[5] recommend the following as components of a rapid cardiovascular assessment:

- heart rate

- blood pressure (volume/strength of central pulses)

- peripheral pulses (volume/strength, present/absent)

- skin perfusion (capillary refill time, temperature, colour, presence of mottling)

- central nervous system (responsiveness, recognition of parents, muscle tone, pupil size, and body posturing).

It is important, in addition, to listen to parents who are the experts on the subject of their child, as they may detect subtle changes in their child before these are obvious to health-care staff. This is especially true of children with complex, chronic, or multiple abnormalities.

Urinary output

In a well hydrated state (according to Hazinski[4]):

- infant = 2 ml/kg body weight/h

- child = 1–2 ml/kg body weight/h

- adult = 0.5–1 ml/kg body weight/h

Urinary output should be measured carefully for the majority of children in the PICU. If the child has a urethral catheter *in situ*, the catheter should be connected to a collection device to facilitate the assessment of hourly urine volume. Where no urinary catheter is in use, urine output can be assessed by weighing the baby's nappies, taking care to weight each individual nappy before use as wide variation exists between the weight of single nappies of the same size and brand.

RESPIRATORY ASSESSMENT

In addition to counting the rate of breaths taken each minute by the child in her care, the PICU nurse must include the effort of breathing, the presence of nasal flaring, subcostal and intercostal recession or cricoid tug in her assessment of the child's respiratory pattern. The nurse should note also in

her assessment, the colour of the child, for example pale, cyanosed or mottled appearance.

The facial expression of any child tells much more than words can explain—a worried or alarmed expression on the infant's face coupled with physical signs of respiratory compromise suggest to the PICU nurse that respiratory assistance is needed urgently.

The nurse will observe, also, how the child copes with coughing, the sounds made on inspiration and expiration, symmetry or otherwise of movement of the chest as the child breathes, the sounds which are heard when she listens to the child's lung field air entry and will be conversant with the clinical signs of airway obstruction by oedema or by foreign body.

She will be aware, also, of the need to observe the type of pharyngeal or endotracheal secretions produced, their colour, consistency and whether the child is able to expectorate these or is swallowing them.

Assessment of the work of breathing is important in the respiratory assessment of ill children. The nurse must appreciate that in childhood the ribs and sternum support the lungs keeping them expanded, and air moves into the lungs due to changes in intrathoracic pressure brought about by contraction of the intercostal muscles and the diaphragm. Airway obstruction or increase in lung stiffness results in extra use of intercostal and suprasternal muscles and diaphragmatic contraction. This is seen as recessions of the rib spaces, above the clavicles, of the lower chest wall and sternum. Where gastric distension has occurred, diaphragmatic movement may be impeded, further compromising the child. Therefore, chest movement should be carefully observed and increased work of breathing reported. Signs of increased work of breathing may be an indication that the child is tiring and may need airway intervention. In the intubated child, they may indicate tube obstruction or displacement.

It must be remembered, also, that where any reduction in airway lumen size occurs resistance increases dramatically. While the child is breathing quietly (laminar air flow), resistance increases by the 4th power of the radius, but if the child is upset and crying resistance increases by the fifth power of the radius (turbulent airflow). Thus, 2 mm of airway narrowing results in a 16-32 fold increase in airway resistance ($2 \times 2 \times 2 \times 2 \times 2$).

It is for this reason that the infant or child with airway obstruction should not be harassed by attempts to provide interventions until such time as the airway can be secured by an experienced anaesthetist using an inhalational anaesthetic technique with 100% oxygen and halothane (see Chapter 5).

Weight

The weight of the child is important for drug dosage calculations, to assess the efficacy of nutrition and the child's fluid balance. Some manufacturers supply particular types of beds and incubators with a weighing function.

Some of the types of monitors described above necessitate the application of adhesive pads to the skin (electrocardiography, peripheral temperature monitoring), the insertion of invasive monitoring lines (arterial blood pressure, central venous pressure, pulmonary artery pressure, and left atrial pressure monitoring) or the application of sensors which generate heat (transcutaneous gas sensors or pulse oximeters), all of which carry special risks for the ill child, for example burns, blistering and infection. Special care must be taken of these sites by frequent observation and regular changes of site where possible. Particular care is required in the immunocompromised child and where peripheral perfusion is poor.

THERMOREGULATION

Increased body temperature in children signifies infection, physiologic stress, drug toxicity or central nervous system disease. Equally, the significance of abnormally low body temperature must be identified and is an important sign in a newly admitted patient in the resuscitation room or in the immediate postoperative period, particularly after open heart or other major surgery. The central nervous control of temperature must be considered along with the difference or gradient between central and peripheral temperature measurements.

The temperature of the environment for children in the PICU is important as shivering and pyrexia both increase oxygen demand. Means to maintain temperature should be used where necessary (e.g. warm air blowers, radiant heaters, electric blankets) taking into account the increased insensible fluid losses which result. Infants and small children have large surface areas in relation to their volume and cannot shiver to generate heat. The neonate can try to generate heat by breaking down brown fat, but this requires increased oxygen consumption.

SO, WHY MONITOR?

Benner[6] described the concept of 'future-think' and expands that expert nurses spend vast amounts of time thinking ahead, anticipating the probable course for a patient based on skill learned from many previous experiences, the vital parameters she witnesses, and instinct. Deviation from this 'anticipated recovery pathway' needs explanation and analysis and often provides the logical basis for adjusting or changing treatment.

ORGANIZATION OF NURSING INTERVENTION

The very fact that nurses provide 24-h patient cover means that they do precisely that, i.e. follow each other on a shift pattern. Skill level and experience vary from nurse to nurse and the care that is delivered to any particular child may be only as skilled and experienced as the nurse delivering it.

This situation highlights the need for some kind of plan or map of care so that the needs of the child and the overall aim of the care interventions can be facilitated. Without such a plan, nursing care is haphazard and uncoordinated.

One such system is that developed by the North American Nursing Diagnosis Association (NANDA),[7] where nursing diagnoses or problems are defined as interactive concepts which should allow the nurse to then determine what interactions she and her patient will have. These are not medical diagnoses, although they may resemble them. Examples from NANDA include pain, impaired gas exchange, and potential for infection.

Practical use of a design of this type means that the nurse interacts with the child and collates some 'data' about the patient. She then calls upon her skill and experience to determine more accurately what the nursing diagnosis or nursing problem is. She may then determine specific goals for outcome and consequently, specific interventions which will take the child closer to the desired outcome. All interventions are set within a time frame at which point the effectiveness of the intervention is evaluated and the plan revised if necessary. This process is a form of audit cycle.

An example of this is shown below:

(1) collection of data (pain assessment) leading to the nursing diagnosis—pain;

(2) desired outcome—the child will be pain-free while being able to move around in bed;

(3) nursing interventions: continuous assessment of the child's pain using an appropriate pain scoring system; administration of pharmacological analgesics as prescribed; use of non-pharmacological interventions as determined by the age and wishes of the child, e.g. music, distraction, play; involvement of the child's parents and family;

(4) evaluation—at a specific time, progress towards the outcome will be reassessed and the plan modified if required.

The use of nursing language and terminology may assist in increasing conceptual clarity, improving the dissemination of nusing knowledge and, by focusing intervention on the *overall* needs of the child and his family, moves

a step closer towards a truly patient focused approach to care. This close emphasis on nursing must also encompass the other disciplines involved in the care of the critically ill child.

THE PICU NURSE'S ROLE IN CARING FOR THE CHILD IN PAIN

Any student nurse will be able to recall being taught that 'pain is what the patient says it is'. Many children in the PICU, however, cannot communicate directly that they are in pain. It is vital, therefore, that nurses caring for children in the PICU must develop skills in observing both verbal and non-verbal signs of pain.

Buckingham[8] described how analysis of a series of behaviours and physiological parameters can assist nurses with the assessment and identification of pain in preverbal children. By categorizing behaviours like verbal communication, facial expression, body posture, physiological changes (e.g. heart rate and blood pressure) and alterations in levels of other chosen activities, much of the subjectivity associated with assessment of any kind can be removed. Lawrie *et al.*[9] suggested hourly pain assessment by matching the nurse's assessment to a code, e.g.:

- 0 = no pain
- 1 = not too sore
- 2 = quite sore
- 3 = very sore (crying).

Since it is vital that the analgesic effect is balanced against associated sedative, nausea and respiratory effects of potent analgesics, all of these symptoms should be assessed simultaneously. The chart used should contain guidance for nurses on when and how to summon medical assistance if needed. This score can also be used by the child to 'self-report' their pain if they are able to.

In teaching student nurses about pain assessment, the use of case scenarios may be useful to encourage learners to consider the many things which are potential pain causes, e.g. intravenous infusion sites, chest drains which may tug if the child moves around, myofascial pain from lack of movement, headache from working hard to breathe, sore elbows if a child is leaning over a bed table to play or to ease breathing, pain from tapes which are pulling on hair covered areas of skin, pain from a full bladder, etc. The PICU nurse must be aware of all of these discomforts and use all means in her power to minimize them. Pain identification, treatment and prevention *must* have a high priority in the PICU.

Consider the following scenario: Mohammed, a child of 7 years, had a closure of atrial septal defect. It is his first postoperative day. He had a bolus of morphine intravenously this morning prior to removal of his chest drains. His morphine infusion was then discontinued. He is sitting stiffly, upright in bed. His facial expression is pained and anxious.

Nurse: 'Are you okay?'
Child: (quietly) 'Yes.'
Nurse: 'Are you sore?'
Child: 'No.'
Nurse: 'You will tell me if you're sore, won't you?'
Child: 'Yes.'

The child and nurse have different agendas.

The nurse's agenda, quite correctly, is to question the child to try to find out if he needs some help from her. However, her method of questioning possibly did not help the child to be open with her.

Action for Sick Children[10] suggest that some of the following may be more important to the child:

- will the nurses think I'm a wimp if I say it hurts?

- will they keep me in hospital longer if I say it hurts?

- will I turn into a drug addict?

- shall I wait until the pain gets very bad before I ask for something?

- will I need an injection?

Nurses must learn communication skills for different age groups and clinical situations. Imagine that the scenario had been along these lines, with the nurse saying: 'Hi, Mohammed. I've noticed that you don't look very comfortable sitting in bed and I wondered if you were feeling a bit sore after your operation because most kids do. I'd like it if we could talk about a few things that I can help with if you are a bit sore.'

Encouraging discussion about the pain and using open-ended questioning techniques which allow the child to express his pain, where it hurts, what the pain is like and how much pain he is experiencing are often helpful.

In circumstances where the child is sedated and paralysed by drugs, particular attention must be paid to the child's vital signs as these may be indicative of pain in a child who cannot complain. As a rule to thumb it is better to assume that the child may be in pain in these instances and medicate accordingly. Hamers *et al.*[11] examined factors which may influence nurses' assessment of children's pain and describe that the age of the child and the knowledge and level of experience of the nurse were contributory factors, along with the

nursing workload and interestingly, whether a medically determined diagnosis existed. This medical diagnosis, it seemed legitimized the child's pain. In addition, the study highlighted nurses' very negative views of non-narcotic drugs, e.g. paracetamol, and postulated that the child may, in fact, receive insufficient analgesia purely as a result of these factors.

Care of the child's skin and hair

Children in the PICU are at their most dependent. Even older children have to rely on nurses or parents either to carry out or assist them with normal hygiene activities.

As far as possible, the child's and parents' own preferences with regard to type of soap, shampoo, and fragrances should be met.

Units serving multi-cultural populations face particular challenges in this area. For instance, the hair of African and Afro–Caribbean children can have a tendency to be dry and brittle particularly when the child is ill.

Some African parents moisturize their child's scalp and hair after washing to replace oils removed by shampoo.

Care of hair and skin is a way in which nurses can return some of the parenting role back to the parents. If doubt exists about what is appropriate for any particular child, the child's parents should be consulted.

Parents' first experiences on visiting the PICU

Appropriate preparation for a critical event in life can reduce the stress which accompanies it.[12] This preparation may take the form of discussion or coming to visit the unit to experience what the machines look like and what the place feels like—an opportunity to see, also, that 'normal' things can happen, even in a very 'abnormal' environment, e.g. mothers can cuddle their babies, can feed and wash them, children can have their favourite toys with them or can watch or listen to their favourite audio-cassette tapes or videos.

The way in which these first impressions are formed can have a profound effect on the perceptions of the parents and family during this time.

Consider the following scenario. The parents of Jody, an 18-month-old child, are coming to see the unit on the evening preceding surgery to correct their daughter's congenital heart lesion. Staff from the presurgical ward have already telephoned to ask if it is convenient for the family to visit the unit. As the family arrive on the unit, the nurse approaches them, and says: 'I'm sorry, the unit is very busy at the moment. They shouldn't have sent you just now, but I'll show you round anyway.'

Compare this with the following approach. The nurse says: 'Hello, you must be Jody's mum and dad. I'm Alison, I'm the nurse who will be looking after Jody tomorrow after her operation. Would you like to have a look at the types of machines we'll be using to help Jody after surgery. Just try to

remember that while it all seems very complex, all of the machines are there for a purpose, so that we know precisely and to the second how things are with Jody and also, so that we don't have to disturb her every minute to take her temperature and other things, this way she can rest completely. I'll run through what these things do, but don't forget that I'll be here tomorrow and I can explain again anything you need. Also, sometimes you can't think of questions you want to ask till the time is gone, so if you think of something later, just call the unit. I may be off duty but any of the other nurses will be glad to help.'

First impressions count—a few minutes of opportunity to reassure and inspire with confidence tells parents a great deal about the unit and the commitment of its staff by just a few minutes of advance preparation.

Other strategies which may help to reduce the anxiety of impending surgery for children where the premedication regime allows, are for the child to walk to theatre or to drive there in a toy car or go-kart. The advance use of 'preparing for theatre' videos and booklets, translated where necessary for ethnic groups is helpful. Allowing the child and his parents to formulate questions to be asked when visiting the unit is also useful.

The story, however, is quite different when parents experience the reality of their child being the subject of the monitors, drips and drains. It seems that preparation, while useful, does not completely prepare families for the stark reality which follows. It is simplistic to assume that preparation can totally remove the anxiety of impending life crisis, even the possible loss of the child, but it can help.

THE IMPORTANCE OF COMMUNICATION

Good communication is vital for the smooth running of the PICU and the well-being of patients and families.

Any PICU must reflect the ethnic population which it serves. In most regions of the United Kingdom, a multicultural approach to care is essential.

It is desirable that communication needs of children and families should be assessed when the child is admitted to the unit and that units should hold a list of interpreters who can be contacted when needed. The content of this list should be validated regularly.

It is always easier to arrange interpreter services in advance rather than trying to find appropriate help in a crisis in the middle of the night. A useful means of getting access to interpretation services at short notice is via Languageline (tel.: 0181 981 9981). This is a telephone service which when accessed asks for the particular language and/or dialect required and rapidly connects the caller with an interpreter with the requested language skills.

PICU nurses must learn from children, parents and families through re-flection on their experiences about what is helpful to them and adapt their

interventions accordingly. The focus must be firmly with the child and his family. We must strive to appreciate that each child is unique to his family, with their particular circumstances and beliefs, and attempt to tailor our care individually to offer assistance which is tangible and meaningful.

PARENTING IN THE PICU

Children, generally do not exist in isolation but are members of families, who generally provide care, protection and support for their members. Critical illness is a time of family crisis when families may need even more support from each other. The crisis may affect not only parents, but grandparents and other members of the extended family. It is worthwhile remembering, in addition, that lone parenthood has never been more prevalent than at the present time, and PICU nurses must facilitate any support strategy suggested by the child's main caregivers provided that these are in the best interest of not only that child but others in the unit. In many instances, also, mothers of very young children may be in employment necessitating that care of the child, for some of the time, is delivered by other people, i.e. family members, neighbours, friends or child-minders. All of these individuals may feel involved in the crisis and may wish to visit the child or the family to offer support.

The geography of the unit is an important consideration when deciding with families, who should visit. The PICU manager must lead decision making in this area, in accordance with the unit and hospital philosophies and taking into account the views and beliefs of staff, parents and children themselves before deciding on a unit visiting policy. As with any policy within the PICU, the policy must be flexible and able to take individual differences into account.

The chief aim of the PICU staff is to discharge the child back to the care of his family in a healthier condition than when he came to the unit for care. If this is accepted, then our interventions must reflect this aim and nurses must strive not to interfere unnecessarily with the 'parent' role. It makes no sense to return the child to his home environment cured of one set of problems but with a new set for his family to contend with. In effect, parents should be allowed, indeed encouraged, to provide as much normal love and care as they normally would. This may mean things as simple as washing their child or holding and rocking him to comfort him. A large part of being a parent is making decisions with or on behalf of the child, for example, 'my baby usually has his bath at night', or 'I usually change his nappy after I feed him'. Information about the child's habits and preferences should be recorded by means of an assessment of needs when the child is admitted to the unit.

It must be stressed to parents that they are not 'being a nuisance' and are not 'getting in the nurse's way'.

Parents often report feeling helpless and useless when their child is in intensive care—communication and negotiation between nurses and parents must surely help parents to maintain their parent role during a time when it is so important that parents feel that they are of some practical use to their child. Parents and other family members generally are not used to performing their parenting skills in public and may need support with this. They may, unless experienced parents of chronically ill children, feel embarrassed at singing or reciting rhymes, using pet names, or using baby talk in the presence of nurses and doctors. I suggest that, in this instance, the best way to support them is to join them.

THE DYING CHILD

Nothing is more tragic for a parent than the death of a child.

The loss of the physical presence of their little one and unfulfilled expectations is almost inconceivable. Nurses must endeavour to gain understanding of helpful and unhelpful things to do and say. By speaking to health-care workers who are experienced in the field of bereavement counselling or by attempting to learn from other families who have experienced this type of loss (perhaps at help groups meetings), considerable insight can be gained.

It is estimated that between 3 and 18% of children admitted to PICUs do not survive:[14] this being the case, it is crucial that these stressful events are managed carefully for the benefit of grieving families and, also, for the PICU staff who are involved in that child's care.

Sudden death

Some children, perhaps as a result of trauma, sudden infant death syndrome, or for other reasons, are admitted to PICUs and die shortly afterwards, or indeed, in some instances, are dead on arrival. In these situations, the chances are that the family is not known to the staff of the unit and vice versa. This is a particularly challenging problem for PICU nurses.

Anticipated death

Child patients with chronic illness are often admitted to the PICU to treat an acute deterioration of their illness.

In situations like this, the child and family may have already built up support relationships with nursing staff in other areas of the hospital. Hence, the PICU staff must join in partnership with staff from other areas of the hospital to deliver the very best possible terminal care.

This brings about the following question: if death is inevitable, where is the best place for the child to die? The parents and family may, in fact, have already

given this matter some thought, and may openly express that arrangements be made for transfer of their child to the ward where they are known or, indeed, for transfer home. The wishes of parents must be given due consideration and all assistance given to make the final decision workable within the local legal, ethical, social and cultural framework. In situations of both sudden and anticipated death of a child, nurses can offer certain things which may be helpful. Time and privacy given to parents and other family members with their child may be beneficial if the family wish this.

Alderson[15] suggests that mementos of the child, i.e. photographs, lock of hair, hand prints, patient's name band etc., may all help to reinforce that the child did, in fact, exist. This is particularly relevant in the case of neonatal death, or where the child never left hospital.

It is crucial that support services are set up in the community prior to the family leaving the unit, i.e. help enlisted of the family doctor and health visitor and social services.

Shandor-Miles and Warner[16] suggest the following actions which may be useful for parents of grieving children:

Potentially helpful advice that PICU nurses can discuss with parents who have other children:

- Take care of your and their physical needs, e.g. nutrition, clothes etc.

- Provide time for grieving.

- Deal with feelings of guilt and blame.

- Understand that children grieve in their own way. Support and encourage this—many children are taught that 'big boys don't cry'—they must be assisted to understand that crying is normal and acceptable.

- Lastly, difficult though it will be, allow surviving children independence.

Potentially unhelpful things that nurses can advise about:

- use of trite sayings

- idealizing the deceased child—'X was never naughty'

- comparing surviving siblings with the deceased child

- trying to replace the deceased child with other children.

SELF-HELP GROUPS FOR BEREAVED PARENTS

There is conflicting opinion about the value of self-help groups.

I sought permission from members and attended a meeting of a self-help group specially convened to assist parents who have lost children.

Imagine the following scenario. A bereaved mother and father were attending their first group meeting following the death 3 weeks previously of their daughter, aged four, who had died suddenly at home. The mother told the story of who the child had become ill suddenly, how she had telephoned for an ambulance, but that the child was dead by the time the ambulance had arrived. The parents were huddled close together holding hands while the mother cried. The father took over the story explaining that he was afraid to go into the room in the house where the child died. Another member of the group crossed the room and knelt on the floor in front of the two and told them: '*I know.*'

Such true empathy must surely be beneficial.

However, some other meetings may be singularly unhelpful in that new members, to some of the existing members, were simply new people to tell their sad story to. Where this is the case, the old campaigners, embroiled in their own sadness have little to offer new recruits, who will benefit little and will probably not come back.

Health-care professionals must, therefore, be wary of recommending groups to bereaved parents with which they (the professionals) are unfamiliar. If no suitable group exists locally they may wish to consider setting up a help group enlisting the help of trained specialist counsellors.

EFFECTS ON THE PICU STAFF

Kiger[17] described student nurse images of death on entry to nurse training and then after several months of nursing experience. The anticipation of coping with the death of a patient was, in fact, less frightening that the event itself, and the behaviour of *trained* staff shaped how comfortable the student nurses felt with the experience.

Spencer[18] explained that there is an expectation that nurses, on the death of a patient in an intensive care unit, are 'good at caring' for relatives, but asks the question 'who cares for the nurses?' She further expands that when nurses were asked to give their opinions of what coping strategies existed for them and which were most useful, a majority felt that the informal support networks in existence were useful. Some nurses felt that a more formal support group would be of use. Other nurses felt that the availability of a trained counsellor would be of value and all nurses felt that more training on the subject of how to deal with their own and others' grief would be beneficial.

From these two studies, it follows that students in the broadest sense, i.e. those who are unfamiliar with the death of children and are learning about it, e.g. new medical and nursing staff on the unit, may require guidance and support. Nursing leaders must be sympathetic to this need.

Some parents express that they feel a sense of 'unfinished business' when they leave the PICU after the death of their child. They must be reassured that they can return to the hospital to speak with staff. Some bereaved parents report the need to see their child again after they return home. The must be made aware that this is acceptable and that by contacting the staff on the unit, this can be arranged.

To be able to provide sensitive, personalized care, nurses practising in the PICU must be aware of the religious observances of their patients and patients' families. For instance, among some Chinese families, the child is regarded as being aged 1 year at birth and when a person dies 3 years are added to their age, one for the person, one for the sky and one for the earth. Lack of awareness by staff of such beliefs may lead to confusion and distress for the family. It may be preferable to refer to the child's date of birth for any necessary documentation.

Similarly, the Muslim faith requires that the deceased's body must be washed by a Muslim, either a representative of the mosque or a family member and that where possible, the burial should take place on the day of death. Usually, children can be washed by a Muslim of either sex. Postmortem examinations may give particular problems to some religious groups. It may be possible to achieve a compromise with the coroner or procurator fiscal to perform a limited PM examination e.g. of the chest or abdomen alone which can be helpful for some parents.

It is important, in order to prevent misunderstanding and distress for parents that nurses working in areas with high mortality become familiar with the belief systems of the ethnic groups which their unit serve.

MANAGEMENT IN THE PICU

Some management practices are required for the smooth running of any PICU, so that patients receive high quality specialist nursing care on a round-the-clock basis. Patients in the PICU setting receive care interventions from a variety of sources. Equally, paediatric intensive care nurses do not work in isolation, but as a member of a multidisciplinary team.

The PICU manager has a major role in the promotion of teamwork by working with staff to formulate the goals which are most appropriate for that particular unit.

It is, in fact, impossible to achieve 100% agreement and undying commitment for any innovation, all of the time. Unit staff, however, must agree that any decision altering their practice are workable and good enough to use practically in order that changes can be made with the minimum of disruption to day to day activity within the unit. It falls to the intensive care unit manager to focus and motivate.

The unit's goals should be known and understood by all staff. One way to approach this is through the development of a shared multidisciplinary unit philosophy. An example of such a philosophy might be:

Each child is unique, and as such, shall receive the benefit of individually planned, physical, social, psychological, culturally sensitive, quality health care delivered by trained specialist professionals.

Usually a child is a member of a family and it is acknowledged that health care within the Paediatric Intensive Care Unit will be planned and administered competently and with compassion by means of a partnership to include children and their parents, Nurses and Doctors.

Such an approach reinforces the belief that staff of all disciplines and at all levels are important in the care provision process and will assist staff in focusing on the child, and not on the needs or wishes of nurses, doctors, or others.

NURSE STAFFING IN THE PICU

The Paediatric Intensive Care Society[19] defines that in order adequately to nurse patients in a PICU, a minimum ratio of one nurse to one patient is essential throughout the entire 24-h period, and that all senior nursing staff employed within the unit will be experienced PICU nurses.

In the United States a myriad of new roles, e.g. patient care assistants, patient care technicians, care pair teams (two-man teams consisting of one trained nurse and a lesser trained nurse's assistant) are emerging in an attempt to try to control escalating health-care costs.

CONCLUSION

Benner's[6] 'expert practitioner' status is the goal.

Traditionally, in the United Kingdom, newly appointed staff nurses take their place dutifully at the bedside and learn there. They are, however, Benner's 'novices'. In order to progress professionally, few career paths exist for nurses where they can remain in the clinical setting beyond the level of senior sister or clinical nurse co-ordinator.

Usually, the attainment of seniority means taking a step away from the bedside towards either management or education.

In the United States, however, a new breed of nurse, educated to masters level, has emerged—the nurse consultant.

Wright *et al.*[20] accept that while consultation with fellow nurses and other disciplines is part of the function of all professional nurses, 'the Consultant

Nurse is able to act as a leader in his or her field, helping to set a vision for nursing and motivate nurses towards it, and to facilitate the process of change as it becomes necessary.'

Other qualities which consultant nurses are required to possess in order to fulfill their function are sound communication skills, mature judgment and problem-solving skills, psychological stamina, political awareness, analytical thinking, and a high level of commitment to nursing. On the other hand, not all nurses wish to develop in this way. Many nurses actually derive a great deal of professional satisfaction from beside care in the PICU and would not wish to function as a consultant, but still wish to develop professionally and build on their PICU nursing abilities.

The unit manager has a role here, in that nurses who choose not to become career nurses may, and should, in fact, continue to develop in a variety of other ways. They can, actually, improve the range of services offered by a particular unit. This may be by perhaps becoming proficient in a new skill, i.e. peripheral intravenous cannulation, or even by learning a new language. Such personal development plans may be a means to influence staff morale, reduce staff stress, and retain staff. Financial reward must be linked to the level of commitment, willingness to develop professionally, and services offered by the unit generally.

Actively encourage nurses to develop, but do not undermine the value of clinical skills.

What is the way forward? A holistic approach encompassing advanced practice, research, balanced management and appropriate education will be of greatest benefit to critically ill children. A properly organized paediatric intensive care service allows nurses in the PICU to develop their professional status and to progress towards excellence.

LEARNING POINTS

1. The PICU nurse has particular skills which require specialized training to acquire.

2. A holistic, child and family centred care plan is helpful.

3. PICU nurses can extend their role with appropriate training and supervision.

4. All PICU nurses should have resuscitation training and certified skills.

5. All PICU nurses should be trained in care of the dying child and their family and should have available a staff counselling service.

REFERENCES

1   United Kingdom Central Council for Nursing, Midwifery and Health Visiting. *Code of professional conduct*. UKCC, London, 1992.

2   United Kingdom Central Council for Nursing, Midwifery and Health Visiting. *The scope of professional practice*. UKCC, London, 1992.

3   Heaf D. Organisation of paediatric intensive care. *Care of the Critically Ill* 1986; **2**: 141–142.

4   Hazinski MF. *Nursing care of the critically ill child*. CV Mosby, Baltimore, 1992.

5   American Heart Association/American Academy of Paediatrics. *Textbook of paediatric advanced life support*. American Heart Association, Dallas, 1990.

6   Benner P. *From novice to expert*. Addison Wesley, Menlo Park, California, 1984.

7   Gettrust KV, Ryan SC, Engleman DS. *Applied nursing diagnosis. Guides for comprehensive care planning*. Wiley Medical, New York, 1985.

8   Buckingham S. Pain scales for toddlers. *Nursing Standard* 1993; **7**: 12–13.

9   Lawrie SC, Forbes DW, Akhtar TM *et al*. Patient controlled analgesia in children. *Anaesthesia* 1990; **45**: 1074–1076.

10 Action for Sick Children. *Children and pain*. Action for Sick Children—National Association for the Welfare of Children in Hospital, London, 1992.

11 Hamers JPH, Juijer Abu-Saad H, Halfens RGH *et al*. Factors influencing nurses pain assessment and interventions in children. *Journal of Advanced Nursing* 1994; **20**: 853–860.

12 Stewart EJ, Algren C, Arnold S. Preparing children for a surgical experience. *Today's Operating Room Nurse* 1994; **Mar/Apr**.

13 European Resuscitation Council. Guidelines for paediatric life support. *Resuscitation* 1994; **17**: 91–105.

14 Pollack MM, Ruttiman UE, Getson PR. Accurate prediction of the outcome of paediatric intensive care. *New England Journal of Medicine* 1987; **316**: 314.

15 Alderson P. *Saying goodbuy to your baby*. Stillbirth and Neonatal Death Society, London, 1986.

16 Shandor-Miles M, Warner JB. The dying child in the intensive care unit. In *Nursing care of the critically ill child* (ed. MF Hazinski). Baltimore, CV Mosby, 1992.

17 Kiger AM. Student Nurses involvement with death: the image and the experience. *Journal of Advanced Nursing* 1994; **20**: 679–686.

18 Spencer L. How do Nurses deal with their own grief when a patient dies on an Intensive Care Unit, and what help can be given to enable them to overcome their grief effectively? *Journal of Advanced Nursing* 1994; **19**: 1141–1150.

19 Paediatric Intensive Care Society (UK) Standards for Paediatric Intensive Care, 1990.

20 Wright S, Johnson MLJ, Purdy E. The nurse as a consultant. *Nursing Standard* 1991; **20**: 31–34.

13

Legal and ethical aspects of paediatric intensive care

N.S. Morton

The legal and ethical framework for decision-making in paediatric intensive care is more complex than in adult practice. Although the primary duty of care is to the child, the decisions usually involve parents or guardians acting as advocates for the child. It is important that good lines of communication are established as soon as possible between the paediatric intensive care unit staff and the parents or guardians because changes in the child's condition can happen very rapidly. The paediatric intensive care unit environment is complex and fraught with risks. Interventions must often be immediate before informed consent can be obtained. Allocations of intensive care resources, consent to treatment, withholding or withdrawing intensive care, diagnosis of brain death, organ donation and medical accidents all give problems. Each case must be considered individually with the overriding principle of acting at all times in the best interests of the child within the prevailing locally determined medical, social and legal rules.

RESOURCES FOR PAEDIATRIC INTENSIVE CARE

Centralization of paediatric intensive care expertise in large tertiary referral centres has been shown to result in improved outcome for the sickest children. It is more cost-effective to centralize care than to duplicate facilities on multiple sites. In the United Kingdom, audit data concerning the performance of paediatric intensive care units are neither accurate nor comprehensive enough to ensure diversion of funds to the best units. With around half of all critically ill children in the United Kingdom being looked after without paediatric intensive care units, the public and the government remain to be convinced about the benefits of centralization. Another concern is whether the overall provision of paediatric intensive care unit facilities is adequate for the needs of the population. It has been suggested that the United Kingdom needs 12 large paediatric intensive care units and that all critically ill children should be managed in these units. This will require a major reorganization of the resources for paediatric intensive care.

CONSENT TO TREATMENT IN THE PAEDIATRIC INTENSIVE CARE UNIT

Parents have legal authority to make decisions on behalf of their child as long as this power is exercised reasonably and in the best interests of the child. It is good practice to keep parents fully informed about their child's condition and the level of life support required. Some invasive procedures are regarded as routine in paediatric intensive care (e.g. intubation, ventilatory support, insertion of intravascular monitoring lines). The list of 'conventional' treatment interventions is expanding all the time to include new modes of ventilation, extracorporeal life support, nitric oxide and surfactant. Specific verbal or written consent is usually sought for these newer treatments and risks and benefits have to be discussed with parents. When techniques are part of a clinical trial, specific written informed consent is necessary. In such trials, control patients are usually offered conventional therapy and study patients receive the new treatment. If clear benefit is demonstrated, then it becomes ethically difficult to complete the study, i.e. the new treatment has become conventional. Parents may not be happy that their child is randomized to the group who will not receive the promising new treatment and may withhold consent. This is a difficult area as unless well conducted trials with sufficient patient numbers are performed, false clinical impressions of benefit may be gained and risks may not be revealed. The 'ethical window' for conducting such studies may only be open for a short time as new innovations are rapidly incorporated into clinical practice. It then becomes difficult not to use the technique if it is available and may be of benefit.

Often in paediatric intensive care, life-saving measures have to be undertaken without specific consent because parents are not immediately available. Parents should be forewarned that this problem may occur during their child's stay in the unit. A good example is the need for emergency insertion of a chest drain for relief of a tension pneumothorax. The law will support such an intervention without specific written or verbal consent as it will assume that any reasonable parent would have given their consent. Where it is not possible to gain consent in such a situation, the reasons should be noted in the case record and a confirmatory note from a second doctor is advisable. For non-life-saving interventions, parental consent should be sought. In most situations this is not a problem after risks and benefits are explained but what if the parent refuses? Parental refusal of life-saving treatment should be overruled by the child's right to live, but only in an emergency situation. Otherwise, the courts will have to decide.

In some situations, such as elective admission to intensive care of an older child who is adjudged to be able to understand fully the nature and consequences of a treatment, it is appropriate to seek the *child's* consent. Usually the parent or guardian will have to be a party to the discussions and will

usually be asked for their consent also. The doctor must judge whether the child is competent to give consent. When the doctor assesses that the child lacks the required competence, consent by a person with parental responsibility permits treatment to take place. This responsibility can rest with either parent if they are married to each other, with the mother alone if unmarried or with others by court order, care order or emergency protection order.

WITHHOLDING OR WITHDRAWING INTENSIVE CARE IN CHILDREN

Beneficial treatment should be started and not withdrawn. Non-beneficial or futile treatment should not be started. Obtaining agreement that the situation is futile for an individual child may take some time to achieve, while the intervention needed is often urgent. To allow time for clarification that the situation is futile and to reach a consensus amongst staff and agreement with parents or guardians, treatment may have to be started but may be withdrawn later. However, difficulties can arise if agreement cannot be achieved. Disagreement between medical staff about the prognosis, disagreement between parents or between staff and parents may all lead to problems which can only be resolved with legal guidance or intervention. Parental pressure in favour of futile treatment should not be allowed to override the best interests of the child as determined by local medical, social and legal rules. It is best if an agreement between staff and parents can be achieved and documented but for difficult cases, the courts should be involved.

Withdrawal of intensive care when it will not benefit the patient is acceptable ethically but must be fully discussed with relatives and staff and must be carried out tactfully and compassionately. A good unit will involve counsellors, religious advisors, support volunteers and support groups and will arrange follow up contact with the family. Where withdrawal of intensive care is appropriate, the comfort of the child should be the first priority in the care given. Warmth, cleanliness, hygiene, oral feeds or fluids, human touch and pain relief are all essential components of comfort. These comforting measures may prolong the dying process but the quality of the process will be enhanced and the extra time for parents to adapt to the inevitable can be helpful. In some cases, parents may ask to take their child home to die and if possible this request should be accommodated.

DIAGNOSIS OF BRAINSTEM DEATH IN CHILDREN

The criteria for establishing brainstem death are in principle the same in children over 2 months of age as in adults. Preconditions for applying the tests of brainstem death must be satisfied. In a patient who is comatose and

mechanically ventilated for apnoea and in whom the diagnosis of structural brain damage has been established or in whom the immediate cause of coma is known, tests of brainstem function may be performed provided hypothermia, neuromuscular blockade, drug-induced coma, endocrine, and metabolic disturbances have been excluded. Measurement of blood concentrations of sedatives and use of a nerve stimulator to exclude residual neuromuscular blockade are helpful in those children who have received sedatives and muscle relaxants. The tests of brainstem death should be performed by senior staff on two separate occasions. The pupillary response to light, corneal reflex, vestibulo-ocular reflex, doll's eye reflex, motor response to pain in the distribution of the fifth cranial nerve, gag reflex in response to suctioning and apnoea in the presence of normal arterial oxygen and high arterial carbon dioxide levels are all checked.

It is rarely possible to diagnose brainstem death in infants less than 2 months of age and for babies less than 37 weeks' post-conceptual age, the concept of brainstem death is probably inappropriate.

ORGAN DONATION IN CHILDREN

Organ retrieval from children for donation is only possible if the child has been diagnosed as brainstem dead. Thus organ retrieval is unlikely to be achievable from children less than 2 months old. Harvesting of organs from anencephalic donors is also not regarded as being acceptable in most countries because of the difficulty in defining brainstem death in these infants.

For healthy children to be allowed to act as donors of organs, the risks and benefits must be carefully discussed. The risk assessment depends upon the regenerative capacity of the tissue or organ being donated. Thus donating blood is less risky than donating bone marrow, skin, a kidney or a lobe of liver. These procedures are not therapeutic as far as the donor is concerned and are potentially harmful to the donor. The consideration that the donor may suffer some psychological harm if the donation does not proceed has also been taken into account in previous cases and the donor's level of understanding and ability to consent must also be considered. In the United Kingdom and some other countries, donation of non-regenerative organs from children is not regarded as being ethically acceptable. With regard to partial liver donations, most authorities advise that the risks to the donor of the surgical resection may outweigh the benefits although these procedures are now being peformed in the United States, the United Kingdom and Europe.

COMPLICATIONS OF TREATMENT AND MEDICAL ACCIDENTS IN THE PAEDIATRIC INTENSIVE CARE UNIT

The paediatric intensive care unit environment is potentially hazardous with invasive treatments being used on critically ill children. Complex equipment, use of potent drugs and multiple infusions are all potential sources of technical or human error. Should an incident occur, it is important that a clear truthful explanation in plain language is given to the parent or guardian and that both this discussion and details of the incident are clearly documented in the case record, signed and witnessed. Where possible, a case discussion as part of a unit audit meeting is helpful in identifying avoidable factors so that staff can learn from such episodes.

LEARNING POINTS

1. Good communication is vital in overcoming problems of consent, complications of treatment and medical accidents.

2. Treatment may have to be started which subsequently is agreed to be futile and may be withdrawn.

3. Brainstem death cannot usually be diagnosed in those infants less than 2 months of age.

4. The courts have to be involved where disagreements occur or when the clinical situation requires clarification.

FURTHER READING

British Medical Association. *Medical ethics today.* BMJ Publishing Group, London, 1993.
British Paediatric Association. *Working party report on the diagnosis of brainstem death in children.* British Paediatric Association, London, 1990.
British Paediatric Association. *Guidelines for the ethical conduct of medical research involving children.* British Paediatric Association, London, 1992.
Pace N, Maclean S. *Law and ethics in intensive care.* Oxford University Press, Oxford, 1996.

Index

abdomen
  abnormalities 115–16
  in children 110
  injuries 33, 79
  wall defects 115
  X-rays 238
abscess
  peritonsillar 104
  retropharyngeal 127–8
accessory muscles of breathing 114
accidents, medical 292
acetylcholine receptors, nicotinic 246
acid–base status, monitoring 219–21
acute respiratory distress syndrome (ARDS)
  12, 123–4, 238
Addenbrooke's Sedation Scale 242
adenosine 65
adrenaline 159, 161
  in croup 9, 101–2, 125
  in neonatal resuscitation 71
  in postextubation distress 99
  in resuscitation 60, 61, 63
adrenoceptor activating drugs 158–63
adult respiratory distress syndrome (ARDS)
  12, 123–4, 238
advanced life support 48, 53, 53–72
afterload 153
air transport 262
airway
  advanced life support 53–7
  anatomy and physiology 81–2, 109–10
  basic life support 49
  care in ventilated patients 146–7
  management 81–106
  nasopharyngeal 84
  obstruction, see upper airway,
    obstruction
  oropharyngeal 56, 83–4
  pharyngeal 83–4
  pressure monitoring 219
  rapid assessment 41–2, 48
  suctioning 146
    complications 147
    in neonatal resuscitation 70
  tubes, assessing position 236
  upper, see upper airway
albumin, plasma 190

Alder-Hey Sedation Scale 242
alfentanil 88–9
alprostadil (PGE$_1$) 160, 169
ambulances 262
amino acids 192, 200, 204
anaemia, pulse oximetry in 215
anaesthetic agents, in endotracheal intubation
  86–9
anaesthetic breathing system 57, 58, 83
analgesia 241–55
  goals 241
  intravenous agents 250–3
  monitoring 241–3
  non-pharmacological alternatives 243,
    244
  in trauma 79
analgesics 244–50
anti-arrhythmic drugs 62, 64
antibiotics
  in catheter-related sepsis 203
  choice 30
anticoagulation, patients on ECMO
  176–7
antidiuretic hormone 145
antihistamines 252
Apgar score 69
apnoea monitors 216
ARDS (acute respiratory distress syndrome)
  12, 123–4, 238
arrhythmias 66
  pulse oximetry in 214
arterial blood gas analysis 219–21
arterial pressure monitoring 223–4, 271
assessment
  of child
    augmented rapid 43
    rapid 41–3, 47–8, 258–9
    reassessment and trends 43
    in trauma 78–9
  newborn infant 67–9
  nutritional 189–90
asthma 11–12, 128–9
asystole 45
  treatment protocol 63–4
  atelectasis 122, 147, 237
atracurium 90, 244, 253–4
atrial natriuretic factor 145

atropine
  in endotracheal intubation 89, 91
  in resuscitation 61, 62

bacteraemia, nosocomial 37
bag and mask ventilation 53, 55, 70–1, 83
bags, resuscitation 57–8, 83
barbiturates 250–1
  see also pentobarbitone; phenobarbitone;
    thiopentone
barotrauma 149
base excess/deficit 221
basic life support 48, 49–52
benzodiazepines 247–8
  in endotracheal intubation 88
  with opioids 250
bereavement 281–3
bicarbonate, sodium
  in diabetic ketoacidosis 209
  in neonatal resuscitation 71
  in resuscitation 60, 61, 62, 64
bleeding, *see* haemorrhage/bleeding
blood gas analysis 219–21
blood pressure monitoring 223–6,
    271–2
  invasive methods 223–6, 271
  non-invasive (NIBP) methods 223,
    271
blood products 210–11
  patients on ECMO 177
blood transfusion 210–11
blood volume 17, 157
bradycardia 89, 91
brain growth 189
brainstem death 290–1
breast milk, human 192, 195
breathing
  advanced life support 57–8
  assessing work of 42, 47, 212, 273
  basic life support 50–1
  control of 110–11
  noisy 99, 118
  periodic 42
  rapid assessment 41–2, 48
bretylium 64
bronchiolitis 10–11, 120
bronchopleural fistula 117
bronchopulmonary dysplasia (BPD) 8–9
burn injuries 186

calcium chloride 61, 62
Candida albicans 203
capillary blood gas analysis 221
capillary return 222
capnography 216–19
  mainstream sensors 218–19
  principles 216–17
  sidestream analysers 217–18

carbohydrates
  in parenteral solutions 199–200
  requirements 192
carbon dioxide
  end-tidal monitoring 216–19
  principles of measurement 216–17
  tension, arterial blood ($PaCO_2$) 219–21
  transcutaneous monitoring 216
carbon monoxide 124
cardiac arrest 4, 45
  aetiology 45, 46
  outcome 73
  signs of impending 47–8
  treatment, *see* resuscitation
cardiac disease
  congenital, *see* congenital heart disease
  ventilation in 131–2
cardiac failure 4, 6, 153–5
cardiac massage 51, 71
cardiac output 153–4
  effects of mechanical ventilation 144
  measurement 4, 228–9
cardiac surgery 1, 2
  pulmonary artery catheters after 228
  ventilation after 131–2
cardiogenic shock 153–5
cardiopulmonary bypass 186
cardiopulmonary resuscitation, *see*
    resuscitation
cardiovascular system 4–6
  clinical assessment 221–2
  development 5
  effects of mechanical ventilation 144–5
  instability, endotracheal intubation in 96
  monitoring 221–9, 271–2
cardioversion 66
carnitine 201
carotid artery cannulation 172, 175
central nervous system (CNS) 13–16
  development 13
  monitoring 229–34
central venous catheters
  in circulatory support 169
  complications of placement 226
  insertion techniques 224–6
  occlusion 204
  in parenteral nutrition 198–9
  in resuscitation 58
  septic complications 203–4
  thrombotic complications 204
  X-ray assessment 226, 236
central venous pressure (CVP) monitoring
    158, 224–6
cerebral blood flow 233
cerebral function analysing monitor (CFAM)
    232
cerebral oedema 27
cervical fascial space infections 102–3

cervical spine instability
  endotracheal intubation 96–7
  precautions 78
charcoal, activated 36–7
chest
  compressions 51, 71
  drains 116–17, 236
  trauma 33, 79
  wall 7–8, 110
    abnormalities 115–16
    compliance 111
chest physiotherapy 146–7
  complications 147
  patients on ECMO 176
chest X-rays 235–8
  central venous lines 226, 236
  in respiratory failure 115, 116, 122, 123
child abuse 33–4
chloral hydrate 252
choking 53
cholestasis 204–5
circulation
  advanced life support 58–9
  basic life support 51–2
  duct-dependent 156
  rapid assessment 42–3, 48
  transitional neonatal 5
circulatory failure (shock) 152–6
  cardiac arrest in 45, 46
  cardiogenic 153–5
  clinical features 47
  early recognition 41–3, 258–9
  hypovolaemic 96, 152
  septic 27–31, 153
circulatory support 152–82
  general measures 156
  mechanical 170–81
  pharmacological 158–70
  volume expansion, *see* fluid, support
Clark PO₂ electrode 220
clinical trials 289
Clostridium difficile 38
coagulation disorders 210–11
Cole endotracheal tube 85
colloid solutions 157, 158, 187
coma 13, 232
communication
  between referring/receiving hospitals
    259–60
  in PICU 279–80
compliance
  effects of mechanical ventilation 144
  lung/chest wall 111
congenital heart disease 4
  duct-dependent circulation 156
  functional effects 6
  PICU admissions 1
  ventilation in 131–2

consent
  by child 289–90
  to treatment 289–90
continuous arteriovenous haemofiltration
    (CAVH) 18, 207
continuous positive airways pressure (CPAP)
    99, 139
  differential 143
  in viral pneumonia 120
continuous venovenous haemofiltration
    (CVVH) 18, 31
convulsions, febrile 14–15
corticosteroids
  in asthma 11
  in croup 9, 101, 125–6
  in postextubation distress 99
CPAP, *see* continuous positive airways
    pressure
cranial ultrasound 239
creatinine, serum 234
cricoid pressure 94
cricothyrotomy 105
critically ill child
  early recognition 41–4, 258–9
  recognition 47–8
  transport 73, 258–65
croup (laryngotracheobronchitis) 9, 101–2,
    125–6
cryoprecipitate 211
crystalloid solutions 157, 187
CT scan 32, 239
cyanide 124, 165
cyanosis 6, 42, 222
  central 212, 222
  peripheral 222
cyclic AMP/GMP 163–4
cytomegalovirus pneumonia 120

death
  anticipated 281–2
  brainstem 290–1
  causes of 45, 46
  effects on PICU staff 283–4
  grief reactions 38
  sudden 281
defibrillation 61, 64
dehydration 18
  in diabetic ketoacidosis 26
  in diarrhoea 24
  in respiratory failure 114
development 189
dextrose, *see* glucose
diabetic ketoacidosis (DKA) 26–7, 208–10
dialysis 206–7
diaphragm 110
diaphragmatic hernia, congenital 23, 115–16
diarrhoea 24, 196–7
diazepam 15, 247

Dinamap 223
dinoprostone (PGE$_2$) 160, 169
diphtheria 104
discomfort, causes of 243
dobutamine 61, 159, 161, 163
donation, organ 291
dopamine 61, 159, 161, 162
Doppler techniques, cardiac output
        measurement 229
drowning, near-miss 33
drugs 35–7
    accidental poisoning 2, 36–7
    in circulatory support 158–70
    distribution 35, 245
    endotracheal delivery 60
    in endotracheal intubation 86–91
    excretion 35–6, 246
    infusions
        administration 169
        compatibilities 170
        prescribing/making up 169–70
    intraosseous delivery 60
    metabolism 35, 145, 246
    in neonatal resuscitation 71–2
    pharmacodynamics 36, 246
    pharmacokinetics 35–6, 245–6
    in resuscitation 60–2
    routes/techniques of administration 246–7
    sedative/analgesic 244–50
    for transport 264–5
ductus arteriosus 5, 156
    drugs maintaining patency 168–9
dye dilution method 229
dying child 281–4, 290

ECG monitoring 222
ECMO, *see* extracorporeal membrane
        oxygenation
EEG (electroencephalogram) 231–2, 242
electrolytes
    abnormalities 188
    balance 17–18, 187–8
    in diabetic ketoacidosis 209
    requirements 187
electromechanical dissociation 65–6
elemental feeds 196
emphysema, subcutaneous 117
empyema 117
encephalopathy
    haemorrhagic shock 31
    hepatic 21
endobronchial intubation, inadvertant 98,
        109–10, 235–6
endocrine disorders 208–10
endotracheal intubation 84–99
    accidental extubation 98
    in cardiovascular instability 96
    in cervical spine instability 96–7

complications 98–9, 148–9
difficult 98
drugs facilitating 86–91
emergency 56–7
in epiglottitis 9–10, 101
equipment 84–6
extubation 99
in head injury 130
nasotracheal 93, 97
neonates 71
orotracheal (OTT) 91–2, 97
patients with full stomach 93–5
in raised intracranial pressure 96
techniques 91–3
in upper airway obstruction 99–104
endotracheal tubes 85–6
    assessing position 235–6
    drug administration via 58
    obstruction 98
    paediatric anatomy and 7, 81–2
    securing 93
    size/length 57, 61, 86, 87
energy
    expenditure, resting (REE) 190, 191
    requirements 190–1
    reserves 188–9
enoximone 159, 164
enteral feeding 24, 192–7
    complications 196–7
    continuous/bolus administration 194–5
    delivery system 193–4
    feed types 195–6
    monitoring 196
    starter regimes 195
Entonox 253
epiglottis 7, 81, 109
epiglottitis (supraglottitis), acute 9–10,
        100–1, 126–7
epilepsy
    traumatic 32, 232
    see also seizures
epoprostenol (prostacyclin) 160, 166–7
Escherichia coli, verotoxin-producing 20
ethical aspects 288–92
extracorporeal carbon dioxide removal 143
    low-frequency positive pressure ventilation
        with (LFPPV-ECCO2R) 172
extracorporeal membrane oxygenation
        (ECMO) 142–3, 170–9, 248
    cannulae 173
    circuit 173–4, 177–8
    decannulation 178
    diseases treated 171
    emergency removal from 178–9
    patient selection 171
    practicalities 175–9
    trouble-shooting 179
    types 172

veno-arterial 142, 172, 178
veno-venous 142, 172, 178
weaning 178

face masks 55, 82, 83
family, *see* parents
fat
  body 35, 184, 185
  in parenteral solutions 200–2
  requirements 192
fatty acids, essential 192, 200
fear, causes of 243
febrile convulsions 14–15
femoral vein cannulation 226
fentanyl 88–9, 244, 249–50
Fick method 229
Finapres 223
fluid
  balance 17–18, 187–8
  body, composition 17, 184, 185
  deficit, *see* dehydration
  extracellular 17, 184, 185
  intracellular 185
  normal losses 185, 186
  requirements 17–18, 185–7
  restriction 18, 19, 185, 186
  retention 19, 154, 177
  support 157–8, 184–8
    developmental factors 184–5
    in diabetic ketoacidosis 26–7, 209
    dose 18, 158
    in haemorrhage 158
    monitoring 158
    in neonatal resuscitation 71
    in resuscitation 61, 62–3
    in septic shock 28, 30–1
    solutions used 157, 187
    in trauma 78
foreign body inhalation 49, 51–5, 129–30
Frank–Starling curve 154
functional residual capacity (FRC) 111,
  144

GABA receptors 246
gag reflex, impaired 118
gallbladder sludge/stones 205
gastrointestinal tract 21–5
  development 22
  effects of mechanical ventilation 145
  mucosal integrity 193
gastroschisis 115
gastrostomy, percutaneous endoscopic (PEG)
  194
Glasgow Coma Scale (GCS) 14, 230–1
  modified for infants 231
Glasgow meningococcal septicaemia
    prognostic score (GMSPS) 30
glomerular filtration rate (GFR) 17, 145

glucose
  disorders of metabolism 208–10
  in hypoglycaemia 210
  in parenteral solutions 199–200
  requirements 187, 192
  in resuscitation 62
glyceryl trinitrate (GTN) 160, 166
glycopyrrolate 90
glycosuria 234
great vessels, congenital anomalies 127
grief reactions 38
growth 189
  charts 190
grunting 42, 111, 114
Guedel oropharyngeal airway 56, 83–4

haemodialysis 207
haemofiltration
  continuous arteriovenous (CAVH) 18, 207
  continuous venovenous (CVVH) 18, 31
haemoglobinaemia 177
haemoglobinuria 234
haemolytic uraemic syndrome (HUS) 19–20
Haemophilus influenzae 15, 119
  type B (HIB) 9, 15–16, 100, 126
haemorrhage/bleeding
  management 158, 210–11
  periventricular (PVH) 13
haemorrhagic shock encephalopathy 31
haemothorax 118
hair care 278
hand-washing 38
head box 82
head circumference 190, 196, 205
head injury 32, 79–80
  EEG monitoring 232
  endotracheal intubation 130
  Glasgow Coma Scale in 230
  transport in 261
  ventilation in 130–1
Head's paradoxical reflex 110
head tilt–chin lift manoeuvre 49, 50
heart rate 43, 153, 271
heat injury, respiratory tract 124
height 190
Heimlich manoeuvre 53
helicopters 262
heparin 176–7
hepatic encephalopathy 21
hepatic failure
  acute 20
  chronic 20
  fulminant 21
  liver support 207
Hering Breuer reflex 110
herpes simplex
  encephalitis 232
  pneumonia 120

hospital-acquired infections 37–8, 150
humidification, of inspired gas 147
hydrocarbon pneumonia 121–2
hyperammonaemia 25–6
hyperbilirubinaemia
    neonatal 20
    parenteral nutrition and 201
hypercapnia/hypercarbia
    clinical signs 212–13
    mental effects 114
    patients on ECMO 179
    ventilatory responses 111
hyperkalaemia 89, 188
hypertension, patients on ECMO 177
hypoglycaemia 25–6, 210
hypokalaemia 188
hyponatraemia 18, 188
hypophosphataemia 205
hypovolaemia/hypovolaemic shock 96, 152
hypoxia/hypoxaemia
    airway suctioning and 147
    blood gas analysis 220–1
    mental effects 114
    parenteral nutrition and 202
    patients on ECMO 179
    ventilatory responses 111

ileus, paralytic 145
iliac vein 172
imaging techniques 235–9
inborn errors of metabolism 25–6, 207–8
induction
    inhalational 95
    rapid sequence intravenous (crash) 94–5
infant formula feeds 195
infections
    central venous catheter–related 203–4
    cervical fascial space 102–3
    enteral feeding and 196
    nosocomial 37–8, 150
    respiratory tract 9–11, 112
    retropharyngeal 127–8
    see also sepsis
infra-red spectrography 217
infusions
    drug, see drugs, infusions
    safety procedures 211
    see also fluid, support
inhalational anaesthetic agents 95, 252
injuries, see trauma
inotropic drugs 71
inotropism 153
inspiratory:expiratory (I:E) ratio 135, 146
inspiratory pressure, peak 146
inspiratory retractions 113
insulin infusions 26–7, 209
intensive care units (ICUs)
    adult 1, 2–3

paediatric, see paediatric intensive care
    units
intercostal muscles 110
intercostal retraction 113
interleukin-1 (IL-1) 28
internal jugular vein cannulation 172, 175, 224–5
interpreters 279
intra-aortic balloon pumps 180–1
intracranial pressure (ICP)
    effects of mechanical ventilation 145
    monitoring 233
    raised
        drug use in 250–1
        endotracheal intubation in 96
        transport of children with 259
Intralipid 200
intraosseous access 59
intravascular oxygenation (IVOX) 143
intravenous induction agents
    in crash induction 94–5
    in endotracheal intubation 86–8
intraventricular catheters 233
ipecacuanha 36
isoflurane 252
isoprenaline 61, 159, 161, 163

jaundice, physiological neonatal 20
jaw thrust manoeuvre 49, 50
jejunostomy tube 194
junior doctors, psychological stress 38–9

ketamine 244, 251
    in crash induction 95
    in endotracheal intubation 88, 96
ketoacidosis, diabetic (DKA) 26–7, 208–10
ketonuria 234

Laerdal resuscitation bag 55, 83
language problems 279
laryngeal web 100
laryngomalacia 100
laryngoscopes 85
    curved blade 91, 92
    fibreoptic 98
    straight blade 92
laryngotracheobronchitis
    membranous (bacterial tracheitis) 9, 102, 126
    viral (croup) 9, 101–2, 125–6
larynx 7, 81, 109
laudanosine 254
left atrial pressure 228
left ventricular assist devices 181
left ventricular failure 155
legal aspects 288–92
Legionella pneumonia 121

lignocaine
  in endotracheal intubation 91, 96
  in resuscitation 62, 64
lipid, *see* fat
liver
  development 20
  drug metabolism 35, 246
  failure, *see* hepatic failure
  lobe donation 291
local analgesia 253
low-frequency positive pressure ventilation
    with extracorporeal carbon dioxide
    removal (LFPPV-ECCO2R) 172
Ludwig's angina 102–3
lumbar puncture (LP) 15, 16
lung
  closing volume 111
  compliance 111
  development 7–8, 111–12
  hypoplasia 23
  mechanics 111
  parenchymal diseases 119–25

magnetic resonance imaging (MRI) 239
management, PICU 284–5
manganese 202
mannitol 210
meconium aspiration 70
medium chain acyl-coA dehydrogenase
    (MCAD) 26
meningitis 15–16
  monitoring 232, 233
meningococcal disease 2, 16
meningococcal septicaemia 28–31
mental changes, in respiratory failure 114
metabolic rate 110, 185
metabolic support 205–10
metabolism, inborn errors of 25–6, 207–8
methaemoglobin, serum 165, 168
mid-arm circumference 190
midazolam 244, 247–8
  in crash induction 95
  in endotracheal intubation 88
  withdrawal 248
milk, human breast 192, 195
milrinone 164
minerals 192, 202
modular feeds 196
monitoring 212–40
  body temperature 235
  cardiovascular system 221–9, 271–2
  central nervous system 229–34
  drug therapy 169
  during transport 260
  ECMO 176
  enteral feeding 196
  nurse's role 269–74
  parenteral nutrition 205, 206

rationale 274
renal function 234–5
respiratory system 212–21
sedation and analgesia 241–3
vital signs 271–2
volume expansion 158
morphine 244, 248–9
mouth-to-mouth ventilation 50–1
multiple organ dysfunction syndrome
    (MODS) 27–8
muscle relaxants, *see* neuromuscular blocking
    agents
myoglobinuria 234

naloxone 71
nasal cannulae 82
nasal flaring 42, 114
nasoduodenal/jejunal tubes 194
nasogastric tubes
  enteral feeds via 193
  gastric aspiration 94, 210
  X-ray assessment 237
necrotizing enterocolitis (NEC) 23–4, 193
Neisseria meningitidis 15
  see also meningococcal disease
neostigmine 90
nervous system, central, *see* central nervous
    system
neurological assessment 13
neurological failure, early recognition 41, 43,
    258–9
neuromuscular blocking agents (NMB) 36,
    244, 246, 253–4
  in crash induction 95
  depolarizing 89–90
  in endotracheal intubation 89–90
  monitoring 234, 254
  non-depolarizing 90
neuromuscular disorders 118–19
nitric oxide (NO) 167–8
  inhaled 131, 166, 168
nitroprusside, sodium (SNP) 159, 165–6
non-accidental injuries 32, 33–4
non-steroidal anti-inflammatory drugs
    (NSAIDs) 252–3
noradrenaline 61, 159, 161–2
North American Nursing Diagnosis
    Association (NANDA) 275
nosocomial infections 37–8, 150
nostrils, flaring of 42, 114
nurse consultant 285–6
nurses, PICU 267–8
  care of parents 278–81, 282–3
  effect of child's death on 283–4
  initial impressions 270
  observations/assessment 269–74
  pain assessment 276–8
  psychological stress 38–9

nurses, PICU (*cont.*):
  respiratory assessment 272–3
  role in resuscitation 269
  scope of practice 268–9
  skin and hair care 278
  staffing levels 285
  vital signs monitoring 271–2
nursing, PICU 267–86
  dying child 281–4
  organization 275–6
  philosophy 267–8
nutrient requirements 189
nutrition 24–5
  assessment of status 189–90
  in ECMO 176
  enteral 24, 192–7
  requirements 190–2
  reserves 188–9
  total parenteral (TPN), *see* parenteral
      nutrition, total
nutritional support 188–205
nutritional therapy 25

observations
  PICU nurse's role 269–74
  respiratory system 212–13, 272–3
oedema
  causes 222
  patients on ECMO 177
  pulmonary 122, 123, 238
oliguria 18
omphalocele 115
opioid receptors 246
opioids 88–9, 247, 248–50
  with benzodiazepines 250
organ donation 291
organic acidaemias 25–6, 208
orogastric tubes 193
osmolarity, urinary 18–19
oxygen
  administration 82–3
    in asthma 11
    in neonatal resuscitation 70
  concentration of inspired 146, 219
  consumption 8
  exchange in ECMO 174
  tension, in arterial blood (PaO$_2$)
      219–21
  toxicity 149
  transcutaneous monitoring 215
oxygenation
  extracorporeal membrane, *see*
      extracorporeal membrane
      oxygenation
  flows, in ECMO 175
  index 142
  intravascular (IVOX) 143
  weaning from ventilator and 148

paediatric intensive care
  aims 2
  resources available 288
  withholding/withdrawing 290
paediatric intensive care units (PICU) 1–3
  causes of admission 1–2
  current status 3–4
  historical perspective 3
  management 284–5
  medical accidents in 292
  nurse staffing 285
  philosophy 285
pain 13
  nurse's assessment 276–8
  relief, *see* analgesia
paracetamol 252–3
paralytic ileus 145
parenteral nutrition, total (TPN) 24, 193,
      197–205
  complications 202–5
  indications 197
  infusion pumps 199
  monitoring 205, 206
  solutions 25, 199–202
  vascular access 197–9
parents
  bereaved 281–3
  communication with 279–80
  consent to treatment 289
  during transport of child 260
  of dying child 281–2
  preoperative visits to PICU 268, 278–9
  psychological stress 38
  role in PICU 280–1
  withholding/withdrawing treatment and
      290
particulate matter, inhaled 124
Ped-el 202
PEEP, *see* positive end expiratory pressure
pentobarbitone 244, 251
peripheral nerve stimulator 233–4, 254
peripheral perfusion
  assessment 42, 222
  pulse oximetry and 214–15
peripheral venous access
  in parenteral nutrition 197
  in resuscitation 60
peritoneal dialysis 206–7
peritonsillar abscess 103–4
periventricular haemorrhage (PVH) 13
pH
  blood 221
  electrode, Sanz 220
pharmacodynamics 36, 246
pharmacokinetics 35–6, 245–6
phenobarbitone 15
phenytoin 15
phosphodiesterase inhibitors 163–4

photoacoustic spectrography (PAS) 217
physiotherapy, chest, *see* chest physiotherapy
PICU, *see* paediatric intensive care units
plasma, fresh frozen 210–11
platelet transfusions 210–11
pleural abnormalities 116–18
pleural effusion 117, 238
Pneumocystis pneumonia 120–1
pneumomediastinum 117
pneumonia 10–11
  bacterial 119–20
  community-acquired 10
  hydrocarbon 121–2
  Legionella 121
  mycoplasma 10
  nosocomial 37–8, 150
  Pneumocystis 120–1
  viral 10–11, 120
pneumopericardium 117
pneumothorax 116–17, 235
  iatrogenic causes 116
  primary spontaneous 116
  secondary spontaneous 116
  tension 116
poisoning, accidental 2, 36–7
polyneuropathy, neuromuscular blocking
    agent-induced 253
pores of Kohn 111–12, 116
positive end expiratory pressure (PEEP)
    138–9
  in cardiac disease 131
  intrinsic 144
  selective 143
postmortem examinations 284
posture, and ventilation 144
potassium
  abnormalities 188
  in diabetic ketoacidosis 209
  requirements 187
preload 153
promethazine 252
propofol 252
prostacyclin (PGI$_2$) 160, 166–7
prostaglandin E$_1$ (PGE$_1$) 160, 169
prostaglandin E$_2$ (PGE$_2$) 160, 169
Prostin (PGE$_1$) 160, 169
proteins
  drug binding 245–6
  in parenteral solutions 200
  plasma 190
  requirements 192
psychological stress 38–9
pulmonary artery catheters 227–9
  cardiac output measurement 4, 228–9
  complications 228
  indications 228
  X-rays 236
pulmonary artery wedge pressure 227

pulmonary capillary wedge pressure 228
pulmonary hypertension 6, 131, 155–6
  acute postoperative 155–6, 166
  persistent, of newborn 166, 167
pulmonary oedema 122, 123, 238
pulmonary vascular obstructive disease 6,
    155
pulmonary vascular resistance (PVR) 5
pulmonary vasodilators 166–8
pulseless electrical activity (electromechanical
    dissociation) 65–6
pulse oximetry 47, 213–15, 260
  clinical uses 215
  technical/clinical influences 214–15
pulses
  central 43
  peripheral 43, 222
pyrexia 186

quinsy 104

rashes, skin 42–3
religious beliefs 284
renal failure
  acute (ARF) 16–17, 18–19
  fluid requirements 186
  support measures 205–7
renal function 17, 35–6, 184, 246
  effects of mechanical ventilation 145
  monitoring 234–5
renal system 16–20
  development 17
Rendell-Baker Soucek face mask 83
renin 145, 154, 177
resources, paediatric intensive care 288
respiratory arrest 72
  signs of imminent 115
respiratory distress syndrome
  adult (acute; ARDS) 12, 123–4, 238
  of newborn 8
respiratory failure 1, 112–30
  cardiac arrest in 45, 46
  causes 115–30
  clinical features 47, 213
  early recognition 41–2, 258–9
  evaluation 112–15
  pathophysiology 112, 113
respiratory rate 113, 212
  assessment 42
respiratory syncytial virus (RSV) 9, 10–11,
    38, 120
respiratory system 7–12
  anatomy and physiology 109–12
  clinical observation 212–13, 272–3
  development 7–8
  effects of mechanical ventilation 144
  monitoring 212–21
respiratory tract infections 9–11, 112

resuscitation 4, 45–73
    bags 55, 57–8, 83
    care after 72–3
    discontinuation 67
    drugs in 60–2
    neonatal 67–9
    nurse's role 269
    outcome 73
    techniques 48–58
    in trauma 78–9
    treatment algorithms 63–6
retropharyngeal infections 127–8
retropharyngeal/prevertebral space 103
Reye's syndrome 26, 233
Ribavirin 11
right ventricular dysfunction 131
right ventricular failure 155
rocuronium 90, 95
rotavirus diarrhoea 24

salbutamol 11
salt, *see* sodium
Sanz pH electrode 220
scoliosis 115
sea transport 262
sedation 241–55
    in ECMO 176
    in endotracheal intubation 86–9
    goals 241
    intravenous agents 250–3
    monitoring 241–3
    non-pharmacological alternatives 243,
        244
    scales 242
sedatives 244–50
seizures 1, 2, 13–15
selenium 202
self-help groups, bereaved parents 282–3
Sellick's manoeuvre 94
semi-elemental feeds 195–6
sepsis
    central venous catheter-related 203–4
    management 28
    syndrome 27–31
    see also infections
septicaemia, meningococcal 28–31
septic shock 27–31, 153
Severinghaus PCO₂ electrode 220
shock, *see* circulatory failure
shunts, circulatory 6
skin care 278
skinfold thickness, triceps 190
skin rashes 42–3
smoke inhalation injury 124–5
sodium
    balance 184
    deficit 18, 188
    in diabetic ketoacidosis 209

    requirements 187
    retention 154, 177, 188
    urinary 18–19
sodium nitroprusside (SNP) 159, 165–6
Solivito 202
sphygmomanometer, mercury 223
staphylococcal pneumonia 119
Staphylococcus aureus 203
status asthmaticus 128–9
status epilepticus 14, 15, 232
steroids, *see* corticosteroids
stomach
    aspiration of contents 94, 210
    full, endotracheal intubation in 93–5
Streptococcus pneumoniae 15, 119
stress
    psychological 38–9
    response 191
stridor 42, 47, 113–14, 212
    expiratory 99, 114
    inspiratory 9, 99, 113
    postextubation 99
stroke volume 154
subclavian approach, central venous lines
        225–6
submandibular space infections 102–3
succinylcholine (suxamethonium) 89–90,
        95
sudden infant death syndrome (SIDS) 26
suppurative parotitis 103
suprasternal retraction 113
surfactant 8
suxamethonium 89–90, 95
swallowing, impaired 118
sympathomimetic drugs 158–62
systemic inflammatory response syndrome
        (SIRS) 27–8, 29
systemic vascular resistance (SVR) 5

tachycardia
    in respiratory failure 114
    supraventricular 66
taurine 204
teams, transport 260–1
temperature
    body 235
    regulation 259, 274
    skin 222
thermodilution method 229
thermoregulation 259, 274
thiocyanate 165
thiopentone 244, 250
    in crash induction 95
    in endotracheal intubation 86–8, 96
thoracocentesis 116–17
thoracostomy 116–17, 236
thorax, *see* chest
thrombosis, central vein 204

tidal volume 113, 146, 148
tolazoline 160, 167
tonsillar obstruction 128
toxic shock syndrome 31
T-piece, anaesthetic 57, 58, 83
trace elements 192, 202
trachea, iatrogenic injury 147
tracheitis, bacterial 9, 102, 126
tracheoesophageal fistula 22
tracheomalacia 100
tracheostomy 104–5
  complications 149
  tube assessment 236
train of four (TOF) response monitoring
    234, 254
transcutaneous carbon dioxide monitoring
    216
transcutaneous oxygen monitoring
    215
transferrin, plasma 190
transport 73, 258–65
  diseases requiring 259
  drugs checklist 264–5
  equipment checklist 262–4
  in head injury 261
  modes of 262
  monitoring during 260
  organization/referral protocols 260–1
  priorities before 259–60
trauma 31–4, 78–80
  assessment 78–9
  head, *see* head injury
  life-threatening 79
  non-accidental 32, 33–4
  PICU admissions 1, 2
  post-resuscitation care 73
  resuscitation 78–9
treatment
  complications 292
  consent to 289–90
  withholding/withdrawing 290
triceps skinfold thickness 190
triglycerides, medium chain (MCT) 195–6,
    197
trimeprazine 252
tumour necrosis factor (TNF) 28

ultrasound scanning 235, 239
United Kingdom Central Council for
    Nursing, Midwifery and Health
    Visiting 268
upper airway
  anatomy 7
  obstruction
    basic life support 49, 51–5
    causes 125–8
    cricothyrotomy 105
    management 99–104

urea cycle defects 25–6, 208
urine output 188, 234, 272
urokinase 203–4

vascular access
  in neonatal resuscitation 71–2
  in parenteral nutrition 197–9
  in resuscitation 60
  in trauma 78
vasoconstriction, pulse oximetry in
    214–15
vasodilators 165–6
  pulmonary 166–8
vecuronium 36, 90, 95, 244, 253
ventilation 109–50
  airway pressure release (APRV; BIPAP)
    139–40
  in ARDS 12
  in asthma 11–12, 129
  bag and mask 53, 55–6, 70–1, 83
  in cardiac disease 131–2
  controlled mechanical (CMV)
    135
  differential lung 143–4
  during transport 260, 261
  in head injury 130–1
  high-frequency (HFV) 141–2
  high-frequency jet (HFJV) 141
  high-frequency oscillation (HFO) 141,
    142
  high-frequency positive pressure (HFPPV)
    141
  humidification of inspired gas 147
  indications 112, 115
  intermittent mandatory (IMV)
    136
  inverse ratio (IRV) 140–1
  mandatory minute (MMV) 136–7
  mouth-to-mouth 50–1
  in neonatal resuscitation 70–1
  physiological effects 144–5
  physiotherapy/airway care 146–7
  postoperative 1, 2, 131–2
  posture and 144
  pressure controlled inverse ratio (PCIRV)
    140–1
  pressure support (PSV) 137–8
  resuscitation bag 55, 57–8
  sequelae 148–50
  starting 145–6
  strategies 135–44
  synchronous intermittent mandatory
    (SIMV) 136
  volume support 138
  weaning methods 147–8
ventilators 132–5
  characteristics of ideal 132
  classification 132–5

cycling from inspiration to expiration
    133–5
flow cycling 135
flow generators 133
inspiratory phase 132–3
microprocessor controlled 133
oxygen monitors 219
ventilators (*cont.*):
    pressure cycling 134–5
    pressure generators 132
    pressure limited 134
    pressure monitoring 219
    rest settings, in ECMO 175
    time cycling 134
    volume cycling 133–4
    volumes, monitoring 219
ventricular fibrillation (VF) 4, 45
    treatment protocol 64–5
ventricular outflow tract obstruction 6

visits
    to child in PICU 280
    preoperative 268, 278–9
vital capacity 148
vitamins 192, 202
Vitlipid 202
volume expansion, *see* fluid,
        support
volutrauma 149

water, total body 17, 184
weight 189–90, 273
    fluid balance and 18
    in nutritional support 196, 205
wheezing 42, 47, 114

X-rays
    abdominal 238
    chest, *see* chest X-rays

Printed in the United Kingdom
by Lightning Source UK Ltd.
103992UKS00001B/82-84